Artificial Insemination in Bovine and Livestock Management

Co-Editors

Dr. Deepak Sharma
Assistant Professor
Department of Animal Genetics & Breeding
College of Veterinary Sciences & Animal Husbandry
Uttar Pradesh Pandit Deen Dayal Upadhyaya Pashu Chikitsa
Vigyan Vishwavidyalaya Evam Go-Anusandhan Sansthan,
Mathura-281 001

Dr. Anuj Kumar
Assistant Professor
Department of Veterinary Gynecology & Obstetrics
College of Veterinary Sciences & Animal Husbandry
Uttar Pradesh Pandit Deen Dayal Upadhyaya Pashu Chikitsa
Vigyan Vishwavidyalaya Evam Go-Anusandhan Sansthan,
Mathura-281 001

Dr. Gulshan Kumar
Assistant Professor
Department of Veterinary Surgery & Radiology
College of Veterinary Sciences & Animal Husbandry
Uttar Pradesh Pandit Deen Dayal Upadhyaya Pashu Chikitsa
Vigyan Vishwavidyalaya Evam Go-Anusandhan Sansthan,
Mathura-281 001

Artificial Insemination in Bovine and Livestock Management

Dr. Sanjeev Kumar Singh
Associate Professor & Incharge
Department of Veterinary & Animal Husbandry Extension
College of Veterinary Sciences & Animal Husbandry
Uttar Pradesh Pandit Deen Dayal Upadhyaya Pashu Chikitsa
Vigyan Vishwavidyalaya Evam Go-Anusandhan Sansthan,
Mathura-281 001

Prof. Satish Kumar Garg
Dean, College of Veterinary Sciences & Animal Husbandry
Uttar Pradesh Pandit Deen Dayal Upadhyaya Pashu Chikitsa
Vigyan Vishwavidyalaya Evam Go-Anusandhan Sansthan,
Mathura-281 001

SSPH

SATISH SERIAL PUBLISHING HOUSE
403, Express Tower, Commercial Complex
Azadpur, Delhi-110033 (India)
Telefax : 011 - 47073040
e-mail : info@satishserial.com, hkjain1975@yahoo.com
Website : www.satishserial.com

Published by :

SATISH SERIAL PUBLISHING HOUSE
403, Express Tower, Commercial Complex, Azadpur, Delhi-110033 (India)
Telefax : 47073040
E-mail : info@satishserial.com, hkjain1975@yahoo.com

ISBN 978-93-88020-18-3

Composed, Designed & Printed in India

Preface

Where land is shrinking day-by-day, animal husbandry has the potential to become a sustainable engine of rural economic growth and social empowerment. For animal husbandry to prosper, it is necessary that the livestock owners adopt the recent technologies along with age old ancient knowledge which has even been accepted by scientific community. Selective breeding using quality sires and dams should be protected for optimum production, and resistance to diseases. Artificial insemination is one of the easiest methods and easily adoptable for selective mating and upgrading on non-descriptive cattle and buffaloes. This book throws light on various aspects of artificial insemination for better understanding of the subject. This book not only discusses about importance of female genitalia and reproductive health, but also other aspects including systemic diseases, use of antimicrobials, foot-health and lameness, etc. and their impact on the fertility in animals. The standard protocols and intricacies involved in production of semen straws and their preservation have been discussed in detail. Similarly, thawing under optimal conditions is must for successful insemination, using frozen semen apart from initial handling and evaluation of semen, loading of semen straw in artificial insemination guns, precautions to be observed before, during and after insemination, etc. Gross anatomy and physiology of the female genitalia, anomalies of the female genitalia and their diagnosis with the help of ultrasound and other techniques, pregnancy diagnosis and fetal health using ultrasonography have also been discussed in detail.

This book also includes chapters on basic health examination of dairy animals, selection of animals to have an elite herd, basics of animal nutrition, preparation of balanced ration, methods of livestock management, prevention and treatment of various diseased animals, bacterial, viral and parasitic diseases, etc. In addition this book also covers the basic aspects of livestock economics, livestock entrepreneurship, strategies to improve livestock production and other important aspects of animal husbandry extension.

This book is the product of identification of real problems, practices in vogue, needs of the veterinarians and livestock industry based on direct interaction of the authors with various stakeholders during kisan/ pashu melas, kisan/krishak goshthis, farmers' trainings, inseminators' training, training of the veterinarians and personnels involved in semen production. We hope, this book would be of immense use to all the readers, to academicians, practitioners, progressive farmers and entrepreneurs.

Editors

Contents

Chapter 1

Indigenous Breeds and Its Importance in Conservation

Deepak Sharma Madhu Ti ari and Sat endra Pal Singh

Department of Animal Genetics and Breeding, College of Veterinary Science and Animal Husbandry, Uttar Pradesh Pandit Deen Dayal Upadhyaya Pashu Chikitsa Vigyan Vishwavidhyalaya Evam Go Anusandhan Sansthan, Mathura

India have diverse climate, land topography, soil, water, vegetation and other natural resources and possesses almost all domesticated animal species, landraces and crops evolved under different production systems. The livestock sector, with its huge Animal Genetic Resource (AnGR) base has emerged as the fastest growing sector, contributing substantially in the GDP as well as in the food and nutritional security of the country. The contribution of livestock sector in country GDP at the current rate was 4.4 to national GDP and 2 6.9 in GDP from Agriculture in the year 2015-16. Among the livestock and their products milk contributed maximum (66.7) as a single commodity. India ranks first in the world for milk production for more than last 20 years. During the year 2015-16, country produced 155.5 million tons of milk with 337 ml per capita availability. India possesses vast variety of livestock wealth, as it maintains 11 of the total world livestock population. According to 19th livestock census, India possessed 512.05 million of livestock comprising of 190.90 million cattle, 108.70 million buffaloes, 65.07 million sheep, 135.17 million goats, 10.29 million pigs and the rest being constituted by other species such as yak, mithun, camel, horse, donkey and mule. All the breeds of indigenous livestock have a long evolutionary history and the natural selection, which essentially led to their establishment in their respective ecological niche. All of these breeds are distinguished from each other by certain morphological as well as production parameters.

The Indian livestock, irrespective of the species, is an admixture of two or more genetic variants/breeds and is generally referred to as non-descript or desi and thus, cannot be precisely allocated to any documented breed. The numerous lesser known breeds, strains and new genetic populations of different farm animal species exist which have not been properly studied and documented. The native farm Animal Genetic Resources possesses unique genes or combinations of genes, which are responsible for like disease resistance, stress resistance, quality animal products, feed efficiency and many more traits of economic and environmental importance. Indigenous bovines are rich in variability and excellent in desirable attributes for different environment and production systems.

Cattle genetic resources of India includes 41 well-defined recognized breeds, which constitute around 18 of the total cattle population in the country and rest 82 of the cattle are exotic/cross-bred (22) and non-descript type (60). Among descript breeds very few are maintained for milk production (Sahiwal, Gir, Tharparkar and Red Sindhi), some are dual-purpose breeds (Deoni, Hariana, ankrej and Rathi, etc.), while the rest are draft purpose breeds of cattle that are maintained by farmers for bullocks. The small, marginal and landless farmers are reared in small herd size of 2-3 animals mainly by of different socio-economic level under different ecologies.

G B

The Indian zebu cattle (*Bos indicus*) evolved over centuries in traditional animal husbandry under low levels of selection. Indian zebu cattle are well adapted to harsh native environment, resistance to external parasites and tropical diseases and sustenance on grasses and low quality roughages. The Indigenous breeds of cattle have lower metabolic rate, which is well suits in hot climates and also comparatively better utilize of low quality roughage. The different breeds of cattle are economically well adopted in the areas where they present. The divergent range of agro-ecological zones in India have helped to develop number of cattle populations. The cattle breeds can be classified as on the basis of its horn size, body size and utility. The cattle breeds can be classified as on the basis of its body size Vechur, Malnad Gidda, Punganur, Motu, Purnea, osali and Hill cattle are known as small type. The breeds Bachaur, Bargur, Binjharpuri, Dangi, Gaolao, Ghumsuri, Tho-Tho, Pullikulam, enkatha, hariar, rishna Valley, Nimari, Rathi, Siri, Umblachery, and herigarh are of medium size. The large size breeds include Ongole, Gir, Hariana, Deoni, Mewati, Nagori, Tharparkar, ankrej, Malvi, angayam, Red Sindhi, Sahiwal, hillar, Hallikar, Amritmahal, Gangatiri.

The cattle breeds can be classified as on the basis of horn size ankrej had the thickest horns. Long horns were available in Hallikar, Bargur, hillar, Pullikulam, angayam, Amritmahal, rishna Valley breeds. The short type horns breeds are Hariana, Siri, Rathi, Ongole, Bachaur, Nagori, Gaolao, Mewati, rishna Valley, Ponwar, Binjharpuri and Gangatiri.

B G R I

Buffalo is a matter of pride for the country, as it is a multi-purpose animal supporting in several aspects. Buffalo provides milk, meat and draught power, in addition to several minor products. The original domesticated stock of buffaloes is believed to have been derived from the Indian wild buffalo, *Bubalus arnee*. Riverine and Swamp buffaloes were domesticated almost together (around 2000 BC), former in the Indus Valley Civilization and the latter in the angtze Valley. Riverine and Swamp which differ in terms of chromosome number (50 vs 48), body size (heavy vs medium built), the main purpose (milk draft vs draft meat), behaviour and body colour.

Buffalo has been rightly christened as a black gold-mine of India. Indeed, it has been widely recognized as more efficient producer of milk (buffaloes count less than half of bovines but produce more than half the country s milk), producing more nutritious milk (at least some available food-fat for the calorie-deficit society), more efficient converter of whatever available roughages and forages, showing more load-carrying-capacity and, of course, more dependability in the day-to-day rural life. In India, buffaloes are spread over almost all parts of the country with varying population density, the majority (72) being concentrated in the north and western states where most of the milch breeds of buffaloes are found viz. Haryana, Punjab, Uttar Pradesh, Rajasthan, Gujarat and Maharashtra. During the last 10 years, there has been a continuous growth of this species in the north-western region at the rate of about 2.1 per annum as against the average growth rate of approximately 1 in the country. Per cent growth in buffalo population was recorded highest in Haryana followed by Gujarat and Rajasthan. Other states that possess a large population of non-descript buffaloes also have shown higher growth rate during the period viz. Madhya Pradesh, Bihar and Jammu & ashmir. Some states with large buffalo population have shown a negative growth rate, e.g. Tamil Nadu, Odisha, arnataka, West Bengal, Assam and Chhattisgarh.

As per 19th livestock census, India possessed 21.23 of the livestock population in India comprised, buffaloes. Presently, the buffaloes are contributing 76.2 m MT (2016) of milk in the country which is about 49 of total milk produced, thus making it economically viable milch species. Moreover, the butterfat percentage is quite high among buffaloes with an average of 6.5 fat. There are 13 registered buffalo breeds -Murrah, Nili-Ravi, Jaffarabadi, Mehsana, Nagpuri, Pandharpuri, Bhadawari, Surti, Toda, Banni, Chilika and alahandi. Murrah is acknowledged as best breed in the world and imported by many countries. Bhadawari is known for high fat in milk.

India possesses a superior genetic resource of buffalo species and excellent milch breeds like Murrah, Mehsana, Surti, Nili Ravi and Jaffarabadi are present in sufficient numbers and are spatially distributed. Murrah is the predominant buffalo breed and is the breed of choice included in breeding programme of most of the Indian states, for upgrading the non-descript /local buffaloes followed by Surti, Mehsana and Jaffarabadi. Toda and Bhadawari are the two breeds that are threatened to extinction. The total buffalo population in the country is 108 million, out of which 17.05 population is pure belong to registered breeds and 39.53 buffaloes are grades of purebred buffaloes.

Buffalo breeds of India, based on their phenotype can be classified into six distinct groups as: (i) *Murrah group* comprising Murrah, Murrah grades and Nili-Ravi (ii) *Gujarat group* comprising Banni, Jaffarabadi, Surti, Mehsana and their grades (iii) *Uttar Pradesh group* has Bhadawari (iv) *Central India* group includes Nagpuri, Pandharpuri and Marathwadi breeds in Maharashtra, alahandi and Chilika breed in Odisha (v) *South India group* comprises Toda (vi) *North astern group* includes Swamp buffaloes mainly distributed in Manipur and Assam.

G

Domestic animal diversity is under threat, globally. Almost one breed is being extinct every month in world, as per FAO (FAO 2013). Situation is much grave in developing countries like in India, where rapid urbanization and mechanization and high production pressure in lieu of bourgeoning demand of rapidly expanding human population has almost altered the conventional utility pattern of indigenous livestock and today, exceptions for few, most of the native breeds of farm animals are facing serious threat in absence of any conservation efforts. In recent time, most of the well-known draught breeds of cattle have become vulnerable due to becoming extraneous after fast farm mechanization in most part of the country. Similarly, high demand of milk and meat has attracted high producing exotic breeds of livestock species, which further, caused dilution of our genetic stock very rapidly. Needless to say by losing a breed, we will lose the specific gene pool generated through long term evolution in specific ecological niche. It is imperative, the breeds loosing utility are nowhere to stand, unless some important measures are not being taken to protect them. Phenomenon of decline of these indigenous farm animal breeds can be averted through their sustainable utilization. Efforts like identifying unique biomolecules, producing high quality products with value addition could be more important as a measure of transforming the utility or making indigenous livestock more utilizable in today s context, which is the only way to conserve our indigenous germplasm, for longer time. Thus, a deeper knowledge of the genetic diversity and population structure can provide a rational basis for the need of conservation and possible use of native breeds as genetic resources to meet potential future demand of adaptation to changing environment or production needs.

Many of livestock breeds have potential of surviving and also to sustain production, reproduction and draught power under various harsh climatic conditions and some breeds have unique attributes. The Indian native cattle *viz.* Gir, Tharparkar, Sahiwal, Rathi, Hariana and Nagori, etc. can survive in extremes of agroclimatic. ankrej an important cattle breed, is known for its adaptability to high temperature, resistance to tick borne disease and powerful draught capacity. Similarly, India has excellent and diverse buffalo germplasm, Murrah is known for high yield and Bhadawari is very high milk fat per cent while Chilika is adaptaed to brackish water and salinity conditions and Banni is known for drought tolerant, adapted to hot-dry climate and nocturnal grazing- buffaloes of utch Gujarat excellent draught power- Swamp buffaloes of northeast India. The indigenous sheep breeds also have remarkable diversity. Garole sheep is known world over for its high prolificacy and adaptation to mangrove ecology. On the other hand, Malpura, Marwari, Chokla sheep and many other breeds from arid zones are well adapted to desert conditions. Many breeds of goat are also adapted to different ecological niche with high temperature, humidity or both for example Andaman goat is adapted to saline conditions, Changthangi is adapted to higher altitude temperate condition, whereas Jakhrana is well acclimatized to semi-arid condition. Further, Zanskari, Spiti breeds of horses, ponies and double hump camel are well known for working ability under hypoxic conditions at higher. Several native populations of poultry *viz.*, Ankleshwar, Assel, adaknath, Punjab brown, etc. are known respectively for their unique qualities in their respective native habitats.

L

During the recent past, there has been a net loss of diversity because of an increased rate of disappearance of some of the traditional breeds of livestock (FAO 2007). It is also contemplated that species involved in production and marketing systems with fast structural change show high proportions of breeds currently at-risk and already extinct. This includes 38 of chicken breeds, 35 of pig, 33 of horse, and 31 of cattle breeds (FAO, 2009). Worldwide there are roughly 3000 breeds of the seven major mammalian species *viz.*, cattle, pig, sheep, goat, horse, donkey and buffalo. It is estimated that in the 20th century, about 600 breeds have already been lost (Hall and Ruane 1993). This situation is even more alarming as per FAO estimates, where it is expected that every week at least one traditional breed of livestock becomes extinct. On the poultry side, the picture is even worse as over half the breeds of the five major species chicken, domestic duck, muscovy duck, goose and turkey are thought to be endangered or critical (FAO 2007). The scenario for India and other developing countries would be of concern, as many of the breeds would be lost without ever having been adequately characterized or studied (FAO 2009).

The national livestock diversity currently under threat from several sources. Intensification of agriculture in developed countries and the pursuits of higher production targets have led to greater reliance on a few breeds and the consequent neglect of the remainder. In developing countries, the major threats to genetic diversity are the extensive use of artificial selection, intensification of agriculture, indiscriminate cross breeding of local breeds with less adaptable exotic germplasm. In addition, introduction of highly productive breeds and demographic pressure are also contributing to the loss of valuable traits or decrease in population of local breeds.

A G R

The conservation of AnGR is now a multi-dimensional activity, which encompasses not only preservation and maintenance of existing breeds but also their improvement and proper management. Two types of conservation strategies are adopted- *in situ* conservation or as *ex situ* conservation. *In situ* conservation is one of the best ways of maintaining a breed and if the sample size is fairly large, sufficient genetic diversity in the breed population can be maintained. In India, *In situ* model of conservation has been developed by the Government agencies by providing technical inputs and incentives to the farmers/ breeders in the breeding tract of respective farm animal breeds and has been adopted under Network Project through the State Agricultural and Veterinary universities/State Animal Husbandry Departments/ ICAR Institutes and NGOs. *In situ* conservation schemes on Tharparkar cattle Toda buffalo Nilgiri, Magra and ilakarsal sheep Beetal and Surti goat and Spiti horse have been established and some success stories conserving native breeds have shown the path. Similar models for other livestock breeds in active partnership with govt. and non-govt. research and development agencies need to be developed and replicated. *x situ* conservation involves conservation of animal germplasm *in vivo*, but out of the environment in which it was developed, and *in vitro* including, the cryo conservation of semen, oocytes, embryos, cells or tissues. A National Animal Gene Bank is established and currently maintains more than 1,20,000 cryo preserved semen doses representing important and endangered breeds viz. Punganur, Amrit Mahal, Hariana, Gir, angayam, Dangi, Sahiwal, Tharparker, Red Sindhi and rishna-Valley breeds of cattle Bhadawari, Tarai, Surti, Murrah, Nili Ravi, Pandharpuri, Jaffarabadi and Assameese breeds/ population of buffalo Garole breed of sheep Chegu and Black Bengal breeds of goat and Jaisalmeri breed of camel. Besides this, large number of cryo preserved semen doses particularly of indigenous cattle and buffalo improver breeds is available with development agencies and are being used for breeding. Animal Genomic Resource Bank is established, which has collection of genomic DNA from almost all well descript livestock and poultry breeds.

P
A G R

Many of the ecologies/regions rich in flora and fauna diversity are in the process of becoming fragile both in terms of biodiversity as well as in economic development of its inhabitants. These ecologies, therefore, need to be protected, strengthened and their resources also need to be exploited judiciously by:

- Empowering the native livestock keepers through developing their economies by judicious utilization of local genetic resources, providing benefit sharing of their rights for genetic resources and associated traditional knowledge.
- Appropriate livestock policy and institutional reforms.
- Enabling them and their production system and environment for maintaining and sustainable utilization of genetic resources.
- Unraveling the unique genes and bio-prospecting the special utility traits, biomolecules, products for commercial exploitation of native Animal Genetic Resources.
- Linking of traditional breed conservation and productivity enhancement activities with overall economic development of animal keepers. Looking for conservation for specific breeds and their genes which provide bio-alternatives rather only conventional utility products.
- Live Animal Gene Banks need to be established for all the breeds of livestock and poultry, preferably for threatened breeds.
- Value addition and better marketing facilities for animals, animal products and byproducts to increase the sustainability of breeds and profitability of the producers.

R

Hall S. J. G. and Ruane J. 1993. Livestock breeds and their conservation a global overview. Cons Biol 7: 815 825.

FAO. 2007. The State of the World s Animal Genetic Resources for Food and Agriculture, edited by Barbara Rischkowsky and Dafydd Pilling. Rome.

FAO. 2009. Status and trends report on animal genetic resources 2008. CGRFA/WG-AnGR-5/09/Inf. 7.

FAO. 2013. In vivo conservation of Animal Genetic Resources. FAO Animal Production and Health Guidelines No. 14. Rome.

❑❑❑

Chapter 2

Preparation of Balanced Ration for Dair Animals at arm

inod Kumar Raju Kush aha and Shalini as ani

Department of Animal Nutrition, College of Veterinary Science and Animal Husbandry, Uttar Pradesh Pandit Deen Dayal Upadhyaya Pashu Chikitsa Vigyan Vishwavidhyalaya Evam Go Anusandhan Sansthan, Mathura

I

Dairy animal s productivity depends on many factors like genetic ability, feeding strategies, farm management and health. For higher productivity, efforts were made to genetically improve indigenous breed by cross-breeding and selection. As the effort to improve the cows genetically continues, we must also improve nutrition and management to allow the cow to produce to her inherited potential. A good dairy feeding program must consider the quantity, suitability of the feed and a time bound feeding programs. Imbalanced in feeding of dairy animals in particular leads to excess feeding of some nutrients, whilst others remain deficient. To ensure improved productivity, it is necessary to augment and secure feed resources through short and long term planning. Here are few examples of imbalance feeding in our feeding schedule and their bad effects: (1) Excessive grain feeding, (2) Oil cake (as *sani* alone (3) Feeding of particular type of green or dry fodder in excess, when in plenty (4) No supplementation of minerals supplement to compensate milk production requirement. All these feeding mismanagement leads to a number of production diseases in dairy animals.

Balancing the ration of a dairy animal warrant proper knowledge of its (i) maintenance, growth and production requirements, (ii) feed ingredients option available for feeding (iii) nowledge of nutrient composition (iv) a sound feeding strategies for low cost. All these factors are keys to feeding a productive or transition animal for preventing production disease and higher production. In following paragraph, there is an outline of nutrient requirements of dairy animals and means to achieve a balance ration.

Nutrient requirement of dairy animals

The major nutrient requirements for dairy animals include water, energy (TDN), protein (CP), minerals (calcium, phosphorus, magnesium, potassium, sodium, and trace elements) and vitamins (especially vitamins A, D and E). The specific nutritional requirements for individual animals differ due to differences in genetic make-up, age, capacity, growth rate and desired gain or production, pregnancy, lactation, work, stresses, sickness, etc. the requirement for maintenance, growth and production of particular animal is calculated for dry matter (DM), total digestible nutrients (TDN), crude protein (CP), minerals and carotene. Requirements are met by giving available feed and fodder in a particular area to meet the requirement. The difference between nutrients in feeds fed and the actual requirements of the cattle must be made up of extra feed or supplements. The best quality feeds and pastures are reserved for the fast-growing and high-producing animals.

Energ : Energy is an important nutritional factor related to poor reproductive function in animals. The metabolic use of available energy in ruminants ranking each physiological state in order of importance are as follows: 1) basal metabolism, 2) activity, 3) growth, 4) energy reserves, 5) pregnancy, 6) lactation, 7) additional energy reserves, 8) estrous cycles and initiation of pregnancy, and 9) excess energy reserves (Ryan *et al.*, 1992). Energy content in diet of Indian animals is measured as total digestible nutrient (kg) or metabolizable energy or net energy. On an average for a crossbred animal, a daily maintenance requirement of energy for lactating animal is about 30 g TDN and 107.0 cal ME/$W^{0.75}$kg and milk production requirement for per kg 4 FCM, energy requirement are 436 g TDN and 1082 cal ME. Out of which, about 45 energy is partitioned for maintenance and rest 55 for milk production (Saha *et al.*, 2013). The maintenance requirement lactating Indian cattle as TDN was 39.5 g/kg $W^{0.75}$ and for milk production and weight gain were 332 g/kg FCM and 1.78 g/g body weight gain, respectively (Paul *et al.*, 2004). In tropical condition, low quality fodders predominates feeding regimen of lactating animal, as a result deficiency of energy in diet leads to adverse effect on health and production. Negative energy balance during early lactation in dairy cows leads to an altered metabolic state that has major effects on the production of IGF family members. Low IGF-I concentrations are associated with poor fertility. Metabolites and metabolic hormones that change in relation to negative energy balance, insulin-like growth factor-I (IGF-I) is strongly associated with the calving to conception interval and pregnancy outcome and their effect on oocyte (Leroy *et al.*, 2006), ovary (Llewellyn *et al.*, 2007), uterus (Butler, 2001) and oviduct (Fenwick *et al.*, 2008) effects embryo development, contributing to the high rates of embryonic mortality in dairy cows.

Protein : A deficiency or excess of dietary protein has adverse effect on reproduction. Overfeeding of protein has been associated with decreased pregnancy rates in female dairy cows (Blanchard *et al.*, 1990) and buffaloes (ureshi *et al.*, 2002). The exposure to high levels of ammonia or urea may impair maturation of oocyte and subsequent fertilization or maturation of developing embryos. Overfeeding of protein during the breeding season and early gestation, particularly if the rumen receives an inadequate supply of energy may be associated with decreased in fertility (Dunn and Moss, 1992). This decrease in fertility may result from decreased uterine pH during the luteal phase of the estrous cycle in cattle fed high levels of degradable protein (mustard cake *sani*). Energy costs for detoxifying ammonia into urea (waste product resulting from excess protein) may aggravate an existing energy shortage resulting in reduced ovarian activity. This means that excess protein requires extra energy to remove it from the body. If cows are in a negative energy balance and are losing weight, they will lose even more weight because of the excessively high protein. Cows that lose excessive weight have a harder time re-breeding and probably won t until their weight begins to come back. Cows fed excess protein (more than 10-15 above requirements) required more services per conception and had longer calving intervals. The maintenance requirement of CP was estimated to be 6.27 g/kg $W^{0.75}$, whereas, CP requirements for milk production and weight gain were 82.3 g/kg FCM and 0.44 g/g body weight gain, respectively (Paul *et al.*, 2004). For example, a cow weighing 350 kg, producing 10 liter of FCM need 1290 g CP and 6.6 kg TDN daily. Approximately dry matter intake of cow is 10 kg diet of cow should have 10-13 protein and 65 TDN. This has to be met by feeding good quality fodders and concentrate to avoid production problems.

at : Cows receiving high level of energy during the postpartum period had increased LH pulse frequency and decreased the period from parturition to ovulation (Perry *et al.*, 1991). Fatty acids and cholesterol are substrates for reproductive hormone synthesis (progesterone, prostaglandins). Therefore, the effects of fat may be independent to those of increased energy availability. In subcontinent, animal diets usually contain 2 to 3 fat. Supplementing fat to improve reproduction was initially attempted to increase the energy density in the diet. High fat diets for cattle contain 5 to 8 fat. Exceeding these dietary fat levels 8 impairs rumen function. For example, a 400 kg body weight cow consuming 10 kg dry matter have about 300 g crude fat in their diet, thus there is scope of adding upto 500 g fat in daily diet for high yielders without any detrimental effect on rumen fermentation. Feeding high fat diets to cycling heifers and postpartum cows increased progesterone production and the lifespan of the corpus luteum (CL). Higher progesterone levels during the luteal phase generally result in improved fertility. Increasing dietary fat also results in increased follicular growth. Fat content of the diet should be increased above the typical 3 of diet DM for cows in the early postpartum period in order to meet the energy requirement. Feeding calcium salts of long chain fatty acids also improved pregnancy or conception rates (Thatcher and Staples, 2000).

Minerals Minerals play an important role in nutrient utilization and several biochemical functions concerning production and reproduction. The availability of minerals to cattle depends upon the production system, feeding practices, and environment (Singh and Bohra, 2005). Macro-minerals include: calcium, phosphorus, magnesium, potassium, sulphur and salt are needed in relatively large amounts in the body. The trace minerals include: cobalt, copper, iodine, iron, manganese, selenium and zinc and are needed in very small or trace amounts in the body. Animals obtained minerals through the consumption of natural feeds, fodders and supplementation of inorganic salts in the ration. Mineral deficiencies and imbalances have long been held responsible for low production among cattle and buffaloes fed on crop residues in tropical agro-climatic condition. Mineral deficiencies and imbalances are often cited as causes of poor reproduction. It is clear that adequate amounts of minerals must be provided, but little is known about the effects of marginal deficiencies and imbalances. The same is true of excessive intakes of minerals which may indeed be harmful.

An important concept surrounding macro mineral balance is dietary cation-anion difference (DCAD). DCAD measures the level of four macro minerals: sodium and potassium, which are cations and carry a positive charge, and chloride and sulphur, which are anions and carry a negative charge. The DCAD of diet can be calculated by equation of Tucker *et al.* (1992) using the quantities of the salts administered and the measured mineral concentrations and dry matter intake of all feeds.

DCAD (mEq/100 g DM) (Na) (Cl S).

Research shows that a negative DCAD prior to calving help in improving Ca homeostasis of periparturient cow, decreasing the incidence of metabolic disorders postpartum and increasing early lactation production. A positive DCAD (20 mEq/100 g DM) have been recommonded for Indian cow and buffaloes (Mohanrao *et al.*, 2015). Shahzad *et al.* (2008a) reported that a diet having 33 mEq/100 g DM DCAD has promoted feed consumption, water intake and resulted in greater milk yield and milk fat in early lactating buffaloes.

Calcium Ca Ca plays a very important role in structural and physiological functions. Ratio of Ca: P between 1.5:1 and 2.5:1 for lactating cows caused no problems. Lactating cows must be provided with adequate amounts of Ca to maximize production and minimize health problems. Other function of calcium is to allow the muscle contraction. A reduction in muscle contractility affects rumen function lower dry matter intake, thus negative energy balance. This results in increase in fat mobilization leading to fatty liver syndrome and ketosis. It has been shown that plasma calcium concentration of 5mg/ml reduces abomasal mortility by 70 and the strength of the contraction by 50 . Low calcium concentrations also prevent insulin production, further exacerbating this situation (Goff, 1999). Muscle tone in the uterus will also be adversely affected with cows experiencing prolonged calving and retained placenta. Uterine involution may also be impaired giving rise to fertility problems. A major concern in the mineral feeding of dry cows relates to providing optimum levels of Ca and P in order to decrease the occurrence of milk fever. Indian lactating cows need about 0.40 to 0.60 to low yielders and ration containing 0.75 to 0.80 per cent Ca on DM basis should be provided to high producing cows.

Phosphorus P It is the second most abundant mineral element in the body with 80 to 85 of P in the body being found in the teeth and bones. Essentially, P is involved in metabolic reaction and energy transfer within the body. It is required for normal milk production, growth, and efficient use of feed and by the rumen micro-organisms in the digestion of cellulose and synthesis of microbial protein. A decreased fertility rate, feed intake, milk production, decreased ovarian activity, irregular estrous cycles, increased occurrence of cystic ovaries, delayed sexual maturity and low conception rates have been reported, when phosphorus intakes are low (Cromwell, 1997). In a field study, when heifers received only 70-80 of their phosphorus requirements and serum P levels were low, fertility was impaired (3.7 services per conception). Services per conception were reduced to 1.3 after adequate P was supplemented. Increasing P supplementation from 0.4 to 0.6 of the ration had no effect on days to first estrus or services per conception. However, in some instances, responses have been reported in the field, when phosphorus supplementation was increased to 0.5 or 0.6 . Increasing the dietary concentration of P above requirement does not improve reproductive performance. Scientists have found that reproductive performance was not different on the lower but adequate concentration of phosphorus, when compared to cows fed a higher concentration (above requirements) of dietary phosphorus. Thus, increasing the concentration of dietary P above requirement (more than 0.38-0.40) does not improve reproductive performance (Amaral-Philips, 2011).

Selenium Se Se is involved in normal spermatogenesis and is an essential component of a range of selenoproteins, including glutathione peroxidase, thioredoxin reductase and iodothyronine deiodinase. Se with GPx also appears to be involved as a structural protein to provide normal sperm motility. Both deficiency and excessive Selenium have been demonstrated to be detrimental to normal spermatogenesis (Wiltbank *et al.*, 2007). There are two major sources of Se for animals: (1) Se naturally originating from plants, in the form of seleno-amino acids, including selenomethionine and selenocysteine (2) inorganic Se in the form of selenate or selenite. Even if the physiological requirement for Se is low in an animal, if this is not met, the anti-oxidant system is compromised, with subsequent detrimental consequences in terms of animal health (Spears, 2000). A marginal Se deficiency in pregnant animals will lead to abortion, or calves will be weak and unable to stand or suckle. Se supplementation reduces the incidence of retained placentas, cystic ovaries, mastitis and metritis. Compromised selenium status has also been associated

with poor uterine involution, and weak or silent heats. In males, Se supplementation has been shown to increase semen quality. Symptoms of chronic Se toxicity include lameness, sore feet, deformed claws and loss of hairs from tail. In pregnant animals, Se toxicity will produce abortions, stillbirth and weak and lethargic calves as Se accumulate in the fetus at the expense of the cow (Patterson *et al.*, 2003). The dietary requirement for Se by most species is about 0.1 ppm. Revised requirement of Se for better immune response in dairy animals is 0.3 ppm (Weiss, 2002).

inc n Zn is an essential component of over 200 enzyme systems of which the metabolic action include carbohydrate and protein metabolism, protein synthesis, nucleic acid metabolism, epithelial tissue integrity, cell repair and division, and vitamin A and E transport an utilization. In addition, zinc plays a major role in the immune system and certain reproductive hormones (Capuco *et al.*, 1990). Zn is known to be essential for proper sexual maturity, reproductive capacity, and more specifically, onset of estrus. Zn has a critical role in the repair and maintenance of the uterine lining following parturition, speeding return to normal reproductive function and estrus. In bulls, a Zn deficiency results in poor semen quality and reduced testicular size and libido (Daniel, 1983). Zn has also been shown to increase plasma beta carotene level which is correlated to improvement in conception rates and embryonic development (Short and Adams, 1988). Improved Zn status also improves fertility by reducing lameness, resulting in cows more willing to show heat and improved mobility and performance of bulls. Severe Zn deficiency in cattle results in reduced growth, feed intake, loss of hair, skin lesions that are most severe on the legs, neck, head and around the nostrils, excessive salivation, swollen feed with open, scaly lesions, and impaired reproduction. A deficiency of Zn in males reduces testicular development and sperm production. In females, cycling and conception rate are decreased by Zn deficiency. Severe Zn deficiency is rare, but has been observed in ruminants grazing forages. Based on Zn supplementation studies, subclinical Zn deficiency can result in impaired reproduction and decreased weight gains (Spears, 1994). The recommended dietary content of Zn for dairy cattle is typically between 18 and 73ppm depending upon the stage of lifecycle and dry matter intake. Cu, Cd, Ca and Fe reduce Zn absorption and interfere with Zn metabolism (Patterson *et al.*, 2003). Requirement of Zn in diet of dairy cows is 40 ppm (NRC, 2001).

Copper Cu Cu is a necessary component of number of enzymes including superoxide dismutase, lysyl oxidase and thioloxidase (Halliwell and Gutteridge, 1999). Cu has an important role in the immune system, where its compounds are involved in reducing infections and diseases. Cu deficiency in cattle is generally due to the presence of dietary antagonists, such as sulphur, molybdenum and iron (Fe) that reduce Cu bioavailability (Spears, 2003). Dietary requirements for Cu are greatly increased by high concentrations of molybdenum and sulphur. Deficiencies of copper have also been associated with retained placenta, embryonic death and decreased conception rates. Inadequate Cu status may be related to an increased incidence of infections at calving, increased severity of infections and a higher SCC than that seen in Cu-adequate cattle. Reproductive problems that relate to Cu deficiency manifest themselves in inhibited conception rate even though estrus may be normal. Weak and silent heats have been reported. Dairy cows with higher serum Cu levels had significantly less days to first service, fewer services per conception and fewer days to open. Proper Cu supplementation of the sire is needed for production of quality semen. Feeding a total of 10 to 15 ppm Cu in the ration dry matter or supplementing with 10 ppm Cu should meet dairy cattle needs. If rations contain antagonists, such as elevated iron, sulphur, or molybdenum, replacing 35 per cent of supplemental Cu with organic Cu sources could improve Cu availability. The following mineral ratios may be helpful in maintaining Cu levels in blood: Zn: Cu 4:1, Cu: Mo 6:1 and Fe: Cu 40:1 (Hutjens, 2000).

Manganese Mn Mn is a required nutrient for dairy cows however, clinical deficiencies are extremely rare because most feedstuffs contain at least marginally adequate concentrations of Mn. Mn is an activator of enzyme systems in the metabolism of carbohydrate, fats, protein and nucleic acids. Mn appears to have a vital role in reproduction. It is necessary for cholesterol synthesis (appel and Zidenberg, 1999), which in turn is required for synthesis of the steroids, estrogen, progesterone and testosterone. Insufficient steroid production results in decreased circulating concentrations of these reproductive hormones resulting in abnormal sperm in males and irregular estrus cycles in females. The corpus luteum has high manganese content and may be affected by level of Mn supplementation. Also, vaginal Mn concentration is higher in cycling than in anoestrous ruminants. A deficiency in Mn may be associated with

suppression of estrus, cyclic ovaries and reduced conception rate (Patterson *et al.*, 2003). The maintenance requirement for absorbed Mn was set at 0.002 mg/kg of body weight (1.2 mg/day for an average Holstein cow), the growth requirement was set at 0.7 mg/kg, pregnancy requirement was set at 0.3 mg/d, and the lactation requirement was set at 0.03 mg/kg of milk (NRC, 2001).

Iodine I Iodine is important in the development of fetus and maintenance of general basal metabolic rate, as it is involved in synthesis of thyroid hormone, thyroxin, which regulates the rate of metabolism. Iodine deficiency leads to delay in puberty, suppressed or irregular estrus (Puls, 1994), failure of fertilization, early embryonic death, still birth with weak calves, abortion, increased frequency of retained placenta in females and decrease in libido and deterioration of semen quality in males (Sathish umar, 2003). Inadequate thyroid function reduces conception rate and ovarian activity. Thus, I deficiency impairs reproduction and iodine supplementation has been recommended, when necessary to insure that cows consume 15-20 mg of I each day. Recently, Excessive I intakes have been associated with various health problems including abortion and decreased resistance to infection and disease. Signs of subclinical I deficiency in breeding females include suppressed estrus, abortions, still births, increased frequency of retained placentas and extended gestation periods (Hess *et al.*, 2008). Calves born to cows that are marginally deficient in iodine are weak and may be hairless.

Cobalt Co Co is needed for proper vitamin B_{12} synthesis. Maintaining adequate vitamin B_{12} status benefits both the dam and offspring. When adequate, sufficient amounts of vitamin B_{12} cross the placenta and are present in colostrums. Milk and colostrums in particular, contain high levels of vitamin B_{12}, which is required for the conversion of propionate to glucose and for folic acid metabolism. Depletion of Co and vitamin B12 at parturition causes depressed milk production and colostrums yield and quality (Patterson *et al.*, 2003). Co deficiency is associated with an increased incidence of silent heats, a delayed onset of puberty, non-functional ovaries, and abortion. Inadequate Co levels in the diet have been correlated with increased early calf mortality. A Co deficiency ultimately results in a vitamin B_{12} deficiency. Mn, Zn, I and monensin may reduce Co deficiency. The required dietary content of Co for dairy cattle is 0.11 ppm (Miller *et al.*, 1988).

Potassium K is the third most abundant mineral element in the animal body, surpassed only by calcium and phosphorus. The requirement for gestating and lactating sows is 0.20 per cent. Potassium requirement increases in diets with higher Na and chloride (Cl) levels. Ruminants have a higher requirement than non-ruminants. is essential for rumen micro-organisms. The single most consistent effect of suboptimal in the ration of ruminants is decreased feed intake. Lactating dairy cattle, particularly high producing cows, require the highest levels of dietary . Under heat stress, their optimal level of dietary can be as high as 1.9 per cent, but the normal National Research Council (NRC) recommendation is 1.0 per cent of dietary dry matter.

Chromium Cr Cr potentiates insulin action, resulting in increased uptake of glucose and amino acids by cells in the body (Short and Adams, 1988). Dietary energy intake in early lactation does not meet energy demands for maintaining body reserves and milk yield (Coppock, 1985). Low serum insulin, high serum glucagon and growth hormone (Herbein *et al.*, 1985), and high plasma NEFA concentrations (Grummer, 1993) in early lactation, dairy cows indicate high catabolic activities and negative energy balance. This leads to increased gluconeogenesis and glycogenolysis in the liver and increased mobilization of protein reserves from muscle tissue (Collier *et al.*, 1984). This metabolic pattern is initiated before parturition (Vazquez-Anon *et al.*, 1994). Several studies reported insulin resistance begins before parturition and continues during early lactation. Thus, during the periparturient period, insulin resistance may be an important factor in the initiation of catabolic activities (Holstenius, 1993). Cr supplementation (0.5 ppm) may enhance the action of insulin and consequently decrease plasma NEFA and liver triglyceride concentrations and improve glucose tolerance, which may result in improvement of performance and production during the periparturient period.

Salt NaCl The daily salt requirements for dairy cattle are met easily by adding 1 per cent salt to a grain mix and offering additional salt free choice. Lactating cows need 2 g salt/kg milk production. Dry cows need 40g salt daily or 0.3 Na per kg DM. Salt deficiencies can affect the efficiency of digestion and indirectly the reproduction performance of cows. Sodium and chloride normally do not appear in feedstuffs in adequate amounts to meet animal requirements and should be provided free choice at all times (Elrod and Butler, 1993).

itamins The vitamin requirements of dairy cows are met by a combination of rumen and tissue synthesis, natural feeds and dietary supplementation. Factory made concentrates containing supplemental vitamins greatly reduces infertility due to a vitamin deficiency. To ensure adequate vitamins intake, animals must be fed with concentrates or mixed in a complete dairy cow ration (Schweigert and Zucker, 1988).

itamin A It is one of the fat soluble vitamins and is known to regulate the development, cellular growth and differentiation, and tissue function. Its metabolites affect ovarian follicular growth, uterine environments and oocyte maturation. Vitamin A is required for maintaining healthy tissue in the reproductive tract. In deficient cattle, delayed sexual maturity, abortion, the birth of dead or weak calves, retained placenta and metritis have been reported (Chawala and aur, 2004). A deficiency of vitamin A has a direct effect on the structure and function of pituitary gland, gonads and uterus. The recommended daily supplementation for dairy cows is 35,000-45,000 units (NRC, 2001). One mg of carotene provides 400 IU vitamin A in dairy ration. Carotene is known to be in high concentrations in fresh green roughages, while grains contain relatively low amounts. Silages, especially alfalfa, contain moderate levels, while corn silage is a poor source. Dry hays, especially alfalfa, are excellent sources of carotene (Schweigert and Zucker, 1988).

itamin D Vitamin D contributes to more than calcium and bone formation in cattle. The active vitamin D hormone also contributes to immune, reproductive, and mammary physiology. Multiple tissues and factors also contribute to vitamin D activity (Nelson and Merriman, 2014). A concentrates containing supplemental vitamin D in amounts sufficient should be provided to meet the cow s requirement of 10,000 IU per day.

itamin E Vitamin E functions as an intra-cellular antioxidant scavenging for free reactive oxygen and lipid hydroperoxidases, and converting them to non-reactive forms, thus maintaining the integrity of membrane phospholipids against oxidative damage and peroxidation. In vitamin E and selenium deficiency condition, these free radicals accumulate and not only damage cell membranes, but also disrupt several processes linked to the synthesis of steroids, prostaglandins, sperm motility and the development of the embryo. The current NRC (2001) requirement for dairy cows is 15 IU/kg of DMI (approximately 150 and 300 IU/d for dry and lactating cows, respectively). The vitamin E (-tocopherol) status of dairy cows is an important component of a well-functioning immune system because of its antioxidant effects on cows (Hogan *et al.*, 1993). Feeding vitamin E during dry periods until 30 days after calving resulted in 80 decrease in clinical mastitis and 60 reduction in intra-mammary infections (Weiss *et al.*, 1997). Supplementation of vitamin E at 1,500 IU daily from 60 days prepartum to 30 days post partum to buffaloes exhibited beneficial effect on plasma α-tocopherol level and total antioxidant activity around parturition and continuation of its supplementation at 1,000 IU d-1 from 30 to 60 days of lactation improved postpartum reproductive performance of buffaloes (Panda *et al.*, 2006).

Balanced ration preparation Typically a balance includes all nutrients required by animal to its optimum levels in ration. Balance ration include concentrate, green and dry fodder in specific ratio as per production status of animal. A good quality concentrate can be made at farm by including cereals, cereal byproduct and oil cake in 1:1:1 ratio i.e. for 100 kg about 32 cereal grain like maize, wheat, barley, bajra, jowar, etc 32 byproduct like brans, chunnies and 33 oilcakes with 2 mineral mixture and 1 salt. One kg of this mixture will provide about 200 g protein and 650-700g energy (TDN) along with minerals and vitamins. A provision of 1 kg concentrate mixture per 3 kg milk production is sufficient to take care of nutrient requirement of lactating animals. Dry animals, heifers, or breeding bull can be easily maintained after supplementation of 2 kg concentrate daily. All lactating animals requires 70 of their nutrient requirement from concentrate rest can be given by green fodder. Dry fodder should always be given as rumen filler or low maintenance fodder. No more than 15 expenditure on ration should be on dry fodder for better nutrient availability.

In traditional feeding practices, mustard cake *sani* is done with green or dry fodder supplementation with little or no energy rich cereal grain mixture. This results in very high degradation of mustard cake in short time leading to excessive ammonia in rumen and blood. This results in loss of energy either as urea synthesis in liver or microbial protein in rumen. Both processes need energy. So, mustard cake *sani* should always be supplemented with 1-2 time cereal grain mixture or good energy source for optimum use of cake. Additional problem of excessive ammonia on reproductive health have already be discussed above. Supplementation of mineral mixture enhances optimum use of resources.

Balance ration has direct or indirect role in production of dairy animals. Supplementation of deficient nutrients in ration of dairy cow not only improves productivity but also potentiate immunity. A good management of transition cows a fortnight before to after parturition helps in prevention of clinical form of production diseases. A good choice has to be made in favour of balance feeding or supplementation feeding for higher production than traditional animal rearing on poor quality roughage with low productivity. nowledge of field worker on balance ration must be objective and easy to apply at farm levels. This paper gives an outline of nutrient requirement under field condition and means to achieve a balanced ration at farm level.

R

Amaral-Philips, D. (2011). Phosphorus important for optimum milk production and reproduction in dairy cattle. Accessed on 08/01/2018 at http://afsdairy.ca.uky.edu/files/extension/nutrition/Phosphorus Important For Optimum Milk Production and Reproduciton in Dairy Cattle.pdf.

Blanchard, T., Ferguson, J., Love, L., Takeda, T., Henderson, B., Hasler, J., Chalupa, W. (1990). Effect of dietary crude protein type on fertilization and embryo quality in dairy cattle. Am. J. Vet. Res. 51: 905-908.

Butler, W.R. (2001). Nutritional effects on resumption of ovarian cyclicity and conception rate in *post partum* dairy cows. *British Society for Animal Science ccasional Publication* : 133 145.

Capuco, A.V., Wood, D.L., Bright, S.A., Miller, R.H. and Britman, J. (1990). Regeneration of teat canal keratin in lactating dairy cows. J. Dairy Sci., 73: 1051-1057.

Chawala, R. and aur, H. (2004): Plasma antioxidant vitamin status of periparturient cows supplemented with a tocopherol and -carotene. Anim. Feed. Sci. Tech. 114:279-285.

Collier, R. J., McNamara, J.P., Wallace, C.R. and Dehoff, M.H. (1984). A review of endocrine regulation of metabolism during lactation. J. Anim. Sci. 59:498 510.

Coppock, C.E. (1985). Energy nutrition and metabolism of the lactating dairy cow. J. Dairy Sci. 68:3403 3410.

Cromwell, G.L. (1997). *andbook of copper compounds and applications*. Pp: 177-202.

Daniel, R.C.W. (1983). Motility of the rumen and abomasums during hypocalcemia, Canadian J. Comp. Med. Vet. Sci., 47: 267-280.

Dunn, T.G. and Moss, G.E (1992). Effects of nutrient deficiencies and excesses on reproductive efficiency of livestock, J. Anim. Sci., 70: 1580-1593.

Elrod, C.C. and Butler, W.R. (1993). Reduction of fertility and alteration of uterine pH in heifers fed excess ruminally degradable protein. J. Anim. Sci., 71: 694-701.

Elrod, C.C., van Amburgh, M. and Butler, W.R. (1993). Alterations of pH in response to increased dietary protein in cattle are unique to the uterus. J. Anim. Sci., 71: 702-706.

Fenwick, M.A., Fitzpatrick, R., enny, D.A., Diskin, M.G., Patton, J., Murphy, J.J., Wathes, D.C. (2008). Inter-relationships between negative energy balance (NEB) and IGF regulation in liver of lactating dairy cows. Domest. Anim. Endocrinol. 34: 31 44.

Goff, JP, Dry cow nutrition and metabolic disease in parturient cows. In: *proceeding western Canadian dairy seminar red deer*.

Grummer, R.R. (1993). Etiology of lipid-related metabolic disorders in periparturient dairy cows. J. Dairy Sci. 76:3882 3896.

Halliwell, B. and Gutteridge, J.M.C. (1999). In: Free Radicals in Biology and Medicine, third ed. Oxford University Press, New ork, USA.

Herbein, J.H., Aiello, R.J., Eckler, L.I., Pearson, R.E. and Akers, R.M. (1985). Glucagon, insulin, growth hormone, and glucose concentrations in plasma of lactating dairy cows. J. Dairy Sci. 68: 320 325.

Hess, B.W., Moss, G.E. and Rule, D.C. (2008). A decade of developments in the area of fat supplementation research with beef cattle and sheep. J. Anim. Sci., 86: 188-204.

Hogan J.S., Weiss W.P., Smith .L. (1993): Role of vitamin E and selenium in host defense against mastitis. J. Dairy Sci., 76: 2795-2803.

Holstenius, P. (1993). Hormonal regulation related to the development of fatty liver and ketosis. Acta Vet. Scand. 89(S): 55 60.

Hutjens, M.F., 2000. Feeding management of the 40 000 pound dairy herds. J. Dairy Sci., Vol. 83, Suppl 1, Abstr 108, p26.

appel, L.C. and Zidenberg, S. (1999). *Manganese: Present Knowledge in nutrition*, In: Brown ML (Ed.), International Life Sciences Institute Nutrition Foundation, Washington, . pp 308.

Leroy, J.L., Vanholder, T., Opsomer, G., Van Soom, A. and de ruif, A. (2006). The *in vitro* development of bovine oocytes after maturation in glucose and beta-hydroxybutyrate concentrations associated with negative energy balance in dairy cows. Reproduction in Domestic Animals. 41: 119 123.

Llewellyn, S., Fitzpatrick, R., enny, D.A., Murphy, J.J., Scaramuzzi, R.J. and Wathes, D.C. (2007). Effect of negative energy balance on the insulin-like growth factor system in pre-recruitment ovarian follicles of postpartum dairy cows. Reproduction. 133: 627 639.

Miller, J. ., N. Ramsey and F.C. Madsen, 1988. The ruminant animal. D.C. Church. Ed. Pp. 342- 400. Prentice Hall, Englewood cliffs, N.J.

Mohanrao, B.A., umar, V., D. Roy, M. umar, M. Srivastava and V.P. Gupta (2015). Influence of dietary cation-anionic difference on hematobiochemical profile, mineral metabolism, postpartum reproductive and productive performance of Hariana cows. Indian J. Anim. Res. 50(4): 497-504

Nelson, C.D. and Merriman, .E. (2014). Vitamin D metabolism in dairy cattle and implications for dietary requirements. Accessed on 23/04/2015 at http://dairy.ifas.ufl.edu/rns/2014/nelson.pdf.

NRC-National Research Council, (2001). Nutrient requirements of dairy cattle, seventh revised ed., National Academic Press, Washington, DC, USA.

Panda, N., aur, H. and Mohanty, T. . (2006). Reproductive performance of dairy buffaloes supplemented with varying levels of vitamin E. Asian-Aust. J. Anim. Sci., 9(1): 19-25.

Patterson, H.H., Adams, D.C., lopfenstein, T.J., Clark, R.T. and Teichert, B. (2003). Supplementation to meet metabolizable protein requirements of primiparous beef heifers: II. Pregnancy and Economics. J. Anim. Sci., 81: 503-570.

Paul, S.S., Mandal, A.B., Mandal, G.P., annan, A. and Pathak, N.N. (2004). Deriving nutrient requirements of lactating Indian cattle under tropical condition using performance and intake data emanated from feeding trials conducted in different research institutes. Asian-Aust. J. Anim. Sci., 17:769-776.

Perry, R.C., Corah, L.R., Cochran, R.C., Beal, W.E., Stevenson, J.S., Minton, J.E., Simms, D.D. and Brrethour, J.R. (1991). Influence of dietary energy on follicular development, serum gonadotropins, and first postpartum ovulation in suckled beef cows. J. Anim. Sci., 69: 3762-3773.

Puls, R., 1994. Mineral level in animal health. Diagnotic data. 2nd ed. Sherpa International, Clearbrook, BC, Canada.

ureshi, M.S., Habib, G., Samad, H.A., Siddiqui, M.M., Ahmad, N. and Syed. M. (2002). Reproduction-nutrition relationship in dairy buffaloes. I. Effect of intake of protein, energy and blood metabolites levels. Asian-Aust. J. Anim. Sci., 15(3): 330-339.

Ropstad, E. and Refsdal, A.O. (1987). Herd reproductive performance related to urea concentration in bulk milk. Acta. Vet. Scnd., 28: 55-63.

Roseler, D. ., Ferguson, J.D., Sniffen, C.J. and Herrema, J. (1993). Dietary protein degradability effects on plasma and milk urea nitrogen and milk nonprotein nitrogen in Holstein cows. J. Dairy Sci., 76: 525-534.

Ryan, D.P., Spoon, R.A. and Williams, G.L. (1992). Ovarian follicular characteristics, embryo recovery, and embryo viability in heifers fed high-fat diets and treated with follicle stimulating hormone, J. Anim. Sci., 70: 3505.

Saha, D., Gupta, R.S. and Baghel, R.P.S. (2013). Energy requirements of lactating crossbred cattle (*Bos indicus*). Inter. J. Adv. Biol. Res., 3(4): 527-529.

Sathish umar (2003). Management of infertility due to mineral deficiency in dairy animals. In: Proceedings of ICAR summer school on Advance diagnostic techniques and therapeutic approaches to metabolic and deficiency diseases in dairy animals . Held at IVRI, Izzatnagar, UP (15th July to 4th Aug.). pp. 128-137.

Schweigert, F.J. and Zucker, H. (1988). Concentration of vitamin A, beta-carotene and vitamin E in individual bovine follicles of different quality. J. Reprod. Fertil., 82: 575-579.

Shahzad, M.A., Sarwar, M. and Nisa, M. (2008a). Influence of altering dietary cation anion difference on milk yield M. and its composition by early lactating *Nili Ravi* buffaloes in summer. Livest. Sci. 113: 133-143.

Short, R.E. and Adams, D.C. (1988). Nutritional and hormonal inter-relationships in beef cattle reproduction. Can. J. Anim. Sci. 68: 29-39.

Singh, V. and Bohra, B. (2005). Livestock feed resources and feeding practices in hill farming system a review. *Indian J. Anim. Sci.,* : 121-127.

Spears, J.W. (1994). Minerals in forages. In: G. C. Fahey, Jr. (Ed.) Forge uality, Evaluation, and Utilization. p 281. American Society of Agronomy, Inc., Madison, WI.

Spears, J.W. (2000). Micronutrients and immune function in cattle. In: Proceedings of the Nutrition Society, 59: 587 594.

Spears, J.W. (2003). Trace mineral bioavailability in ruminants. J. Nutr. 133: 1506S 1509S.

Thatcher, W.W. and Staples, C.R. (2000). Effects of dietary fat supplementation on reproduction in lactating dairy cows. In: Advances in Dairy Technology, 12: 213-232.

Tucker, W.B., Hogue, J.F., Waterman, D.F., Swenson, T.S., in, Z., Hemken, R.W., Jackson, J.A., Adams, G.D. and Spicer, L.J. (1992). Sulphur should be included, when calculating the dietary cation-anion balance of diets for lactating dairy cows. In Animal Science Research Report, Pp. 141 150.

Vazquez-Anon, M., Bertics, S.J., Luck, M. and Grummer, R.R. (1994). Peripartum liver triglyceride and plasma metabolites. J. Dairy Sci. 77: 1521 1528.

Weiss, W.P. (2002). Relationship of mineral and vitamin supplementation with mastitis and milk quality. In: National Mastitis Council Annual Meeting Proceedings. Pp 38-44.

Weiss, W.P., Hogan, J.S., Todhunter, D.A. and Smith, .L. (1997). Effect of vitamin E supplementation in diets with a low concentration of selenium on mammary gland health of dairy cows. J. Dairy Sci. 80: 1728-1737.

Wiltbank, M.C., Weigel, .A. and Caraviello, D.Z. (2007). Recent studies on nutritional factors affecting reproductive efficiency in U.S. dairy herds, *estern Dairy Management Conference.*

❑❑❑

Chapter 3

Balance Ration for Optimum Reproduction and Production in Dair Animals

Muneendra Kumar inod Kumar and Raju Kush aha

Department of Animal Nutrition, College of Veterinary Science and Animal Husbandry, Uttar Pradesh Pandit Deen Dayal Upadhyaya Pashu Chikitsa Vigyan Vishwavidhyalaya Evam Go Anusandhan Sansthan, Mathura

I

A dairy animal is known as one of the most efficient producers of food for man. It can utilize large quantities of feed, much of which is inedible in the natural state. Economical production of milk, however, depends largely upon three main factors-the efficiency of an animal, its nutrition, and management. Field surveys to assess the adequacy of traditional feeding practices in dairy cattle and buffaloes followed by farmers have revealed that most of the feeding practices across the different locations, in India, are imbalanced characterized by under or overfeeding of energy and protein (Mudgal *et al.*, 2003). Shortage of feeds and fodder apart from imbalanced feeding is one of the major constraints for improving the dairy production (Garg and Makkar, 2012). The efficient cow/buffalo are the result of inheritance and improved breeding. Its productivity, however, depends upon the adequate inputs in terms of feed and care.

Imbalanced feeding leads to excess feeding of some nutrients, whilst others remain deficient. This not only reduces milk production and increases costs per kg milk, but also affects various physiological functions including long term animal health, fertility and productivity. To ensure improved productivity, it is necessary to augment and secure feed resources through short and long term planning. It is also essential that milk producers feed their animals the nutrients in amounts that match the physiological needs and objective of keeping the animal. The average daily milk production data at 6.52 kg for crossbreds, 2.10 kg for indigenous cattle and 4.44 kg for buffaloes (NSSO, 2007) suggest that the productivity of these animals is far below their genetic potential. Added to this, the in-milk animals as a percentage of the total breedable population, is also very low, as noted by Basic Animal Husbandry Statistics (BAHS, 2010), which reported that at any one time an average of 46 of the total breedable population were dry. This is attributed in part to the deficiency of critical nutrients in the ration. Low productivity of animals with higher genetic potential can be primarily attributed to the imbalanced and inadequate feeding.

A. Feeding of balance ration for optimum milk production

A good feeding programme for a milking cow should achieve a high peak yield early in lactation and a high total lactation yield, prevent too much weightloss, and enable the cow to go on heat become pregnant and produce a healthy calf and make best use of the feeds available. A lactating cow requires nutrients for: maintenance, growth if she is young (less than 30 months), growth of the unborn calf, if she is pregnant and milk production. The amounts of the different nutrients required will depend on which of the above applies to the cow. Immediately after calving, the cow has a low appetite and will not eat as much feed as the body may require. In addition, the cow needs a lot of nutrients to recondition the body as well as to support milk production. If the cow is not given adequate feed during early lactation, it will not produce as much milk as it could, even if the feed supply is improved later in the lactation. In order to make milk production more economical, feed cows with as much forage as possible before offering concentrates. Ensure the milking cow has constant access to water and regular access to a good quality mineral mix. Lactating cows should be fed as per their stage of lactation as mentioned below:

1. Feeding of dairy cows in early lactation

Early lactation usually refers to the first 100 days of lactation. At the beginning of this phase, cows will achieve peak milk production, feed intake is lagging and cows are usually losing weight. At the end of early lactation, peak dry matter will be achieve and no weightlosses occurring. Rations for lactating dairy cows are usually formulated based on protein and energy requirements. However, to achieve maximum production, dairy rations should be balanced for effective fiber, non-structural carbohydrates, ruminal undegraded protein, soluble protein. Dairy rations are usually formulated to maximize microbial yield and for requirements for ruminal undegraded amino acids. The recommendations for feeding dairy cows in the following discussion is based on the assumption that total mixed rations are fed. Dairy cows should be divided into two groups according to stage of lactation. This implies that two different rations should be fed to the herd, one for the high producing group and the other for the low producing group.

During this period, milk yield increases more rapidly than dry matter intake (peak production). The demand for energy is, therefore, higher than the amount of energy consumed. Thus, the cow mobilizes body reserves and losses weight (negative energy balance). The genetic potential is usually expressed during this period and the cow will be under pressure to produce a large amount of milk. However, the cow at this stage has a limited capacity to ingest the required amount of feed. Thus, it is normal for the cow to mobilize body fat during early lactation. The ability of the dairy cow to mobilize body fats contributed to its genetic potential (cows with higher genetic potential will mobilize body fats for a longer period of time than cows with a lower genetic potential). During this period, the cow could lose as much as 0.7 kg/ day.

Feed intake is the key factor in maintaining high milk production. Cows should be encouraged to maximize their intake during early lactation. Each additional kg of dry mater (DM) consumed can support 2 to 2.4 kg more milk. Feed intake by the dairy cow is influenced by many factors including level of production, forage quantity and quality, feed digestibility, feed processing, feeding frequency, consistency of ration ingredients, etc. Maintaining good rumination is essential in early lactation. Thus, it is important to feed at least 40 of the ration DM as forage. About half of the forage should have a particle length of at least 2.6 cm to effectively stimulate chewing. High quality forage should be fed during this period to improve dry matter intake. Neutral detergent fiber and acid detergent fiber levels should be set at 28 and 19 , respectively to maximize intake. Major ration changes should be avoided. To avoid any digestive problems (e.g. acidosis, depressed intake), concentrates should be added gradually at a rate of about 0.5

to 0.7 kg/day for the first two weeks. Protein is very critical during early lactation as the amount of body protein that can be mobilized is very limited compared with body fat. Thus, in early lactation, a dietary protein content of 17 to 19 is recommended. About 35-30 of dietary protein should be ruminally undegraded protein, while 30 should be soluble protein. A guideline is to feed 0.5 kg of a 34 to 50 protein concentrates for every 5 kg of milk produced above 20 kg of milk.

Other feeding strategies for high producing cows

i) Cows usually eat after milking. Thus, fresh feed should always be available in the feed bunk immediately to encourage feed consumption.

ii) Feed feeds and fodders in the form of total mixed rations (TMR). The concentrate component is usually fed only once or twice daily. This result in non-uniform supply of nutrients and inefficiencies of nutrient utilization can occur. Providing feeds and fodders in the form of TMR may help in uniform supply of nutrients and stabilization of rumen environment.

iii) A TMR or forage combination must be adequately mixed in order to provide a proper nutrient balance. When mixing small quantities of specific ingredients (minerals and vitamins), it may more appropriate to include them in a pre-mix, where larger quantities can be added to the ration.

iv) If concentrates are being fed separately from forages, they should be fed several times a day.

v) Do not feed more than 2.5-3.5 kg of grain per feeding. Limiting the amount of grain fed at one time lowers the risk of creating acidotic conditions in the rumen due to rapid breakdown of carbohydrates in the rumen.

vi) Watch particle size of grain. Finely ground grains breakdown rapidly in the rumen and can lead to acidosis problems.

vii) Protein supplements should be fed with energy sources and/or feed the energy source before protein.

viii) Hay should be fed before grain and/or protein supplement in the morning.

ix) Forage should be checked to make sure, it contains enough long fiber. If two forages are being fed, it is preferable to mix them rather than feed them separately.

x) If intakes are below normal, begin by checking the non-fiber carbohydrate level, forage particle size and water quality.

xi) Avoid large variation in forage quality. Feed forages frequently and push up feed frequently. This practice helps keep feed fresh and encourage cows to eat smaller meals more often. Feed some in the morning before cows have access to concentrate.

xii) Increased feeding frequency reduces daily variations in rumen pH and thus, helps stabilizing the rumen environment. The proper range and consistency of ruminal pH is critical in fiber digestion.

xiii) Feeding frequency affects rumen function and cow performance. Feeding protein (soybean meal) and carbohydrate (corn) supplements together results in higher milk fat percentage than feeding them separately. This is because rumen microbes require both energy and protein to grow.

2. Feeding of dairy cows in mid-lactation

Mid-lactation period is the period from day 100 to day 200 after calving. By the beginning of this phase, cows will have achieved peak production. Peak DM intake has also occurred with no more weight-losses. Cows should reach maximum DM intake no later than 10 weeks after calving. At this point, cows should be eating at least 4 of their body weight. The cow should be fed a ration that will maintain peak production as long as possible. For every 2 kg of expected milk production, large-breed cows should eat at least 1 kg DM. The main target during this period is to maintain peak milk productions as long as possible. For each extra kg of milk at peak production, the average cow will produce 200-225 kg more milk for the entire lactation. Thus, the key strategy during mid-lactation is to maximize DM intake. During this period, the cow should be fed high quality forage (minimum 40 to 45 of the ration DM) and the level of effective fiber should be maintained at a level similar to that of early lactation. Concentrates should not exceed 2.3 of body weight and sources of non-forage fibers, such as beet pulp, distiller s grains and cereal bran can replace part of the starch in the ration to maintain a healthy rumen environment. Protein requirements during mid-lactation are lower than in early lactation. Therefore, rations for dairy cows in mid-lactation should contain 15 to 17 crude protein (CP).

3. Feeding of dairy cows in late-lactation

This phase may begin 200 days after calving and end, when the cow dries off. During this period, milk yield continues to decline and so does feed intake. However, the intake easily matches milk yield. The cow also gains weight during this period to replenish the adipose tissue lost during early lactation. However, as lactation approaches an end, more of the increase in body weight is due to the increased size of the growing fetus. Sources of protein and energy are not very critical during this period. Cheap rations can be formulated with non-protein nitrogen (NPN) like urea and a source of readily fermentable carbohydrates, such as molasses.

B. Feeding of balance ration for optimum reproduction

The relationship between nutrition and reproduction is a topic of increasing importance and concern among dairy producers, veterinarians, feed dealers and extension workers. The interaction between nutrition and reproduction has long been known to have important implications for the reproductive performance (Smith and Chase, 2010). Under nutrition results in the loss of body weight and body condition, delays the onset of puberty, increases the post-partum interval to conception, interferes with normal ovarian cyclicity by decreasing gonadotropin secretion and increases infertility. A more complete understanding of how and when nutrition affects reproduction, may provide an alternative approach to managing reproduction in commercial systems that do not depend on the use of exogenous hormones (Pradhan and Nakaghosi, 2003).

Reproductive performance of dairy cattle is influenced by the way cows are fed during the dry period and early lactation. After parturition, cows should be fed rations balanced to maximize dry matter intake so that body weight losses are minimized. This allows the cow to attain a positive energy balance in a shorter period of time. In addition to feeding more energy in early lactation, perhaps more bypass protein is needed. The nutrient requirements for dairy cattle have suggested 60 to 65 degradable and 35 to 40 bypass in the ration dry matter (NRC, 1989). Also, a slightly higher level of protein has been suggested during the first few weeks of lactation due to less dry matter intake. However, it has been suggested that feeding rations high in protein (18 to 20 of dry matter) over long periods may have an adverse effect on conception rate and days open. Fertility in lactating dairy cows appears to have trended downward in recent years, at a time when rapid advances were being made in milk production.

Dry cow feeding programs should be designed to minimize metabolic problems associated with calving. The body condition of the cow should be monitored. Other suggestions follow:

i) Reach a desired body condition score (BCS) at the time of dry-off for cows, 3.0 to 3.5, and at calving, 3.5 to 4.0.

ii) Separate dry cows into two groups: the early dry period and prepartum period (3 to 4 wks before expected date of calving).

iii) After calving, design the feeding program to maximize energy intake, so a positive energy balance can be achieved early in lactation. Increase the grain energy (amount of concentrate) gradually as lactation advances. Feed 3 to 5 kg of high quality long forage around calving to improve DMI and rumen function.

iv) Avoid high levels of degradable protein in early lactation that increase the amount of nitrogenous nutrients to ruminant tissues that may affect reproduction by toxic effects of ammonia on sperm cell, ova and embryo viability.

v) Consider a fresh cow top dress mixture that contains bypass protein and digestible fiber (soy hulls or citrus pulp) to meet lysine and methionine needs.Feed prepartum cows and early lactating cow s rations containing 35 to 40 bypass protein.

vi) Watch for marginal deficiencies of certain minerals and vitamins that may lower fertility.

vii) Use fat and certain feed additives in early lactation that may have a favourable effect on reproductive performance. Dietary fat supplementation (200 and 400 g/cow/day) has the potency to enhance energy balance and improve milk yield without any adverse effects on milk composition.

viii) Drench with propylene glycol (200 ml) starting 3 to 7 days before calving or feed calcium propionate (150 ml) if subclinical ketosis is occurring.

ix) Dietary supplementation of niacin (6 to 12 g/day) will also helps to reduce incidence of ketosis by lowering blood plasma concentration of non-esterified fatty acid (NEFA) and β-hydroxy butyric acid (BHBA) by increasing the serum glucose levels.

x) Add yeast culture (10 to 120 g/day) to stimulate fiber digestion in rumen.

xi) Feed anionic diet (50 to 150 meq/kg DCAD), which increases tissue responsiveness to parathyroid hormone, thus increasing Ca resorption from bone and prevent incidence of milk fever in high milk producing cows.

xii) Adding a buffer pack (sodium bicarbonate/magnesium oxide/calcium carbonate/potassium carbonate @ 200g/cow/day) during early lactation helps to stabilize rumen pH (5.5 to 6.2) and maintain rumen functioning.

xiii) Supplementation of conjugated linoleic acids (CLA) during the periparturient period is an effective means of potentially decreasing energy demand during early lactation.

xiv) Feeding monensin @ 200mg/cow/day before parturition enhances propionate production, so prevent ketosis.

Since feeding alone accounts for more than 70 of the total cost of milk production, balanced feeding of dairy animals can play a pivotal role in a successful dairy development programme worldwide. To maximize profitability from the animals, one needs to ensure that they receive the required quantity of protein, energy, minerals and vitamins, preferably from locally available feed resources. Dairy animals in India are fed mainly on by-products of various food crops, oilseeds and locally grown fodder. In some situations these by-products, especially oilseed cakes or meals are not available in sufficient quantity to meet the entire demand of the livestock population. Limited land available for meeting the needs of an ever growing human population in developing countries cannot be spared for growing additional green fodder and coarse grains for feeding livestock. Even the available resources are not utilized judiciously, as the majority of the animals in these countries are fed imbalanced rations, resulting in milk yields below their genetic potential. If the increased demand for milk caused by an increase in population, urbanization and buying capacity is to be met, productivity of dairy animals must be improved coupled with greater efficiency of use of the available feed resources.

R

BAHS (Basic Animal Husbandry Statistics), 2010. Ministry of Agriculture, Department of Animal Husbandry, Dairying and Fisheries, Government of India, New Delhi.

Garg, M. R. and Makkar, H. P. S., 2012. Balanced feeding for improving livestock productivity, Increase in milk production and nutrient use efficiency and decrease in methane emission, FAO, Animal Production and Health Paper No. 173. Rome, Italy.

Mudgal, V., Mehta, M. ., Rane, A.S. and Nanavati, S., 2003. A survey on feeding practices and nutritional status of dairy animals in Madhya Pradesh, Indian Journal of Animal Nutrition, 20(2): 217-220.

NRC (National Research Council), 1989. Nutrient Requirements of Dairy Cattle. 6th rev. ed. National Academy Press, Washington DC, USA.

NSSO (National Sample Survey Organization), 2007. National Sample Survey Organization, NSSO 61st Round, Livestock productivity and ownership across operational land holding classes in India, Department of Statistics, Government of India, New Delhi, India.

Pradhan, R. and Nakaghosi, N., 2003. Reproductive disorder in cattle due to nutritional status. Journal of International Development and Cooperation, 14(1): 45-66.

Smith, R.D. and Chase, L.E., 2010. Nutrition and reproduction, Dairy integrated reproductive management.

❑❑❑

Chapter 4

Basics of Animal Nutrition and Use of Common eed Ingredients from Local Resources

Shalini as ani inod Kumar and Muneendra Kumar

Department of Animal Nutrition, College of Veterinary Science and Animal Husbandry, Uttar Pradesh Pandit Deen Dayal Upadhyaya Pashu Chikitsa Vigyan Vishwavidhyalaya Evam Go Anusandhan Sansthan, Mathura

I

Traditionally Animal Nutrition is the science of feeds and feeding that includes preparation of feed and it s feeding to animals, to produce adequate and wholesome edible and non-edible products. It forms the basics of livestock production system. The profit and the productivity from livestock sector are largely dependent on providing optimum and balanced nutrition to livestock. It impacts almost every sector of the livestock production *viz*-animal reproduction, health, animal product safety, quality and welfare. The primary aim of raising livestock and poultry is to profitably produce quality animal products for the consumers use. In order to do so, the livestock should be fed with wholesome feeds and fodder. The objective of animal nutrition is to provide all essential nutrients in adequate amount and in optimum proportions.

General Nutrition Principles

Feed is the source of energy and tissue building constituents. Any food constituents or group of food constituents that have the same general chemical composition and that aids in the support of animal life is called nutrients. There are six classes of nutrients: water, carbohydrates, proteins, fats, minerals and vitamins. The roles of certain feed ingredients in a diet can be divided into groups according to how they function in the body. For instance, corn generally provides the greatest source of carbohydrates (for energy) and soyabean meal is used primarily as a protein source. The structural nutrients also include water, minerals, and proteins as well as fats. The regulatory nutrients include vitamins, water, minerals, and proteins. The nutrients that primarily supply energy are fats and carbohydrates, but sometimes proteins can also be used as energy source. The following are the essential nutrients:

Water

Water is an important constituent of all plants and animal tissues. Approximately 50 to 70 per cent of body mass of adults and upto 90 per cent of body mass of newborn animals is water (Church, and Pond 1995). There are typically two major functions of water: component in metabolism, and factor in controlling body temperature. Some of the biological functions of water include aiding digest transport through the gastrointestinal tract, and solvent in blood, tissue fluids, secretions, and excretions. The access to water may occur through different ways. One major source of water intake is through free access to drinking water. Poor water quality will negatively impact the animal s intake and therefore, reduce animal performance. Water quality can be compromised by high levels of salts, nitrates, sulphates, fluoride, pathogenic micro-organisms, algae, pesticides, dissolved solids, and industrial compounds that may be polluting the water supply (EPA 2006 ellems and Church 2002 Hairston and Stribling 1995). Secondly, water can be consumed through the water content of ingested feedstuffs. The leafy succulent roughages contain about 80 water and green grass about 75 .

Carbohydrates

Carbohydrates comprise the largest proportion of livestock rations by providing energy and bulk in the diet. Chemically, carbohydrates contain carbon, hydrogen, and oxygen. The carbohydrate fraction of plant feedstuffs comprises between 70 to 80 per cent of the dry matter of forages and cereal grains, respectively (ellems and Church 2002). Glucose, lactose, galactose, maltose, sucrose, and starch are the main components of carbohydrates that provide energy. However, in ruminant animal, volatile fatty acids are produced in the digestive system from specific carbohydrates that can be used as a source for energy. The carbohydrates that are used in plants and cereals for structural purposes are cellulose, hemicellulose, and lignin. Energy is the nutrient that most often needs to be supplemented in diets of livestock. Energy requirements for cattle and energy content of feeds are expressed in several different ways-Total digestible nutrients (TDN), metabolizable energy (ME), and net energy (NE). Net energy is more accurate than TDN because it accounts for some losses due to metabolism, and it is sub-divided into maintenance energy and energy used for growth and lactation.

Proteins

Proteins are made up of amino acids, which are called the building blocks of muscle. Chemically, protein contains nitrogen, carbon, hydrogen, oxygen, and may contain sulphur. Protein requirements of cattle and feed content of protein is usually expressed as crude protein (CP). Typically, nitrogen in protein is approximately 16 per cent of the protein molecule therefore, to convert nitrogen in feeds to a crude protein equivalent, the formula is: N 6.25. Specific levels and ratios of amino acids are required by the animal to grow, reproduce, and produce milk and eggs therefore, nutritionists try to formulate diets to contain the correct ratios and levels of the amino acids. This is especially more important for pigs and poultry. For cattle, sheep and goat non-protein nitrogen can be used as source of nitrogen to produce microbial protein in the digestive system by micro-organisms to meet the needs of the animal.

Fats

Fats and oils provide additional energy in the diet and it also aids in the absorption of vitamins. Chemically, fats contain carbon, oxygen, and hydrogen, but they can be arranged in a triglyceride form with different length fatty acid units. The energy value of fats is 2.25 times more as compared to carbohydrates.

Minerals

Minerals, including calcium (Ca), phosphorus (P), magnesium (Mg), sodium (Na), potassium ( ), chlorine (Cl), copper (Cu), iron (Fe), manganese (Mn), selenium (Se), zinc (Zn), etc. are recognized to perform essential functions in the body. They play important role in structural integrity and are critical components for maintaining the ionic balance and metabolic activity of the animal. The elements are classified as major and trace (micro) elements according to their requirement by plants and animals or according to concentration in which they are present in plant or animal tissue. Livestock and poultry usually derive their mineral nutrients from the feeds, forages and the water that they consume. Inorganic sources of minerals are often added to diets to provide the correct level of biologically available sources of minerals and to balance levels of minerals that are in other feed ingredients in the diet.

Vitamins

Vitamins are the chemical entities, which are essential for maintaining the metabolic processes at a normal level in animals. They are provided in small quantities in animal diets to assist in metabolic activities. Certain vitamins can be synthesized in animals however, commercial vitamin mixes are added to the diet for those not synthesized and because normal plant feed sources do not contain sufficient amounts of available vitamins. Some vitamins are metabolic essential, but not dietary essential, for certain species, because they can be synthesized readily from other food or metabolic constituents, e.g. various B-vitamins are essential for normal ruminant metabolism (metabolic essential) but are not needed in the diet (not dietary essential) because of bacterial synthesis in the rumen. Vitamin B_{12} is not dietary essential for ruminants, provided cobalt is present in the diet since bacteria can synthesize it in the rumen. While metabolic needs are similar in most of the animals, dietary needs for the vitamins differ widely among the species.

Classification of Feeds

Livestock feeds are generally classified according to the amount of a specific nutrient, they furnish in the ration. A basic understanding of the classification of feed and the nutrient content of common feeds will make it easier for producers to make feeding decisions. They are divided into two general classes- *Roughages* and *Concentrates*.

Roughages They are bulky feeds containing relatively large amount of less digestible material i.e. crude fibre more than 18 and are low (about 60) in TDN on air-dry basis. They are further sub-divided into two major groups green/succulent and dry, based upon the moisture content: 1) Green / succulent roughages They contain about 60-90 per cent moisture e.g. Pastures, cultivated fodders, tree leaves, root crops and silages. 2) Dry roughages They contain about 10-15 per cent moisture e.g. Straw, Hay and kadbi.

In the absence of sufficient grazing grounds of good quality for maintaining the livestock on pasture all the year round, the importance of growing fodder crops to provide economical feed to livestock is of utmost importance. These cultivated fodders are further classified into two groups-leguminous and non-leguminous. The cowpea, cluster bean are the most common *kharif* leguminous crops. Berseem and lucerne are the two other common leguminous *rabi* fodder in India. Although rich in nutrition profile, both of these fodders are liable to produce bloat if given in large quantities and hence, it is advisable that they should be given along with some dry fodder. Among the non-leguminous fodder jowar, maize and sudan grass are most common *kharif* fodder. The oat and barley are the common *rabi* non-leguminous fodder crop. Non-leguminous perennial fodder crop consist of napier grass, hybrid napier, guinea grass and para grass. Other examples of green roughages are- tuber crops (e.g. turnip, sugarbeet), vegetable/fruit wastes, tree leaves (subabool, ber, kachnar, babool, etc.), silage, etc. The roughages could also be grouped on the basis of their capacity to supply nutrients as: 1) Maintenance type Containing 3-5 per cent DCP e.g. Green maize, oat. 2) Non-maintenance type containing less than 3 per cent DCP e.g. Straw, kadbi. 3) Production type containing more than 5 per cent DCP e.g. Berseem, lucerne.

Concentrates These are the feedstuffs which contain less than 18 per cent crude fibre and more than 60 per cent TDN. They are less bulky and have higher digestibility. They are concentrated source of nutrients and therefore, they have higher nutritive value than roughages. The concentrates are further classified as: 1) Energy Rich Concentrates in which CP content is less than 18 e.g. Cereal grains, cereal grain byproducts, Molasses, Roots and tubers. 2) Protein Rich Concentrates when the CP value exceeds 18 . They are further categorized according to source of origin as i) Plant proteins e.g. Oilseed cake, pulse chunni, Brewer s grains and yeast. ii) Animal proteins e.g. Fish meal, Meat meal, Blood meal and iii) non-protein nitrogen.

Feed Supplements

Feed supplements are the compounds used to improve the nutritional value of the basal feeds so as to take care of any deficiency. Commonly used feed supplements are: 1) Vitamin supplements e.g.

Rovimix, Vitablend, Arovit, etc. 2) Mineral supplements e.g. Minimix, Milk min, Nutrimilk, Aromin, etc.

Feed Additives

Feed additives are the non-nutritive substances usually added to basal feed in small quantity for the fortification in order to improve feed efficiency and productive performance of the animals. Some commonly used feed additives are as below: 1) Antibiotics e.g. Terramycin, Zinc bacitracin, Flavomycin, etc. 2) Enzymes e.g. Amylase, lipase, protease, pepsin, etc. 3) Hormones e.g. Estrogen, progesterone, hexosterol, etc. 4) Thyroprotein e.g. Iodinated casein. 5) Probiotics e.g. Microbial species. Lactobacillus. 6) Biostimulators e.g. Extracts of living organs like spleen, liver, ovary, chick embryo, etc. 7) Antioxidants e.g. Vitamin E (Tocopherols), BHT (Butylated hydroxy toluene). 8) Mold inhibitors e.g. Propionic acid, acetic acid. 9) Pellet binders e.g, molasses, sodium bentonite. 10) Coccidiostats, etc.

Ration Ration is the feed allowed for a given animal during a day of 24 hrs. The feed may be given at a time or in proportion at intervals. Balanced ration, is a ration which provides the essential nutrients to the animal in such proportion and amount that are required for the proper nourishment of particular animal for period of 24 hrs. The ration should be balanced, palatable, fairly laxative, bulky, economical and of good quality.

Formulation of ration for dairy animals

For ration formulation, it is desired to meet the total requirement in terms of dry matter, protein and energy. The requirement of dry matter depends upon the body weight and production level of animal. Cattle will generally eat daily 2.0 to 2.5 kg dry matter for every 100 kg of live weight. Buffaloes and crossbred animals are slightly heavy eaters and their dry matter consumption varies from 2.5 to 3.0 kg daily per 100 kg body weight. The total dry matter allowance (DM) is to be partitioned as roughages and 1/3rd as concentrates. Out of the total roughages offered, 2/3rd will be from dry roughages or 3/4th if sufficient legume is available and 1/3rd as green roughages but if the green fodder is legume, this proportion may be only th of the total roughage ration. Production ration is the additional allowance of ration for milk production over and above the maintenance requirement. For zebu, 1 kg additional amount of concentrate is required for every 2.5 kg of milk over and above the maintenance requirement, while the same amount of concentrate is required for every 2.0 kg of milk for crossbred and buffaloes. The formulation of ideal concentrate mixture includes various types of feed ingredients. The primary aim is to fulfill the requirements of energy and protein content of ration. Following feed ingredients are utilized to formulate the concentrate mixture:

1. Cereal supplements (primary source of energy) includes cereal grains like maize, wheat, etc., millets grains like jowar, milo, etc.
2. Cerealby products (diluents medium energy content and source of minerals) like wheat bran, rice bran, maize, etc.
3. Pulse chunnies (medium protein and energy source) arhar chuni, mung chuni, masoor chuni, etc.
4. Salt
5. Minerals
6. Vitamins

India is basically an agriarian country and its large population lives in villages. Their livelihood is dependent mainly on agriculture and animal husbandry. Though India has a huge livestock population, yet the production of per animal milk and other livestock products is below world s average. The analysis of this situation reveals that one of the main reasons for the low productivity of our livestock is malnutrition, under-nutrition or both, besides the low genetic potential of the animals. Availability, vis-a-vis the requirement of green-fodder crops and concentrates, that there is a huge gap between demand and supply of all kinds of feeds and fodders. On the other hand, if we examine the land resources available for growing fodder and forage crops, it is estimated that the average cultivated area devoted to fodder production is only 4.4 per cent of the total area. The permanent pastures, cultivable wastelands, forests and open grazing land are able to meet the forage requirements of the grazing animals only during the monsoon season. But for the remaining periods of the year, the animals have to be maintained on the crop residues or straws of jowar, bajra, wheat, barley, etc. either in the form of whole straw or a bhusa, supplemented with some green fodder, or as sole feed. The crop residues are available mainly from wheat, paddy, bajra, jowar, sugarcane trash, etc. But now it is essential to explore the methods to increase the nutrient utilization of crop residues as well as non-conventional feeds.

Non-conventional feed resources (NCFR)

The non-conventional feed resources (NCFR) refer to all those feeds that have not been traditionally used in animal feeding and or are not normally used in commercially produced rations for livestock. NCFR include commonly, a variety of feeds from perennial crops and feeds of animal and industrial origin. The term NCFR has been frequently used to describe such new sources of feedstuffs as palm oil by-products, single cell proteins, and feed material derived from agro industrial by-products of plant and animal origin. Poor-quality cellulosic roughages from farm residues, such as stubbles, haulms, vines and from other agro-industrial by-products, such as slaughter-house by-products and those from the processing of sugar, cereal grains, citrus fruits and vegetables from the processing of food for human consumption also comes under category of NCFR.

Need of Non-conventional feed resources

There is an acute shortage of conventional type animal feeds. The grains are required almost exclusively for human consumption. With increasing demand for livestock products as a result of rapid growth in the world economies and shrinking land area, future hopes of feeding the animals and safeguarding their food security will depend on the better utilization of unconventional feed resources, which do not directly compete with human food. The availability of feed resources and their optimum utilization for livestock represents biggest challenge to animal scientists in the world. The situation is acute in numerous developing countries, where chronic annual feed deficits and increasing animal populations are common. Thus, non-conventional feeds could partly fill the gap in the feed supply, decrease competition for food between humans and animals, reduce feed cost, and contribute to self-sufficiency in nutrients from locally available feed sources. It is, therefore, imperative to examine for cheaper non-conventional feed resources that can improve intake and digestibility of low quality forages. Feedstuffs, such as fish offal, duckweed and kitchen leftovers (i.e., potato peel, carrot peel, onion peel, and cabbage leftover), poultry litter, algae/Spirulina, leucaena leaf, local brewery and distillery by-products, cactus, coffee pulp are commonly used in India, and could be invaluable feed resources for small and medium size holders of livestock.

Advantages of NCFR

1. These are end products of production and consumption that have no further use.
2. They are mainly organic and can be in a solid, slurry or liquid form. Their economic value is often very less.
3. Fruit wastes, such as banana rejects and pine apple pulp by comparison have sugars, which are energetically very beneficial.
4. The feeds of crop origin, the majority are bulky poor-quality cellulosic roughages with a high crude fibre and low nitrogen contents, suitable for feeding to ruminants.
5. They have considerable potential as feed materials and their value can be increased.

Agro-industrial b -products Appropriate use of relatively inexpensive agricultural and industrial by-products is of great importance for profitable livestock production. However, high cost and low availability of conventional livestock feedstuffs frequently demand consideration of by-products even if efficiency of utilization is low. Efficient use of by-products relies on their chemical and physical properties, which influence production system outputs. AIBP refer to the by-products derived in the industry due to processing of main products. They are less fibrous, more concentrated, highly nutritious and less costly as compared to crop residues.

Agricultural crop residues and concentrate b -products Most common pulses are Urad (Phascolus radiatus), Moong (P. mungo), Moth (P. aconitifolius), cowpea (Vigna catiang), Masoor (Lensasculenta) and Arhar (Cajanus indicus). The husk of pods with leaves and tender stems are left behind as by products, which can be utilized as fairly nutritious cattle feed. They are fairly good source of digestible protein (Ranjhan, 1993) and may be used for livestock feeding along with the concentrate mixture (Bhatti & han, 1996). Gram husk, arhar, urad, moong and masoor chunies are most commonly available by-products used for feeding the animals (Verma, 1997). Wheat bran is very much-used product in formulating feed for dairy animals. It contains about 10 DCP, 65 TDN, 0.07 calcium and 0.35 phosphorus. Rice polish contains about 3 fiber, 12 fat and 12 to 14 CP. It is excellent source of energy and rich in vitamin B complex. It is good feed for Livestock. However, maize gluten feed is rich source of protein (45 to 48) and very useful for livestock feeding (Verma, 1997).

Sugar industr b -products Molasses provides the major source of fermentable carbohydrate (Cheeke, 1991). It is the readily available source of sugar and phosphorus to the animal body. The urea molasses diet can be successfully fed as a sole ration with little protein supplement and forage to growing calves and lactating animals (Ranjhan, 1993). In concentrate mixture, inclusion of 10 to 15 molasses increases the palatability of the concentrate mixture (Verma, 1997). Sugarcane tops are palatable and cattle can be maintained entirely on them with a little supplement of concentrate mixture or leguminous feeds (Verma, 1997). Cane tops can be converted into a good quality silage or hay for feeding during scarcity of fodder. Sugarcane tops with or without leaves have good feeding value and are readily accepted by ruminants fresh, dried or ensiled (Bhatti & han, 1996). Bagasse is a good source of cellulose but is poor in protein (1.3) and high in lignin (16). It has been used successfully as roughage for ruminants. Press Mud can be used in the formulation of livestock feed because it has a higher CP content than molasses and contains more soluble calcium, which is an important constituent of animal feed (Benerjee, 1993).

Animal b -products Fishmeal is highly nutritious feed supplement obtained from fish usually feed supplement for poultry. It contains about 10 moisture, 55 protein, 6.9 fat and 25 mineral salts particularly 5.4 Ca and 3.4 P. It also contains vitamin A, D and few members of vitamin B-group. It is the richest source of vitamins B12 (Verma, 1997). Sterilized fishmeal should be used for feeding the growing and producing animals. Bone meal is a nutritious substance obtained from sterilized bones. It contains about 7 CP, 30 Ca, 15 P and 3 fat. In growing and producing animals, it is used for supplementing their needs of calcium and phosphorus (Verma, 1997). However, blood meal is a major slaughter house by-product which contains over 80 CP but is poor in Ca and P, which make it unpalatable to animals (Ranjhan, 1993 Verman, 1997). Meat meal is a rich source of animal protein and may be fed in small amounts to the growing and producing animals by mixing with concentrate (Restic & ormanjos, 1992). Poultry slaughter wastes contain 3.42 to 21.35 CP, 0.14 to 17.42 crude fat, 0.54 to 11.31 nitrogen free extract (NFE) and 0.16 to 5.0 ash. Amino acid structure of the proteins indicated that the wastes are valuable raw material for the production of protein feed for cattle (Ristic & ormanjos, 1992). Poultry excreta is rich source of protein, calcium, phosphorus and minerals and can be used as source of nitrogen in the cattle ration (Ranjhan, 1993). However, the use of animal by-products is banned in ruminant rations.

Industrial b -products Guar Gum industry by-products is being used as a cattle feed. Starch industry by-products contain enough of nutrients, especially protein and are quite useful for feeding the animals (Ranjhan, 1993). Lemon grass oil industry by-products contains 0.64 DCP and 49.76 TDN hence has got a better nutritive value than straw (Cheeke, 1991) and can be fed to livestock. Dairy Industries by-products, such as skim milk, buttermilk and whey, etc. are valuable substance obtained as by-products during the manufacture of cream, butter and cheese. These substances are quite rich in nutrients, especially proteins. Hence, they are quite useful for feeding the newly born calves (Verma, 1997). Similarly, other Grains milling by-products from barley, sorghum, rye and oats are valuable and may be used as feed for animals (Cheeke, 1991).

ruit and vegetable b -products Citrus pulp contains high amount of soluble sugars with digestibility of 85 and contains about 6.0 CP. It can replace one-third of a concentrate mixture without ill effects on the health and utilization of nutrients in buffaloes (Ranjhan, 1993 Verma, 1997). Tomato Pomace after drying and grinding can be used as a part of animal feed upto 35 level (Verma, 1997). Pine apple waste can be directly fed or can be ensiled. Mango seed kernels are the by-products and are available after the mangoes have been consumed by the human beings. It contains 6 DCP and 70 TDN. It is rich in tannins, which may vary from 5 to 7 . It can be used as one of the ingredients in Livestock rations (Cheeke, 1991).

Marine astes and a uatic plants b -products Various marine (sea) product wastes are available for animal feeding, such as fish wastes, frog meal, weeds and aquatic plants, etc. Agar-agar is being extracted from sargussan seaweed and its by-products can be used for livestock feeding. This product contains about 33 ash and 10 protein (Verma, 1997).

It is quite essential to have the knowledge of basics of animal nutrition for effective and optimum feeding of livestock. This will ensure better health, enhance production and will turn to be a profitable venture. The main reason for the poor animal production is the inadequate supply and low level of feeding due to serious shortage of feedstuffs. A major gap exists between the requirements and supplies of nutrients for feeding of animal, the non-conventional feeds could partly fill this gap. Several factors may account for their limited use, among which is their low nutritive value, Seasonal availability, high cost of handling and transportation from the production site to the farm, presence of anti-nutritional factors. It is essential to increase feeds by growing more fodders, propagating agro and social forestry, improving the nutritive value of crop residues and utilising other NCFRs.

R

Banerjee, G.C., 1993. Animal Husbandry. Oxford and IBH Publishing Co. Pvt. Ltd., New Delhi.

Bhatti, M.B. and S. han, 1996. Fodder Production in Pakistan. FAO PARC, Islamabad.

Cheeke, P.R., 1991. Applied Animal Nutrition, Feeds and Feeding, New ork.

Hairston, J.E. and L. Stribling, 1995. Drinking water for livestock and poultry. Alabama Cooperative Extension System. ANR-790 2.6. Auburn University, Auburn, AL.

ellems, R.O., and D.C. Church, 2002. Livestock feeds & feeding. 5th ed. Prentice-Hall. Upper Saddle River, NJ.

Pond, W.G., D.C. Church, and .R. Pond, 1995. Basic animal nutrition and feeding. 4th ed. John Wiley and Sons. New ork, N .

Ranjhan, S. ., 1993. Animal Nutrition in Tropics, 3rd, Ed. New Delhi.

Ristic, M. and S. ormanjos, 1992. Non-edible poultry slaughter by products as raw material for producing feed for cattle, Veterinarski Glasnik, 46: 233 8.

□□□

Chapter 5

Basics of Clean Milk Production

D.N. Singh Aja Kumar and Rajneesh Sirohi

Department of Livestock Production Management, College of Veterinary Science and Animal Husbandry, Uttar Pradesh Pandit Deen Dayal Upadhyaya Pashu Chikitsa Vigyan Vishwavidhyalaya Evam Go Anusandhan Sansthan, Mathura

Milk and milk products are a rich and convenient source of nutrients for people in many countries and international trade of milk-based commodities are significant. All foods especially animal products have the potential to cause food borne illness, and milk and milk products are no exception. Dairy animals may carry human pathogens. Such pathogens present in milk may increase the risk of causing food borne illness. Moreover, the milking procedure, subsequent pooling and the storage of milk carry the risks of further contamination from man or the environment or growth of inherent pathogens. Therefore, implementing the proper hygienic control of milk and milk products to ensure the safety and suitability of these foods for their intended use.

The objective of clean milk can be achieved by practical application of science based system, such as Hazard Analysis Critical Control Point (HACCP). Not only it should produce quantum milk, but must also be free from debris, microbes and must remain so, till it is consumed. Raw milk quickly becomes sour, when it is stored for long periods at high ambient temperatures prevalent in tropical and subtropical countries. This is due to the inherent lactic acid bacteria and contaminating micro-organisms from milk vessels or the environment break down the lactose in milk to lactic acid. When sufficient lactic acid has accumulated, the milk becomes sour and coagulates. Raw milk that contains too much lactic acid, even if it does not appear to be curdled, will coagulate when heated. This acidity is known as developed acidity and such milk is not acceptable for sale.

Clean milk is essential for production of good quality dairy products, taste and flavour, free from pathogens and long keeping quality. Good quality dairy products cannot and can never be made from poor quality raw milk. Good quality raw milk must be:

a) Free from dung & debris and sediment.

b) Free from off-flavours.

c) Low in bacterial numbers.

d) Normal composition and acidity.

e) Free of antibiotics and chemical residues.

In order for milk to reach the processor and ultimately the consumer still in good condition, a number of things must be observed right from the farm level to the processing factory, and thereafter to the retailers and consumer.

Strategies for clean milk production

The first step to clean milk production should be education and training of milk producers on hygiene, housekeeping, sanitation, milking methods and good animal husbandry practices.

1. **A areness and training** Educational aids and programmes should be organized for the farmers for making them aware of the importance of clean milk production. This should be in the form of charts/posters displayed at village, society and milk collection centres. Make them aware of the correct handling of the milk from udder to reception dock, maintenance of hygienic environment, clean utensils to availability of milk cooling bulk tanks and coolers.

2. **eeding practices** The feeds and fodder of the animals should not introduce directly or indirectly microbiological or chemical contaminants in the milk in amounts that is unacceptable to health. Feed fodder and silage should be procured from a reliable source and should be stored properly.

3. **Housing management** The shed should be comfortable and clean with suitable arrangement to dispose off dung, urine, feed and fodder residues. There should be proper supply of clean drinking water and electricity. The shed should be washed before

milking.

Sanitation and Disinfection of the Animal Houses

Cleaning and sanitation are complementary. By sanitation we adopt hygienic measures aiming at creating conducive to health of animals and assuring product quality. The measures include proper cleaning of habituation, adequate drainage system, adequate lighting of building and sheds, proper ventilation and proper disinfection measures. It involves cleaning of bedding material like sawdust, paddy, straw, etc. once daily. Watering and feeding material to be thoroughly cleaned.

- In case of mud floor, a top of 12-15 cm soil is removed and replaced with clean soil.
- Cleaning and washing of milk parlours.
- Sloped drains having width of 6-12 inches and 2 inch depth. It should maintain a proper gradient of 1 in 60 for easy flow of drain water.
- Provide adequate lighting.
- Provide proper ventilation.
- Disinfect the houses by washing the houses with boiling water, flame blower or by using suitable disinfectants, such as formaldehyde, phenols, cresols, washing soda, quick lime, bleaching powder, etc.
- The hygiene and sanitation process practiced in a dairy herd can not only keep the animal and surrounding healthy but will also find its way for export of milk and milk products thereby, enhancing the efficiency of livestock and its productivity, survivability and longevity.

4. *an n of n esse s* The milking vessel should be made of stainless steel. It should be cleaned before and after milking with hot water and certified detergents/chemicals. It should have small mouth. The milker should wear clean clothes and maintain personal hygiene. He should wash his hands before milking and should not spit or smoke. Shaving the hair of the hind legs and tail should be carried out routinely. Also the fore milk should be discarded in a proper place.

5. Udder Hygiene

- Effective milking practice is one important criterion in order to produce safe and suitable milk failure of which may introduce contamination of milk. From an ethological perspective, the cow rests in a lying position, which inevitably leads to contact of the udder skin with filth on the bedding surface. As much as 1×10^{10} of total micro-organisms can be found in one gram of filth from the udder surface.
- With unsuitable udder hygiene, the micro-organisms present on the teat skin can contaminate the milk during milking or through the teat tip will penetrate the teat canal increasing the possibility of mastitis. Hence, it is necessary to implement hygienic-prophylactic measures in maintaining cleanliness and udder health before and after milking of dairy herds, with the aid of disinfecting agents.
- There are many procedures for udder hygiene prior to milking, such as:

  Washing by spraying water and wiping of teats.

  Washing of teats with a cloth immersed in warm disinfectant solution and drying with a dry cloth.

  Immersing of teats in disinfectant and wiping with a paper cloth.

  Appropriate hygiene, such as dry cleaning, is necessary for lowering teat contamination, whereas only the substantially soiled udders require washing with water. Therefore, if the udder is not substantially soiled, the teats should be immersed in active foam disinfectant and wiped with disposable paper cloths after 1-2 minutes.

  Disinfection prior to milking by immersing teats in a special cup, containing active foam based on surface active compounds, organic acids and hydrogen peroxide, and disinfection after milking by immersing teats in the agent containing 1.94 linear dodecyl-benzene sulphonic acid (LDBS) and skin care substances.

  The implementation of udder hygiene after milking is a very rational method for maintaining acceptable udder health status, and is conducted by immersing teats in a disinfecting agent. This procedure removes the milk droplets that are left behind, which can serve as a breeding ground for surrounding pathogenic micro-organisms. Subsequent drying of the disinfectant creates a thin layer over the teat orifice, mechanically preventing the incursion of micro-organisms through the teat canal.

6. *ea t ana e ent*: Good animal husbandry practices including regular monitoring of disease, such as mastitis should be a part of the routine work. During milking, using teat dips, and washing of udder should be an ongoing activity of the dairy farm. Sick animal shed should be far away from the milking barn and separated from the healthy ones. The healthy animals must be milked first. Improper use of veterinary drugs should be avoided.

7. *co ect on an trans ortat on* There should be a provision of bulk cooling tanks in order to reduce the bacteriological load in the milk immediately after collection. Introducing differential pricing system based on bacteriological quality of milk will help in overall improvement of milk quality reaching the dairy dock. Other pre-requisites for clean milk production include hygienic norms, good animal husbandry practices and proper handling, storage and transportation of milk are important elements to produce quality milk. The lids of the milk cans should fit tightly preventing from entry of rain and dust. The cans should be stored in an inverted condition on stand. Excessive agitation, while transportation should be avoided. When milk is agitated, the milk fat is destabilised which becomes easily oxidised. The milk tanker should have proper insulation. The number of spoilage bacteria in raw milk depends on the level of hygiene during milking and the cleanliness of the vessels used for storing and transporting the milk. During the first 2 3 hours after milking, raw milk is protected from spoilage by inherent natural antibacterial substances that inhibit the growth of spoilage bacteria. However, if the milk is not cooled, these antibacterial substances break down causing bacteria to multiply rapidly. Cooling milk to less than 10 C may prevent spoilage for upto three days. High storage temperatures result in faster microbial growth and hence, faster milk spoilage.

It is concluded that the dairy organizations whether co-operative or private, concentrate their focus on the animal husbandry practices in general and basics of handling of animal products & clean milk production. For this purpose, the dairy organization should create a taskforce to initiate quality improvement program. This taskforce should undertake benchmark survey in terms of standard plate count and spore counts, and then decide the targets to be achieved in phased manner. It is essential to induct quality control professionals, who can face the challenge of improving substantially the quality of milk and milk products.

❑❑❑

Chapter 6

Management Strategies to Improve Production Efficiencies in Dair Animals

Rajneesh Sirohi ajuvendra Singh and D.N. Singh

Department of Livestock Production and Management, College of Veterinary Science and Animal Husbandry, Uttar Pradesh Pandit Deen Dayal Upadhyaya Pashu Chikitsa Vigyan Vishwavidhyalaya Evam Go Anusandhan Sansthan, Mathura

---

Management is the art and science of combining ideas, facilities, processes, materials and labour to produce and market a worthwhile product or service successfully.

Thus, a manager is an organizer and a converter-he converts resources into products. This is just as true for our dairy farm as for our biggest industries. The managers of motor company convert labour, steel, rubber, plastics into falcons. We convert labour, soil, fertility, hay, silage, and other inputs into milk. These transformations do not occur by happen stance. They are the result of a purposeful and pre-meditated force called management, a process we shall examine more closely.

From a general point of view, a manager must perform five major functions he must plan, organise, co-ordinate, direct and control. Another way of expressing these managerial functions is to consider the manager s role as a decision-maker , i.e. who must decide what to do, how to do it and when. This decision-making responsibility distinguishes the manager from the hired worker who awaits to be told. Thus, the functions of management may be outlined as steps in decision-making, sometimes called the management process . For successful performance of these processes, the manager must:

i) **Observe** Gather information about all resources available, new technologies which may apply, alternative market outlets, sources of capital credit needed and other items affecting successful operation.

ii) **Establish goals** Clearly set out the objectives he wants to achieve

iii) **Identif problems** Find the obstacles, or stumbling blocks, which hinder progress towards goals

iv) **Anal se** Compare alternative methods of reaching goals, considering for each plan the income potential, the capital needed, the labour required, etc.

v) **Decide** Choose a plan of action and set out a clear-cut procedure for getting under way

vi) **Act** Put his chosen plan into operation

vii) **Be responsible** Assume responsibility for the consequences of actions taken

viii) **Evaluate** Measure results and compare accomplishments with goals and standards of performance

ix) **Control** eep a careful check on production level, labour efficiency, cost, investments, etc.

x) **Adjust** eep the operating system flexible to take advantage of new development which are applicable.

One will not take time, of course, to work through these processes formally for every decision made. With some practice, however, it may become a way of reasoning and planning, which may be applied to any problem to be solved. For major decisions, such as buying a farm, closing a long-range plan of operation or making a major adjustment in operations, it should be followed carefully, using the appropriate tools outlined below:

Tools of Management

One of our first jobs as a farm manager is to be well-informed about many kinds of information affecting our business. Should decisions cannot be made consistently on the basis of erroneous information Some of the tools which are helpful in acquiring accurate information about our business and in guiding our management decisions are as follows:

1. **arm records** No business of any consequence can be operated successfully without a good system of accounting. For a dairy farm, these accounts should include the following as a minimum:

   a) Complete inventories at the beginning and end of each year-including a summary of all assets, debts and net worth

   b) Production records (including main animal products and their by-products)

   c) Current expenditures and receipts (including quantities sold)

   d) An annual production and financial summary and

   e) An analysis of the year s records to determine strong and weak points of the business and to serve as a guide to wiser adjustments.

2. **Comparative Block Budgeting** : This is a quick and effective way to compare alternative system of organizing our overall farm business from the standpoint of capital, labour requirements, and the net income potential. These budgets are based upon long-run expectations of yields, prices and costs.

3. **Annual budgeting** : This is a must to guide year to year adjustments in an operating system. Annual budgets are based on the current outlook for yields, prices and costs. They give a preview of the coming year s business and often allow one to correct mistakes in judgment before they happen.

4. **Partial budgeting** : This is a shorter process of comparing the costs and returns from alternative adjustments in some part of our business, such as the pros and cons of some new technology.

It is worthwhile repeating that all kinds of budgets used in planning for the future-one of our major responsibilities as a planner-must be based upon reliable information. Careful analysis of our own records, a study of analysis from similar farming operations and an up-to-date knowledge of the results of new research will provide the data needed.

Environmental stress management

Environmental temperatures affect dry matter and water consumption of cows and buffaloes, which subsequently affect animal productivity. The animals should be provided *ad libitum* water during hot-dry and hot-humid months so that the requirement of milk synthesis can be met. The roughage intake of cows during summer reduces due to more heat of fermentation generated in rumen from fibrous feed. In fact, heat also reduces total DM intake. Therefore, animals should be fed lush green fodder and adequate concentrate during summer. Crossbred cows can resist the rigours of high temperature for longer periods without adverse effect on dry matter intake, milk production and the production of fat, protein and lactose, if *adlib* water and green fodder are made available during hot-dry months of May-June.

- Provision of wallowing tank for buffaloes during summer and hot-humid season further improves their reproductive behaviour and milk production.
- Through adoption of eco-friendly housing system (uccha floor, sand bedding) problems of hoof diseases can be minimized. Besides, introduction of forced water and fan cooling can sustain the body temperature of crossbreds cow at a temperature levels ranging between 38.4 to 38.6^{0}C. The average body temperature of cows can be reduced from 39.62 to 38.40^{0}C in hot-humid season during daytime. The process of sustaining body temperature close to normal range 38.4 to 38.8^{0}C increases average daily milk yield of crossbred cows by 2.86 and 2.26 g in hot-dry and hot-humid season, respectively.
- In winter season, adequate protection from the cold stress also improves milk productivity by 2.6 g/day/cow. Buffaloes have remarkable capacity to adopt themselves to the most adverse climatic conditions from 4 to 40^{0}C. Appropriate nutritional/ feeding approaches like offering the fresh feeds during evening/ night or cool hours should be adopted. The lactating animals should be offered succulent green fodder along with high amounts of concentrate. The animal should be offered adequate salt and sodium bicarbonate to maintain the sodium and potassium levels of blood.

Milking management

- Lactating animals should be milked completely and at regular milking intervals. For complete letdown of milk proper and adequate milking stimulus should be given to buffaloes. Washing with lukewarm water improves milk letdown time. Improper preparation of the lactating animal leads to incomplete evacuation of milk, which in turn increases the amount of residual milk and decreases the intensity and amount of milk secretion.
- If more number of animals are to be milked in a organized dairy farm, use of single cloth for washing the udder and teats should not be done, as it spreads pathogens between cows. The towel cloth should never be dipped in bucket after it has been in contact with a cow.
- Hands of the milder, his dress and milking instruments should be clean and properly sanitized. It is the duty of every milker to regularly inspect the udder, teats and milk for any injury/ abnormality. Any change should be recorded and treatment followed.
- It has been observed that comfortable and congenial environment during milking leads to more milk yield from the animals than that of roughly handled and excited ones (Release of oxytocin is inhibited in stressed animals). Therefore, attempt should be made to make milking a pleasant experience for the cows to ensure more milk flow. Overcrowding of animals in milking place should be stopped, as it also causes stress.

Tips for clean milk production

- Production of clean milk is one of the most important factors in dairy industry.
- Animal housing should be clean and free from any contaminants.
- Milking place should be separate and suitably comfortable.
- Washing of teats/udder before milking.
- Animal should be healthy and free from any disease. Milk drawn from a healthy animal already contains some bacteria.
- Milker hand should be clean/properly washed.

- Milker should be healthy and free from any infection or disease.
- Milking machine, milking utensils/collection vessels should be clean to lower the bacteriological counts of milk.
- Storage tank of milk should be washed with cleaning detergent daily.
- Milk should be stored at 4^0C immediately till milking operations are over.
- A clean and good quality muslin cloth may be used to remove foreign particles of milk.
- Milk tankers should be cleaned at regular intervals and milk transport to the plant should be within 1 hour of milking.
- Milk with high Somatic Cell Counts (SCC) or mastitis should be discarded. Cows producing such milk require immediate attention for mastitis control.

Concetrate feeding

Concentrate is used to supplement roughages to meet milk production requirement and is essential even for maintenance, when poor quality roughages are fed. The grain should be grinded to atleast of the raw size so that it may not pass off undigested in dung. To further enhance digestibility and palatability, concentrate mixture can be made wet with water and sweetener (Gur) for atleast 4-6 hrs. before mixing with dry feed hay. The ingredients of the concentrate mixture should be of standard quality and free from fungus (aflatoxins), weeds, molds, and dust.

- Concentrate mixture is given at the rate of 2.5 kg per kg milk for animals yielding milk of high fat percentage, in addition to maintenance ration.

Milk production kg	Concentrate kg
5.0	2.0
10.0	4.0
15.0	6.0

- Concentrate mixture is given at the rate of one kg per 1.5-2.0 kg milk for buffaloes.

- The detailed composition of the concentrate is given below:

Composition of the eed Materials	Parts
Maize	16
Barley/wheat/oats or combination	15
G.N. Cake (oiled)	18
Mustard Cake (oiled)	8
Cotton seed cake	7
Wheat bran	15
De-oiled Rice bran	8
Mineral Mixture (BIS standard)	2
Common salt	1
BIS Standard for eed ualit	
Crude Protein not less than	20
Crude Fibre not more than	10
Acid Insoluble Ash not more than	2.5
Crude Fat not less than	4.5
Moisture not more than	10

Buffaoes

Milk production kg	Concentrate kg
5	2.5
10	5
15	7.5
20	10

- The amount of concentrate mixture can be altered based on the type of feed i.e., green or straw and the dry matter content. However, more grain intake relative to the forage often result in off-feed problems, metabolic acidosis and decline in milk production.

Rations for dair co s eighing kgs ith kg milk ield	
Green fodder (25 DM)	10 kg
Wheat Bhusa	4 kg
Concentrate mixture	5 kg
Or	
Green Berseem (12 DM)	12 kg
Wheat Bhusa	5 kg
Concentrate mixture	5 kg

Cow- 450 LW, 20 kg milk (4% fat)

A ration on a leguminous fodder, such as berseem as the chief roughage is given below:

eedstuffs	**uantit**	**DM**	**TDN**	**CP**
Berseem fodder, kg	80	9.6	6.144	1.344
Concentrate, kg	6.5	5.85	4.095	0.819
TDN 70				
CP 20				
Total nutrients, kg		15.45	10.239	2.163

10 kg of berseem should be replaced by wheat/rice straw, equivalent to its DM for avoiding bloat condition, and to keep the animal warm during winter, as straw generates more heat during fermentation.

A combination of a leguminous and a non-leguminous fodder, as the basic roughage can be used as part of the ration as given below:

eedstuffs	**uantit**	**DM**	**TDN**	**CP**
Berseem fodder, kg	55	6.6	4.224	0.924
Oats fodder, kg	25	5	3.2	0.5
Concentrate, kg	4.3	3.87	2.709	0.774
TDN 70				
CP 20				
Total nutrients, kg		15.47	10.133	2.198

Cow-450 kg LW, 38 kg milk (4% fat)

Maintenance of lactation

High protein die with highly degradable protein is avoided at the initiation of lactation. An extra allowance of 1-1.5 kg concentrate mixture over and above the calculated amount for a period of 2 months can be given to encourage the cows to produce more milk. Increasing the bypass protein of the diet without increasing the total protein intake can prove economically beneficial to high yielding animals.

The composition of the concentrate mixture is given below:

Ingredients		Percentage Part
1.	Ground Nut/Cotton Seed/Mustard Cake	33
2.	Maize grain/Oats/Wheat	31
3.	Wheat bran/Rice Bran	33
4.	Mineral mixture	2
5.	Common salt	1

Feeding during dry period

During lactation, the animal exhibit heat symptoms and passes through the various stages of reproductive events and becomes pregnant. During the last 2-3 months of pregnancy, a concentrate supplementation over and above maintenance is given at the rate of 1-2 kg/cow/day and 1.5-3.0 kg/buffalo/day with the composition as described above. The requirement of the buffaloes differs from that of cattle, as they are heavier in body weight than cattle, have more feed capacity (0.5), possess better capacity to utilize crop residue and have more fat in milk. Therefore, buffalo is less temperamental with respect to feeding of crop residue based diets.

Type of fodder and feeding

- The fodder can be fed fresh as such or in preserved form like hay or silage. Non-leguminous fodder substantially meets the maintenance requirement but is limiting in protein content, while leguminous fodder are rich in protein, calcium and phosphorus but is limiting in terms of dry matter (and thereby TDN) because of high moisture content. Therefore, a combination of both leguminous and non-leguminous fodder is best to meet the maintenance and production requirement of animals.

- Split feeding day and night during summer and hot-humid months improves milk production. Non-availability of water restricts the total DM intake of lactation animals and could limit peak milk yield. The reports indicate that even a one pound increase in peak yield translates into a 200 pound increase in milk production over the entire lactation.

Dr matter re uirement and milk production fat NRC

Production level kg	DM intake L
10	2.1
10	2.55
15	3
20	3.4
25	3.75
30	4.15
35	4.6
40	5.05

- Portable and clean water should be provided *adlib* during summer months, as it is one of the most essential input for milk production.
- Lactating animal feed should contain at least 17 crude fiber. The low fiber diet along with high intake of concentrate during hot-humid season leads to drop in milk fat per cent, a condition called low fat syndrome . The changes occur due to altered ratio of Acetate: Propionate as a result of less feed intake and more of concentrate. On the other hand, high fiber and low quality fodder always limit intake of animals, and this is very true during hot-humid conditions. The quantity of crop residues offered during hot-humid season should be minimum to relieve the animal of extra heat load, as a result of higher heat of fermentation from crop residues. This can also increase the energetic efficiency for milk production.

R

Sastry, N.S.R. and Thomas,C. .In Livestock Production Management By alyani Publications, New Delhi.

❑❑❑

Chapter 7

Health E amination of Animals

Mukesh Srivastava

Department of Veterinary Medicine, College of Veterinary Science and Animal Husbandry, Uttar Pradesh Pandit Deen Dayal Upadhyaya Pashu Chikitsa Vigyan Vishwavidhyalaya Evam Go Anusandhan Sansthan, Mathura

In the investigation of any animal disease problem, the veterinarian must, of necessity, undertake a careful and thorough clinical examination with the object of recognizing the nature of the affection, so that effective treatment and, where practicable, control measures are adopted. The situation is rendered complex by the necessity to deal with a variety of species of domestic animals and birds. Increasing specialization on the part of practising veterinarians will resolve some of the apparent problems, thus presented. In general, however, the same principles may be applied in all cases to deal with the diverse difficulties that clinical diagnosis presents. The organs or systems involved, the location, type of lesion present, the pathophysiological processes occurring and the severity of the disease can be deduced from the information gained during the clinical examination. Without a proficient clinical examination and an accurate diagnosis, it is unlikely that the control, prognosis and welfare of animals will be optimized.

The success of clinical examination relies heavily on the knowledge of the clinician and usually assumes a single condition is responsible for the abnormalities. Many clinicians begin their examination by performing a general examination, which includes a broad search for abnormalities. The system or region involved is identified and is then examined in greater detail using either a complete or a problem oriented examination. For this sound knowledge of Anatomy, Physiology, Pathology and Animal behaviour, skills in the methods and techniques of clinical examination, knowledge of etiology, clinical sign and pathogenesis of the diseases are the basic requirements for clinician to make diagnosis. This manual is a practical guideline for veterinary practitioner with the following objectives:

- Guide to apply methods of animal handling/restraint and ability to take history.
- A guide for general and systemic physical clinical examination for further diagnosis, treatment and take practicable control and prevention measures on identified disease.
- Having knowledge on preparation and administration of veterinary drugs.
- Gives skills on veterinary laboratory sampling.

History Taking (Anamnesis) : Disease problems in veterinary medicine are invariably presented to the clinician through the medium of the owner s complaint, which is a request for professional assistance. For completeness and accuracy of history taking, the following points should be well considered (Patient data, Immediate/Present history, Past history, Management and Environment history):

- Art of getting essential information relating to the circumstances of the immediate disease problem from the owner by mean of appropriate questioning.
- Whenever possible leading question should be avoided and an attempt should be made to establishing good rapport by exhibiting a friendly manner.
- The owner or attendant must be handled with diplomacy and tact.
- Local language should be preferred, technical terms should be avoided as owner likely to get confused by these terms.

Patient data

This data is essential for accurate identification of the patient and includes:

- Name and address of owner.
- Identification of animal marking /tags / branding
- Species of animals.
- Breed of animal.
- Sex of animal.
- Age of animal.

- Use of animal.
- Colour
- Parity
- Pregnancy status and lactation

a) Present history

This relates to the sequence of events associated with the period of time that the animal has been ill the chronological order. e.g In Parvo virus infection first dullness, then vomiting followed by diarrhea and in last hemorrhagic diarrhea. Points to be focus in present history are:

- Duration of the disease: whether it is peracute, acute, subacute or chronic,
- Specific question should be centered on aspects like appetite for food or drink, defecation, urination, respiration, sweating, physical activity, milk production, growth, gait, posture, voice, odour, etc.).
- The question should be designed to certain the degree and nature of departure from normal,
- That may have been observed in any of these function,
- Information related to any surgical, therapeutic or prophylactic procedure, such as docking,
- Castration, vaccination, de-worming, topical paraciticide should be obtained,
- Treatment given: determine whether any treatment has, in fact, been given before calling for assistance. Due consideration must be given to effect of treatment modifying the clinical sign of disease also their effect on laboratory investigation,
- Nature of disease can be determined by:

  Morbidity rate : It is usually expressed as the percentage of animals which are clinically affected to the total number of animals of the species exposed to same risks.

  Case fatality rate : It is the percentage of affected animals which died.

  Population mortality rate: It is the percentage of the all animals exposed which died.

b) Past history

In this respect, information should be obtained relating to the nature and timing of any previous illness, which had affected the individual animal or group. Details regarding clinical features, diagnosis, treatments, morbidity and mortality rates, post mortem observations, laboratory test, etc., should be obtained.

System of animal replacement- this information is used to determine either herd is closed or animals are frequently added at a regular interval. Newly introduced animal:

- Can be carrier of disease (from earlier environment)
- Can get infection during transit.
- Can get infection in new environment for which he is not immune (endemic disease of new environment).
- May have not been adopted to mental stressor like altitude, temperature, new feeding practice.
- May have not been accustomed to poisonous plant of new area.
- Prophylactic and control measure: this include vaccination schedule, de-worming, course of chemo-prophylactic drugs (specially in neonatal calves and piglets), use of diet containing growth promoter and laboratory monitoring to determine the resistance pattern of environmental pathogenic bacteria.
- Culling rate : due consideration should be given to reason for culling like failure to grow, poor productivity, short productive life, these consideration will suggest a no. of chronic disease including some caused by infectious agent and some by nutritional deficiency and some by poison.
- Transit : The possibility of infection during transit is always potential risk and presale certificate of health may be of value if an animal has passed through a sale barn. Highly infectious diseases may be transmitted via trucks, rail, road, cars or other accommodation contaminated by previous inhabitant.

c) General history / Managemental history

- This includes nutrition, breeding, climate, and general management of animals.

1. Nutrition

- Nutrition: uantity and quality of feed will determine the level of nutrition
- a- Animals on pasture-
- Diet of livestock at pasture is less controlled, so difficult to access.
- Risk of parasitic infestation and some infectious disease is more on pasture feeding.
- Enquiry should be made for:

  Composition of pasture

  Probable nutritive value of pasture

  Recent change brought by rain or drought

  Method of grazing (rotational/ random)

  Fertilizer program

  Top dressing with mineral mixture and trace elements.
- b- Animal on Stall feeding/ Hand feeding
- They are subjected to more or less controlled feed supply
- Examples of human mistake for dietary errors are osteodystrohia fibrosa in horse on diet containing excess bran, azuturia in horse on high carbohydrate diet in period of rest and acid indigestion in cattle.
- Source of dietary ingredient : It is very important factor because grains from some area are often much heavier and contain much greater proportion of starch to husk ratio.
- Digestive capacity: Digestive capacity of newborn animal is most efficient in the digestion of whole milk, so use of non-milk source of carbohydrate and protein in the formulation of milk replacer may result in diarrhea.
- Processing of feed: it may lead to change in value in case of-

  Overheating/ cooking of feed can reduce their vitamin content

  Pressure extraction of linseed can leave considerable residues of HCN in the residual oilcake.

- Feeding practice: Pig fed in large No. with inadequate space is likely to be affected by overeating or inanition depending on their size and vigor.
- uality of conserve fodder: It may be caused of ragwort, moldy sweet cover, horsetail and ergot poisoning.
- Ensiled grasses are cause of primary ketosis as high content of butyric acid.
- Silage which has not undergone complete fermentation may allow multiplication of Listeria spp., which can cause out break of listeriosis (Silage disease).
- Food stuff of animal origin is possible source of FMD, African swine fever, Anthrax, and Salmonellosis.

2. Breeding/ Reproductive performance

- In the examination of single animal the breeding and parturition history may suggest or eliminate some diagnostic possibilities like:

  Pregnancy toxemia in sheep occurs in late pregnancy.

  etosis in dairy cow occurs between 2-6 weeks after parturition.

  Acute septic metritis may occur in few days after post-partum.

  Incidence of milk fever increases with parity.

- A general relationship between selection for high productivity and susceptibility to certain disease is apparent in many breeds of animal.(Crossbred animals are more susceptible for FMD, haemoprotozoan and production diseases).
- Possibilities of genetotrophic diseases (inheritance for greater requirement of a specific nutrient) should be considered.
- Reproductive history will comprise of-

  Mean length of interval between parturition and conception.

  Mean No. of service per conception (conception rate).

  Average length of reproductive life.

  Percentage mortality of young ones over a period of 4- 8 weeks. 3-Climate.

- Foot rot (caused by Spherophorus necrophorus) in cattle has peak incidence in warm wet summer.
- Hypomagnesic tetany mostly occurs in cool, wet season.
- Anhidrosis (non sweating syndrome or puff disease or dry coat) in equine occurs in hot, humid climate.
- Mild damp season may be responsible for appearance of rachitogenic effect in young grazing animal because of high content on carotene in lush pasture.
- High rainfall is associated with fasciola infestation in sheep and cattle.
- Haemorrhagic septicemia occurs during monsoon.

3. General Management

Important factor for consideration in general management are:

- Hygiene particularly in milking parlour, parturition and rearing stall.
- Adequacy of housing in terms of space, ventilation and drainage.
- Opportunity for exercise.

d) Environmental history

It can be divided into two parts:

A- Outdoor environment B-Indoor environment

A- Outdoor environment

1- Topography and soil type

- Flat treeless plains offering no protection from wind predisposes cattle for lactation tetany.
- Low marshy area facilitates the spread of insect borne diseases and soil borne infections requiring damp condition like leptospirosis, Johne s disease, liver fluke and lung worm pneumonia.
- High rainfall area dense low shrubs associated with vector borne diseases like looping ill, Babesia, Anaplasma, Trypanosoma, Blue tongue.

- Cobalt and Copper deficiencies are most common on littoral soil.
- Co deficiency and Md excess occurs on peat soil.
- Poor drainage resulting in sea of mud following heavy rainfall leads to wetting of feet udder resulting in mastitis and foot rot in cattle.

2. Feed and water supply

- Decrease supply of water causes salt poisoning in swine.
- Increase water consumption (cold) by calves during summer may cause water intoxication.
- Fluorine is present in high concentration in artesian and sub-artesian well.
- Nitrate concentration is very high in drain off water rich in organic matter or water contaminated with silage.
- Algae in stagnant water, pond, and shallow lakes may be source neurotoxic and hepatotoxic substances.
- Faecal contamination of rivers or streams with slurry is a recognized source of salmonella infection.

B-Indoor environment

1-Housing design

- Communal surface drainage system is more likely to spread infection through out animal house via faeces and urine.
- Tubular partition between pens permits the spread of infectious agent than solid division.
- Concrete floor causes bruising of sole of feet with consequent lameness, also it increases the incidence of mastitis.

2. Stocking density

High stocking density causes:

Excess build up of urine and feces, which increases the level of infection.

Inadequate space for animal movement causes fight and cannibalism.

Difficult detection of animal in heat or sick animal.

3. Ventilation

- Important factors are relative humidity and No. of air exchange per unit of time.
- Low temperature, high humidity and inadequate ventilation increase the chances of enzootic pneumonia of pigs and calves.

4. Light

- Proper light is necessary for maintenance of sanitation and hygiene, recognition of sick animal and to minimize the error in general management.

5. Floor

- Improper flooring is main cause of diseases of musculo-skeletal system.
- Use of saw dust or shaving in the loose housing system for dairy cattle may be associated with outbreaks of coliform mastitis in cattle.
- Wet bedding in winter is associated with endemic pneumatic in calves.

6. Hygiene

- Accumulation of feces and urine not only lead to buildup of pathogenic bacteria but also makes condition favourable for their spread.
- Environmental mastitis (E. coli, Str. Dysgalactiae and Uberis) may be due to saw dust or wood shaving.
- Occupation time (total length of time which animal have occupied the pen without cleaning and disinfection) should be less for good health of the herd.

E P

Clinical Examination of animal comprise of three parts.

A- General inspection [Distant examination]

- General appearance

Demeanor, Posture, Gait, Physical condition, Conformation and Skin

- General Behaviour

Eating, Defecation, Urination and Voice

B. General clinical examination (Physical examination)

- Pulse
- Respiration
- Temperature
- Palpation
- Percussion
- Auscultation
- State of hydration

C. Regional / systemic clinical examination

By using various clinical methodologies (Sensory & Physical)

Should be performed on the basis of interpretation of finding of general inspection and general clinical examination together with history of case.

- Head/neck
- Thorax
- Abdomen
- Urinary system
- Cardio-vascular system
- Reproductive system
- Integumentry system
- Digestive system
- Hepatobillary system
- Endocrine system
- Sensory organs
- Blood & blood forming organ
- Nervous system
- Musculo-skeletal system

A- General Inspection

1. Distinguishing mark

Purpose	1-Vetrolegal purpose
	2-Epidemiological purpose (for record of disease)
Cattle	Branding, ear tag, ear tattoo Permanent (scar, proganthism, visual defect) Horned/polled
Horse	Color of hoof, presence of wall eye (unpigmented iris)
	Habit of showing white sclera of eye Size & shape of chestnut
Dog	type of coat (long, curly, smooth/wire hair) Form of ear (pendulous, erect or cropped) State of tail (natural length/docked)

2. General appearance

a) Physical condition

Done by simple inspection (but not accurate in case of long haired or woolled animal. So, in this condition by running the hand over certain part of body) rib, spine, shoulder, pelvis, etc.

Normal : All prominent part of skeleton are covered with flesh giving the body a rounded appearance.

Lean / thin: Various parts of body are readily identified (ribs, pelvis) and Supra orbital fossa is deepened but the animal is physiologically normal.

Emaciated : Extent of leanness/thinness, when it affect physiology of animal

Coat is lusterless, dry

Elasticity of skin is reduced (hide bound) become leathery

M.M. become pale & watery

Reduced work performance/production

- Severe wasting is common finding in old age, severe parasitism, extensive/diffuse neoplasm & malnutrition.
- Primary emaciation : When ration is qualitatively or quantitavely inadequate.

- Secondary emaciation : Due to illness which affect appetite of animal or its ability to take and digest and assimilate nutrients.

Case of poor body condition

1. Too little food / food of poor quality
2. Ingested food improperly digested / absorbed or insufficiently utilized after absorption. (dietary error / loss of power to ingest because of pain)
3. Chronic wasting disease (J.D., cobalt deficiency, parasitic gastroenteritis)
4. Disease arising from disturbances of metabolism like diabetes mellitus
5. Inadequate indigestion like E.P.I.
6. Hereditary (because of influence of high productive capacity, which is the cause of leanness in dairy cow)
7. Emaciation in spite of good appetite e.g. Chronic nephritis, E.P.I.

Extreme emaciation generally result of chronic process but in subacute grass sickness in horse, it may develop within a week.

Fattiness : Excessive deposition of body fat e.g.-Hypothyroidism, castration in males , spaying in females.

Obesity : Extent of fattiness which causes systemic disturbance (dyspnea or difficulty in walking, etc.)

The deposition of fat may be throughout the body or only in certain parts like crest of stallion or at base of tail in fat tailed sheep. Different scores can be given for individual animal and can further classified as normal, fatty, lean/thin, emaciation.

Condition Score 1 : Very thin : This animal s skeletal structure is very prominent. Notice the deep depressions next to the spine, between the pelvis and rib cage, between the hooks and pins, and around the tail head.

Condition Score 2 : Thin : The animal s skeleton is still very apparent. The individual spinous processes are clearly visible, but there is a small amount of fat tissue over the spine, hooks, and pins.

Condition Score 3 : Medium (Normal body condition) : The animal appears smooth over the spine, ribs, and pelvis and the skeletal structure can be easily palpated. The hooks and pins are still discernible, with a moderate, rather deep depression between the pelvis and rib cage, hooks and pins, and around the tail-head.

Condition Score 4 : Fat : There are no spinous processes detectable, and no depression in the loin area, which gives the top-line of the animal a flat, tabletop appearance. The ribs can no longer be felt, and the pelvis can only be felt with firm pressure. The hooks and pins have a rounded appearance due to areas of fat covering.

Condition Score 5 : Very Fat : The animal appears rounded and smooth with a square-shaped appearance, because of the amount of fat filling in the loin. The skeletal structure is no longer visible, and can only be palpated with excessive pressure.

b) Demeanor

It is response of animal for external stimuli, such as movement & noise. Sensory motor aspect (mental status is regulated by RAS (cerebrum) and brain stem.

1. Bright/Normal : response will be in the form of elevating head , ears, turning towards & directing the attention at the source of stimuli or walking away or showing the sign of attack.
2. Decreased : Dullness/apathy - sluggish reaction, animal exhibits relatively indifference to normal stimuli. Feature of febrile and toxemic condition e.g. Grain overload.

Dummy/wooden horse : advance degree of failure to respond to external stimuli (although animal capable of standing & perform sluggish unco-ordinated movement) e.g. Advance hepatic fibrosis, encephalomyelitis, listeriosis, lead poisoning, ketosis in cattle

Coma : Most advance degree of failure to respond to external stimuli. Animal remain unconscious & fail to respond for even painful stimuli. e.g. Cow in advance stage of milk fever.

3. Increased : Mild (alertness)- animal appear hyperalert, look about constantly but exhibit normal movement. It is indicative for constant pain or other abnormal sensation (early parturient paresis or in recent blindness).

Restlessness : movement in constant & consisting of continuous lying down, rolling, getting up again, other abnormal movement like looking at flank, kicking at belly, rolling, bellowing. Again this demeanor is indicative for pain (sharp constant / intermittent) & early phase of contagious pyelonephritis.

Mania : behaviour abnormalities appear to be compulsive & include vigorous licking of some specific part of body surface (in bovine ketosis, psedorabies), pressing forward with head in meningitis, rape poisoning, compulsive walking either in circle or straight line with failure to avoid obstacle (ragwort poisoning, water intoxication and hepatic insufficiency, licking or chewing inanimate objects, e.g. Rabies.

Frenzy : Animals action are uncontrolled so that they are danger to anyone approaching them, this situation may exist in cases of acute lead poisoning hypomagnetic tetany, ketosis in cattle, rabies in most species.

c) Body conformation

Assessment of body conformation done, when physical condition of animal is under consideration. It is based on symmetry, shape & size of different body regions relative to other region. Disproportionate enlargement of abdomen is more usual abnormality of conformation seen in animal. Change in body conformation occurs in dropsy of fetal membrane (hydroamnion in cow), ascites, and exudative peritonitis & in skeletal system in rickets & in nymphomania (from cystic ovary), where part of pelvis & coccygeal vertebrae are prominent. Large swellings on the surface of body occur with subcutaneous haematomas in dog with angiostrongilosis.

d) Examination of skin and appendages

Structures or parts associated with skin as its appendages are hoofs, hairs, horns, quills, claws, nails, sebaceous glands and sweat glands. Assessing the condition of skin and coat to identify clinical signs of skin lesions, such as:

- Condition of the coat
- Elasticity of the coat
- Pruritus
- Primary and secondary skin lesions
- Dermatitis

- Hyperkeratosis or parakeratosis
- Presence of ectoparasites

e) Posture

Posture implies the general appearance of animal from the anatomical aspect. Change in posture takes a variety of form including:

1. Curvature of vertebral column dorsally (kyphosis), ventrally (lordosis) or laterally (scoliosis)
2. High oblique carriage of head & neck
3. Rotation of head
4. Abnormal position of limbs

For abnormal posture (acquired) - disease of bone, joints, ligaments, tendon, tendon sheath, bursae, muscle, nervous system, ear, hoof and claws should be considered e.g. of abnormal posture include:

a) Arching of back with the limbs tucked under the body (feet more closely) or depressing the back & moving the feet more widely apart - indicative for abdominal pain (TRP, pyelonephritis)

b) Abduction of elbow - pain in chest or difficulty in breathing

c) Shifting of weight from one to other limb (horse) - laminitis / early stages of osteodystrophia fibrosa. While in advance laminitis, the unaffected limbs are advanced cranially.

d) Dog setting posture in horse associated with rolling and kicking at belly is usually associated with abdominal pain & pressure on diaphragm, such as occur in acute gastric dilatation after engorgement of grass.

e) Due to hypertonia (increase muscle tone) animal affected with tetanus shows erection and rigidity of ears, restrict limb movements, separation of eyelids (3rd eyelid protrusion) partial elevation & rigidity of tail.

f) Due to hypotonia (decrease muscle tone) animal affected with myasthenia gravis, there is lowering of head & weakness of limbs (also in limber neck - staphylococcal food poisoining)

g) Sheep which are blind as in early pregnancy toxemia assume a listening attitude (head elevated &ear pricked)

h) Sheep in hypocalcemia & cattle with bilateral hip dislocation usually lays sternal recumbency with the hindleg extended behind in a frog like attitude

i) Extended head & neck or held to one side - unilateral painful condition of pharyngeal region

j) Lateral deviation of head - listeriosis, coenurusis

k) Rotation of head - middle ear infection

l) Dog adopting praying posture - gastritis

m) Male dog urinating like bitch cystitis, urolithiasis

n) yphosis of dog (arching of back - acute nephritic pain)

o) Prolong standing in cattle, buffalo & abduction of elbow with extension of head, neck - pneumonia, pleurisy, pericarditis (TRP)

p) Star gazing in sheep - polioencephalomalacia

q) Broad base stance in dogs - CHF

r) Cattle in sternal recumbency with head deviated towards flank - milk fever

s) Cattle affected by unilateral sciatic nerve paralysis or unilateral dislocation of hip joint - the affected limb sticks out in an awkward position.

Head tilt

Vestibular system consists of :

1. Vestibular nuclei in rostral medulla of brain stem
2. Vestibular portion of vestibulo-coclear nerve
3. Receptor in semi-circular canal

Function of this system is to co-ordinate the position & movement of head with that of eyes, trunk, and limbs by detecting linear acceleration & rotation of head.

Head tilt in opposite direction to lesion (in unilateral vestibular).

Other sign : Abnormal nystagmus (fast phase opposite to heat tilt site)

Strabismus in the side of head tilt - peripheral vestibular disease (parallel/horizontal nystagmus), facial nerve paresis/paralysis & Horner s syndrome.

Peripheral	Central
1. Nystagmus horizontal & rotatory	Horizontal / vertical or rotator
2. Mentation - alert but depressed	dull or stupor
3. Other sign sign related to cranial nerve 7	5 , 7 , 9 , 10 , 11

Normal posture - Shoulder width distance b/w thoracic limbs

Hip width distance b/w pelvic limbs

f) Gait

Expression of movement of limb in term of rate, range, force & direction.

It evaluates motor system & sensory system.

In true cerebellar disorder - all 4 qualities are affected.

In looping ill of sheep rate & force is excessive giving a high steeping gait & a bounding form of progression. In arthritis (because of pain in joints) or laminitis (pain in feet), range is diminished & patient has a shuffling or stumbling walk.

Walking in circle : Spasmodically acetonemia & pregnancy toxemia

Permanent - Listeriosis

Circling : One side (either left or right) - Vestibular injury

Brain abscess / cyst / tumor / gid / otitis & listeriosis

Both side : etosis / pregnancy toxemia / hepatic insufficiency, surra (cerebral injury)

Ataxia : Because of:

1. Proprioceptive defect
2. Vestibular
3. Cerebellar defect

Causing in co-ordination, when moving limbs & body.

Seen as swaying from side to side of the pelvis, trunk & sometimes whole body.

It may also appear as wearing of the affected limb during swing phase of stride resulting in abducted or adducted foot placement, crossing of the limbs, or steeping of opposite foot.

Cause : Brain stem, cerebellum, spinal cord (PNS spinal nerve or CNS)

All 3 cause of ataxia cause changes in limb co-ordination but vestibular & cerebellar ataxia. Also produce changes in head & neck movements.

Abnormality in stride (range) Dysmetric (two types)

Hypermetria - lack of direction & increased range of movement seen as over are of limbs with excessive joint movement.

Hypometria - stiff or spastic movement of limbs with little flexion of the joints particularly carpal & tarsal.

Important

1. Compulsive walking or walking directly ahead regardless of obstruction is part of dummy syndrome is a character of encephalomyelitis & hepatic insufficiency.
2. In warbler syndrome, there is initial slight in co-ordination of gait with knuckling over the fetlock with lurking & swaying particularly of hind quarters.

General behaviour

a) Defecation

1. Difficult and painful defecation accompanied with groaning (Tenesmus) - Constipation, paralysis of rectum, colon, ulceration of colon (Colitis), stenosis of rectum.
2. Painful abdominal disease like peritonitis, acute nephritis, acute cystitis & inflammatory condition of anal region, defecation is painful & difficult.
3. Involuntary defecation occur in severe diarrhea & in paralysis of anal sphincter due to injury in lumber part of spinal cord or / & caudal thoracic part.
4. Constipation - Incomplete or difficult defecation with passage of hard dry feces.

5. Constipation - Intractable constipation caused by prolong retention of hard dry feces & defecation.
6. Diarrhea - Increase in frequency, fluidity or volume of feces.
7. Tenesmus/straining - defecation with pain (groaning or grunting) with repeated testing of abdominal musculature.

Quantity of Feces

Horse	15 20 kg
Cattle	25 45 kg
Sheep/Goat	0.5 1.0 kg

When additional fiber are added in diet - amount increased.

Frequency of Defecation

Active healthy horse (Stall fed)	-	8-12 times daily
Grazing	-	16 times a day
Cattle	-	12-16 times a day
Lactating cattle	-	12-24 times
Dog (on pellet diet)	-	1-3 times a day

Alimentary So-journ (Depend on anatomical complexity of GIT)

Length of time taken by ingested feed material to pass through the alimentary tract.

Complex large intestine in horse & capacious stomach compartment of cattle prolong the sojourn for 1-4 & 2-4 days. In Canine and Pig it is about 12-36 hr.

Character of Feces (Consistency & form of feces)

Horse (Stall fed) : yellowish brown with the shape of relatively large balls of somewhat regular shape.

Grazing : Dark green with softer consistency so that ball breaks on striking the ground.

Cattle : Grass fed : Dark green semi- solid

House fed : Dark brown & firmness (no. of firm spherical pellets)

Dog, Cat : Firm elongated cylindrical masses.

Colour of Feces

In herbivore	Green fodder -	green soft
	Beet root -	dark red
	Hay, cereal concentrate - dark brown	
In carnivore	Meat -	dark brown
	Meat Bone -	light grey (but become firm)

Liver Disease (obstructive & toxemic jaundice) - feces become clay coloured

Melena - in S. I. disorder

Haematochzia - L. I. Disorder

Phenothiazine therapy - reddish stool

Incompletely digested cereal grain or hay suggests the possibility of falty mastication due to dental disorder.

Diarrhea	Dysentery
Voluminous fluid feces	Scanty, sticky feces
Blood /mucous/fibrin (no)	Present
Less straining	More straining

In dog : Grey, putty like fowl smelling loose feces Inadequate digestion because of pancreatic insufficiency

- Undigested meat in the feces (Creatorrhoea)
- Large amount of fat (Steatorrhoea) are recognized by pasty consistency.

In cattle

- Pasty feces in rumen stasis/Abomasal displacement

Abnormal Constituent of Feces

- Dark tarry feces - bleeding of stomach & small intestine (ankylostomiasis)
- Red feces - bleeding of large intestine

But if haemorrhage occurs in terminal portion of colon or rectum-blood is not mixed uniformly, it is present irregularly on the surface in clots or liquid form (Colitis). When blood present in feces is in so small amount that it cannot be recognized macroscopically, it is termed as occult blood.

Mucous is normal constituent which gives feces a stringy appearance. This surface coating increase in thickness, when alimentary sojourn is prolonged as in constipation of any cause.

b) Urination

Aspects of urination which are significant are: Posture, frequency & evidence of pain.

1. Posture

- Horse : In both male, female similar posture. Extending for limbs & lowering abdomen, thereby increase intra abdominal pressure.
- Cattle : Female cattle & female pig advances the hind legs, so arching the back and elevate tail. Male cattle urinate while walking, feeding or standing still by allowing the urine to run from penile urethra & then escape from surface.
- Male pig : Void urine in a sequence of spurts, simulating ejaculation.
- Male Dog : Raise & abduct one hind limb & discharge urine against to selected object (Territory marking component). Male dog adopting squatting posture (female like) indicate cystis, urolithiasis. With defect of vertebral column or spinal cord, which interfere with muscular co-ordination will cause to micturate in standing position.

2. Frequency

Depend on quantity of water consumed together with that produced by metabolic process & amount lost by respiration & defecation, milk production.

Horse, Cattle	5-6 times (0.6-2 ml/kg/hr)
Pig	2-3 times
Sheep, Goat	1-3 times

Dog (male): urinate voluntarily (0.5-1.0 ml/kg/hr) at frequent interval

Abnormally frequent urination (Pollakuria) may occur with or without an increase in the volume excreted.

e.g. Cystitis, stone, urethritis & urethral obstruction

POL URIA : Diabetes insipidus, mellitus, hyperadrenocortism, chronic interstitial nephritis, use of diuretics, administration of drug that raise hydrostatic pressure in renal capillaries.

❑❑❑

Chapter 8

eterinar irst Aid of Dair Animals

Shanker Kumar Singh

Department of Veterinary Medicine, College of Veterinary Science and Animal Husbandry, Uttar Pradesh Pandit Deen Dayal Upadhyaya Pashu Chikitsa Vigyan Vishwavidhyalaya Evam Go Anusandhan Sansthan, Mathura

Veterinarians play a keyrole in ensuring dairy farms to have healthy and productive herds. Veterinarians regularly visit the farm to help manage the health and well-being of the herd. Veterinarians work with the dairy producer to develop a health management plan, which becomes part of the guide in caring for the herd. In dairy animal practice, most of the time veterinarian has to visit the animal farm from a long distance, in such situation he should be prepared to handle the emergency condition of the animals. Animals requiring first aid may be encountered in a variety of situations, however, the same decisions or steps are required to assess the situation and determine the best course of action. An animal should only be removed from where it is found, if the animal is expected to respond positively to care within 24 hours. The suffering of an animal should not be prolonged, if the prognosis is poor.

The commonly encountered emergency situations in dairy animal practice are injuries to legs and horns, epistaxis, excess intake of grain rich diet, or fodder may lead to bloat and impaction, milkfever, peracute mastitis, hypomagnesaemia, neuro-trypanosomosis, haemoglobinuria and various poisonings. Necessary treatment should be done immediately or else the animal may be in danger. Before, going for therapeutic management examination of the animal and clinical history taking are the most important part of the dairy animal practice. The common signs of health in dairy animals includes eating with relish and rumination, muzzle and nostrils are moist, no fluctuation in milk yield, the normal temperature 38.3^0 C to 38.8^0 C for cattle while 37.8^0 C to 39.3^0 C for buffaloes, semi-solid dung in consistency with dark green colour and clear and straw coloured urine. Whereas, the common signs of ill health includes serration of animals from the general herd showing weakness and lack of alertness, stoppage of rumination, pyrexia, redness in the eye and lancination, raised on the skin, yellow colour of dung indicating constipation, change in quality and quantity of milk produced is an early indicator of disease, undigested feed particles in the dung indicate that there is some disturbance in the digestive system. Animals which are not taking feed while milking may be suspected for fever or any kind of indigestion.

Some commonly encountered ailments should be managed with first aid. Wounds should be thoroughly cleaned in potassium permanganate solution. Septic wounds should be cleaned with hot saline water. In case of bleeding from the wound, a bandage can be applied with the help of gauze cloth or cotton after applying antimicrobial powder. Maggot infestation can be treated by removing the maggots initially with a forceps and then camphor oil, turmeric powder or custard leaf can be applied. Neem oil can be used as fly repellent. oke gall is a condition characterized by local swelling upon neck caused due to constant irritation of yoke or plough. Camphor mixed in coconut oil should be applied on the affected portion. In case of severe swelling, iodine ointment can be applied. Due to this, it will rupture and then it can be treated like ordinary wound. The animal should not be allowed for carting until the swelling ceases. In case of horn facture, the hanging portion of the horn should be removed. Bleeding can be prevented by applying a bandage with a white cloth dipped in water. Sugar solution can be applied on the bandage. Consult the veterinary doctor for further treatment. In case of sprain, hot fomentations with water should be applied thrice daily on the affected portion. Massage the area with camphor oil. In case if it is possible to tie a bandage, then it should be done with the help of tamarind leaves.

Animals with burns require veterinary attention unless the burn is very mild. When assessing burns on animals the depth (superficial, partial thickness or full thickness), extent (percentage of body burnt) and location of the burn(s) needs to be considered. Cold water or a cold compress (wet cloth) needs to be applied to the burn without overcooling the animal. The animal may also need to be treated for shock, pain and dehydration. Shock is a result of a collapsed circulatory system and can occur due to stress, blood loss, fluid loss, low blood pressure and a damaged heart. Many animals, which are badly injured show signs of shock. Signs of shock include rapid pulse or breathing, hypothermia and pale/white gums. The signs of shock are not always obvious and can develop over time. An animal in shock is usually still, quiet and cold. Treatment for shock should first aim at reducing stress (covering the animal s eyes), stopping any visible signs of bleeding and then making sure the animal is kept warm and quiet. Oral fluids should not be given to animals in shock. Once the animal has been warmed up, warm fluids can be given. Hypothermia is caused by a lowering of the body temperature. Signs of hypothermia include cold skin, lethargy, bradycardia. The animal needs to be gradually warmed with a constant artificial heat source, such as body contact in a handling bag, heat lamp or a hot water bottle. It is preferable that the heat source comes from outside of the holding container and directed at one end, so the animal can move closer to or away from the heat source. If the heat source is inside, the holding container must be padded or shielded to avoid the animal burning itself. Care must be taken not to have any electrical connections or wiring within reach of the animal. Heat can be lethal, so place a small dish of water near the heat source. Always keep a very close watch, as overheating is a danger. Once the animal has been warmed to its normal body temperature, high energy fluids can be offered.

Dehydration is the excessive loss of fluid from the body. It can be life threatening, as it can prevent every system in the body of an animal from functioning properly. To check for signs of dehydration, in mammals, pinch the skin of the animal to check for elasticity. Generally tenting of the skin will occur in a dehydrated animal. Sunken or dry eyes, a glazed look and dry tacky gums are also signs of dehydration. It is important not to offer fluid therapy to an animal until it is warm and its condition has stabilised. The best way to offer fluids to an animal is by placing a shallow container of water in them as long as they cannot tip it and get wet. If they are unable to drink by themselves, one can wet his fingers and touch the animals mouth, this usually results in a swallow response. Never pour water down an animal s throat. The severity of dehydration will determine the most appropriate course of action. In all cases, basic treatment and release as soon as possible is the preferred option. Severe changes can develop rapidly with hyperthermia. Signs of hyperthermia include rapid panting, hypersalivation, congested mucous membranes, tachycardia, diarrhoea and dehydration. The animal must be placed in a cool quiet environment, gradually reducing the body temperature with water and wet towels and cool circulating air.

Bites and stings can be dangerous to an animal, if they are allergic to the venom injected. Signs of bites or stings can include drooling, muscle weakness, difficulty breathing, convulsions, etc. Pressure immobilisation is used for snake and spider bites. Cold compress can be applied to other bites and stings, however, unless threatening the animal s ability to breath or one suspect bite/sting from a venomous animal, treat for shock and re-assess regularly before release. If one suspect a venomous snake or spider bite, then the animal is likely to have a poor prognosis, if left untreated. A decision will need to be made to seek special veterinary treatment. Poisons can be swallowed, inhaled or absorbed through the skin. Signs that an animal has been poisoned include, vomiting/regurgitation, salivation, muscle tremors, unco-ordination of gait, convulsions, paralysis, coma and death. If one suspect poisoning, then the animal is likely to have a poor prognosis, if left untreated.

Impaction, due to over-feeding of fodder without water intake or due to intake of grain rich diet will lead to impaction of rumen. Important symptoms include stoppage of rumination, dry and hard flakes of dung and severe abdominal pain. Stop feeding the animal with any kind of diet. 250 ml. of castor oil can be given as a drench. If it is not subsided in two days, then consult the veterinarian. Bloat can be managed by a mixture of 50 ml of camphor oil and 500 ml of good quality mustered oil should be drenched. Stop feeding the animal till the bloat subsides. Small quantities of rice gruel can be fed. In case of non-specific diarrhoea, animal should be drenched with a mixture of 20 gms of kaolin and 20 gms of crota should be mixed in the gruel and can be fed to the animal. If animal is suffering from milkfever, it should not be allowed to go in lateral recumbency, owner should try to keep the animal in sternal recumbency until the veterinarian came for management of the condition. A veterinary clinician should have the first aid kit having, absorbent cotton adhesive tape antiseptic scrub disposable latex gloves disposable razor duct tape (for bandaging the bottom of hooves) dusting powder epsom salt (for soaking hooves) Farrier s rasp flashlight with extra batteries gauze dressing pads hoof dressing (for thrush/foot rot) isopropyl (rubbing) alcohol lubricant for the thermometer (i.e., petroleum jelly) oral syringe (for dosing medications by mouth) pocket knife rectal thermometer roll gauze safety scissors (for cutting dressings) scissors self-stick elastic bandage sterile saline solution stethoscope syringe (without the needle, for flushing wounds) tweezers udder ointment wire cutters and wound ointment/spray.

❑❑❑

Chapter 9

Collection of Samples for Laborator Diagnosis

Udit ain Singh Parul and Barkha Sharma

[1]Department of Veterinary Public Health, [2]Department of Veterinary Epidemiology and Preventive Medicine, College of Veterinary Science and Animal Husbandry, Uttar Pradesh Pandit Deen Dayal Upadhyaya Pashu Chikitsa Vigyan Vishwavidhyalaya Evam Go Anusandhan Sansthan, Mathura

---

Sample collection is a first as well as crucial point for the laboratory investigations and disease diagnosis. Samples may be taken from animals or the environment for a variety of purposes, such as disease diagnosis, disease surveillance, health certification or monitoring the response to treatment or vaccination. The purpose of samples collection should be clear so that lab diagnosis can reach to a conclusion point. The pre-requisite of diagnostic laboratories is the receiving of appropriate samples in a good condition without any deteoriation.

Relevance of proper sample collection

- To isolate and identify the causative agents
- Forms the backbone of the investigative procedures
- For definitive diagnosis of infectious diseases
- To help in prescribing treatment strategies
- For prevention and control measures

Precautions during sample collection

Before taking the samples, a clear cut strategy should be in mind, about the purpose of sample collection, for which they are required. The skilled person and considerable care are required for correct sampling and dispatch to the laboratory.

The following points need to care:

1. The type and number of samples needed is the first thing to be done correctly during sample collection, which can draw the appropriate results of that investigation.
2. When samples are taken from live animals, care should be taken to avoid injury or distress to the animal or danger to the operator and attendants by using mechanical restraint, tranquillization or anaesthesia to animals.
3. During the collection of biological material, from either live or dead animals, the risk of zoonotic and other infectious disease should be kept in mind and necessary person equiped with protective measure to avoid the human infection.
4. The Post-mortem examinations should be carried out under aseptic conditions as far as practicable and possible.
5. Care should be taken to avoid environmental contamination, or risk of spread of disease through insects or fomites during collection.
6. The samples collected should be true representative of the condition being investigated and the lesions observed.
7. The samples should be carefully packaged, labelled, and transmitted to the laboratory by the fastest practicable method, under the appropriate refrigeration, conditions.
8. If samples are sent to abroad in laboratory, in that condition the particular laboratory should be consulted in advance, before sending the sample and follow their guidelines properly.

G P S
T

A. Guidelines for collecting diagnostic lab purpose samples

1. Collection of specimens for diagnostic bacteriology

i) Collect the specimen before administering the any antimicrobial agents, if possible.

ii) Collect specimen with less contamination from indigenous microbiota and possible to ensure that the sample should be representative of the infected site.

iii) Use sterile equipments and aseptic techniques to collect specimens to prevent the introduction of micro-organisms during invasive procedures.

iv) Clearly label the specimen container with the animals identification number.

v) Develop an understanding of the microbiology laboratory s source identification schemes and also now when to include rule-out request. For example, the laboratory may routinely screen for *Shigella, Salmonella,* and *Campylobacter* species in stool cultures but not for *Yersinia* or *Vibrio* species. Consider geographic location and season, when notifying the laboratory of rule out requests.

vi) Identify the specimen source and/or specific site correctly so that proper culture media will be selected during processing of sample in the laboratory.

vii) If a specimen is to be collected through intact skin, cleanse the skin first. For example, use 70 alcohol followed by iodine solution (1 to 2 tincture of iodine or 10 solution of povidone-iodine).

Collection of anareboic specimen

Anaerobic cultures are best collected by aspirating abscess fluid with a sterile syringe and needle. Syringes can be capped and submitted, or the aspirated fluid can be injected into a vacutainer anaerobic specimen collection. The submission of swabs for anaerobic culture is discouraged, but if swabs is used, it should be placed immediately into anaerobic transport tubes.

2. Collection of specimen for diagnostic virology

Diagnostic virology has played an important role in the effective control of virus diseases. There are 5 main approaches for the diagnosis of viral diseases in a laboratory:

- Isolation and identification of virus.
- Identification of the causal virus using Electron microscope on the clinical specimens.
- Identification of viral antigen in tissue specimens using serological techniques.

- Examination of histopathological changes in the tissue specimen.
- Demonstration of an antibody response.

In the diagnosis of viral diseases, following points should always be borne in mind :

i) Virus titers are negatively affected by the time in transit, temperature, pH and the amount of virus present at the sampling time.

ii) Specimen material should be collected as early as possible in the acute stage of infection, since virus tends to disappear relatively quickly after the onset of disease.

iii) Separate set of sterile instruments should be used for collection of each tissue specimen to avoid cross-contamination. Each tissue should be collected in separate sterile neutral glass vial.

iv) Secondary bacterial infection is quite common in viral disease, hence sample collected from the later stages of the illness or at necropsy is less likely to contain viable virus.

v) When collecting skin scrapings, falling off the blade/scalpel.

vi) The specimen should be rapidly transported to the laboratory in a sterile container placed in wet ice or over frozen cool packs and stored at 4^0C until inoculated into isolating medium (cell culture, eggs, laboratory animals, etc).

vii) For transport to a remote laboratory, specimen can be held at 4^0C for upto 48hrs has without much loss of infectively. It is not advisable to freeze specimens for transport to the laboratory.

viii) If need arises to freeze the specimens (for transport over a long distance or storing the specimens for a long time), it should be done in small volumes as slow rate of freezing leads to greater loss of infectivity. Freezing at -70^0C and shipping in dry ice is advantageous.

ix) The swab tips used for collection may be comprised of cotton, rayon or polyester. The calcium algenate wool, commonly used for bacterial swabs is viricidal for some viruses (IBR virus). The wooden shaft of swab can be replaced with aluminium.

x) Specimen taken in a small amount (swabs and scrapings) are most likely to be affected by ambient conditions and should be placed and transported in a suitable virus transport medium. The ratio of specimen to virus transport medium should be between 1:5 to 1:10. However, when specimen are in larger volume (feces, tissue), most of the requirements for virus stability are met by the specimen itself, but it is advantageous to place a portion of the specimen into virus transport medium.

xi) In diseases where viraemia occurs, the maximum titre of virus often coincides with the peak pyrexia, the blood should be collected during the febrile stage, using heparin (preferably) or EDTA as anticoagulant and submitted on frozen cool packs as soon as possible.

xii) The serum for serological test should be stored at 4^{0}C and sent to laboratory packed on frozen cool packs. No preservative should be added to the serum samples for viral diagnostic purpose. If need arises, antibiotics could be added in appropriate concentration.

3. Collection of Specimens for Diagnostic mycology

i) The affected areas are lightly sponged with 70 ethanol to check the surface contamination.

ii) Using a scalpel or suitable substitute like edge of glass slide, skin scrapping is taken from active periphery of a lesion.

iii) Clipping of nails are collected near the base of nail.

iv) In ringworms of the scalp, forceps should be used to pluck involved hair from the edge of patches.

v) These specimens are kept in covered containers like envelops, disposable petridishes or sterile containers.

4. Collection of specimen for diagnostic toxicology

i) In case of veterolegal cases, the sample should be collected in rectified spirit/alcohol and another container with same preservative, after properly sealing it should be sent to the chemical examined and forensic lab.

ii) The veterinarian must be thorough in selecting and handling the toxicological specimen and must try to get as much information on circumstantial evidence, symptomatic, pathological, chemical experimental before reaching at accurate diagnoses.

iii) List all pesticides known to have been used in the general area, and medications administered within week prior to death.

iv) As a rule blood, urine, vomitus, stomach contents, kidney, liver, should be collected surely in any poisoning case for further analysis.

5. Collection of specimen for diagnostic histopathology

i) Specimen from died or biopsies from ailing animals should be collected for histopathological examination.

ii) Relevant tissues should be sliced in small pieces i.e. upto 2 cm size and 0.5cm thickness.

iii) Samples from all vital organs showing gross lesions and lymphnodes must be collected.

iv) The samples must be preserved in 10 formol saline using a volume, which is about 10 times to that of sample and other useful fixative are Zenker s and vines fluid.

B

I. Sample collection from live animals

i) Blood sample collection

Blood samples may be taken for haematology or for culture and/ or direct examination for bacteria, viruses, or protozoa, in which case it is usual to use anticoagulants, such as ethylene diamine tetra-acetic acid (EDTA) or heparin. Samples may also be taken for serology, it requires a clotted sample. Blood plasma is also used for some procedures.

Site of collection Usually blood sample is taken by venipuncture but the site of collection is different in small and large animals.

In large animals Usually in large animals the jugular vein or a caudal vein is selected, but brachial veins and mammary veins are also used. Vena cava veins are also used in pigs.

In birds, a wing vein (brachial vein) is usually selected. Blood may be taken by syringe and needle or by needle and vacuum tube (not easy in delicate veins but convenient in strong veins). Small quantities of blood are conveniently obtained by pricking with a triangular, solid-pointed needle. Ideally, the skin at the site of venipuncture should first be shaved (plucked) and swabbed with 70 alcohol and allowed to dry.

Blood samples collected with anticoagulant

For samples that are collected with anticoagulant, thorough mixing, using gentle agitation only, is necessary as soon as the sample has been taken. It may also be necessary to make a smear of fresh blood on a microscope slide both thick and thin smears may be prepared. For polymerase chain reactions, EDTA is the preferred anticoagulant.

Blood for haematological studies is collected with anticoagulant

i) Ethylene Diamine Tetra Acetic acid-1-2mg/ml of blood

ii) Sodium citrate (3.8)-1ml/10ml of blood

iii) Heparin- 0.1ml of 1 solution/5ml-10ml blood (commonly used for research purposes).

Serum collection For serum samples, the blood should be collected without anticoagulant and left to stand at ambient temperature (but protected from excessive heat or cold) for 1 2 hours until the clot begins to contract. The clot can then be ringed round with a sterile rod and the bottles placed in a refrigerator at 4 C. After several hours, or overnight, the sample can be centrifuged at about 1000 for 10 15 minutes and the serum can be decanted or removed with a pipette. A clear straw coloured serum gets separated from the clot and is collected in a sterile clean vial.

ii) Faecal sample collection

- At least 10 g of freshly voided faeces should be collected for lab diagnosis.
- Screw top containers or sterile plastic bags should be used for shipment avoid tubes with rubber stoppers, as gas generated can result in blowing the stopper off the tube, ruining the integrity of the sample and contaminating other samples in the package.
- An alternative and sometimes preferable method is to take swabs from the rectum (or cloaca), taking care to swab should properly touched to the mucosal surface.

- The swabs should be visibly coated with faecal material and swabs should be transported in appropriate transport medium however, samples collected with a swab are inadequate for parasitology.
- Faeces are best stored and transported at 4 C.

Faeces samples collection for Parasitological samples

Faeces for parasitological examination should fill the container and be sent to arrive at the laboratory within 24 hrs. If transport times are likely to be longer than 24 hrs, the sample should be sent on ice or refrigerated to prevent the hatching of parasite eggs. Faecal samples for examination of ova cysts and larvae are preferably collected in wide mouth bottle. Refrigeration or 5-10 formal saline is the best method of helminthes preservation. Ectoparasite like mites and fleas may be collected by brushing or combing the fur or hair or feathers over a sheet of white paper and placing them in vial containing 70 alcohol. Common blood protozoan parasites can be visualized in blood smears. Parasites like microfilaria can be examined in hemolysed centrifuged blood and feces for trophozoits are examined immediately after collection.

iii) Genital tract and semen sample collection

Samples may be taken by vaginal or preputial washing, or by the use of suitable swabs from the cervix or urethra. Samples of semen are best obtained using an artificial vagina or by extrusion of the penis and artificial stimulation. The sperm-rich fraction should be present in the sample and contamination by antiseptic washing solutions should be avoided. Specific transport media and conditions are often required.

iv) Sample collection from skin

In diseases producing vesicular lesions, collect, if possible, 2 g of affected epithelial tissue as aseptically as possible and place it in 5 ml phosphate buffered glycerine or Tris-buffered tryptose broth virus transport medium at pH 7.6. Additionally, the vesicular fluid should be sampled, where unruptured vesicles are present, vesicular fluid should be aspirated with a syringe and placed in a separate sterile tube. Plucked hair or wool samples are useful for surface-feeding mites, lice and fungal infections. Deep skin scrapings, using the edge of a scalpel blade, are useful for burrowing mites and, in birds, feather tips can be taken for detection of viral antigen, where Marek s disease is suspected.

v) Sample collection from Eyes

A sample from the conjunctiva can be taken by holding the palpebra apart and gently swabbing the surface. The swab is then put into transport medium. Scrapings may also be taken on to a microscope slide. The handles of metal-handled swabs are useful for this, to ensure that sufficient cells are removed for microscopic examination. Mucopurulent nasal and lacrimal discharges are rarely useful.

vi) Sample collection from Nasal discharge, saliva & tears

Samples may be taken with dacron, cotton or gauze swabs, preferably on wire handles as wood is inflexible and may snap. It may be helpful, if the swab is first moistened with transport medium. The swab should be allowed to remain in contact with the secretions for upto 1 minute, then placed in transport medium and sent to the laboratory without delay at 4 C. Long protected nasopharyngeal swabs should be used to collect samples for some suspected viral infections.

vii) Milk sample collection

Milk samples should be taken after cleansing and drying the tip of the teat, the use of antiseptics should be avoided. The initial stream of milk should be discarded and a tube filled with the next stream(s), a sample of bulk tank milk can be used for some tests. Milk for serological tests should not have been frozen, heated or subjected to violent shaking. If there is going to be a delay in submitting them to the laboratory, preservatives can be added to milk samples that are being collected for serological testing. If necessary, milk for bacterial examination can be frozen.

viii) Pus sample collection

It is collected with the help of sterile cotton swab. It may be preserved in a test tube containing a few drops of sterile normal saline to check drying.

II. Sample collection from dead animal during post-mortem

Samples of tissue from a variety of organs can be taken at post-mortem and the procedures are given below :

- Animal health personnel should be trained in the correct procedures for post-mortem examination of the species of animals with which they work. The equipment required will depend on the size and species of animal, but a knife, saw and cleaver will be required, and also scalpel, forceps and scissors, including scissors with a rounded tip on one blade, for opening intestines.
- A plentiful supply of containers and tubes of transport media appropriate to the nature of the sample required should be available, along with labels and report forms.
- Containers should be fully labelled with the date, tissue and animal identification. Special media may be required for transport of samples from the field.
- If rabies or transmissible spongiform encephalopathies (TSEs) are suspected, it is usual to detach the animal s head. Tissues may be collected for microbiological culture, parasitology, biochemistry, histopathology and/or immuno-histochemistry, and for detection of proteins or genome nucleic acids. Addition to this the buccal, oropharyngeal or rectal (cloacal) swabs may be collected.
- Each piece of tissue should be placed in a fully labelled separate plastic bag or sterile screw-capped jar. Swabs should always be submitted in appropriate transport media.
- Sterile instruments should be used for collecting specimens for microbiological culture and care should be taken not to contaminate tissues with intestinal contents.
- Disinfectants should not be used on or near tissues to be sampled for bacterial culture or virus isolation.
- The tissues may be sent to the laboratory dry or in bacterial or virus transport medium, depending on the type of specimen and the examinations required swabs should be sent in transport medium.
- After collection, the samples for microbiological examination should be refrigerated until shipped. If shipment cannot be made within 48 hours, the samples should be frozen however, prolonged storage at 20 C may be detrimental to virus isolation.

- For histopathology, blocks of tissue not more than 0.5 cm thick and 1 2 cm long are cut and placed in neutral buffered 4 10 formalin, which should be at least ten times the volume of the tissue sample. For certain suspected diseases, larger portions of brain are required the brain is sectioned using a sagittal cut, half is submitted fresh, on ice, and the other half is submitted in 10 buffered formalin.
- Care should be taken to insure that formalin-fixed tissues are not frozen. Once fixed, tissues can be removed from formalin and, as long as they are kept moist and protected (e.g. by wrapping in formalin-soaked paper towels, then sealed in screw-capped jars), they can be forwarded to the laboratory without formalin.
- Store and pack formalin-fixed tissues separately from fresh tissues, blood and smears.

III. Environmental and feed sampling

- Environmental samples are commonly taken from litter or bedding and voided faeces or urine of the animal.
- Swabs may be taken from the surface of ventilation ducts, feed troughs and drains in hatcheries, artificial insemination centres and slaughterhouses in which specialized equipment is maintained.
- Samples may also be taken from animal feed, in troughs or bulk containers.
- Water may be sampled from troughs, drinkers, header tanks or the natural and artificial supply.

3. Selection of specimens in Relation to various diseases

Just any tissue is not adequate for the specific diagnosis of a disease, rather specific material/ specimen is required for the laboratory diagnosis of a particular disease. The following table has been prepared to provide specific information as regards to the type of specimen required for the laboratory diagnosis of different diseases:

Disease	Specimen Morbid Material
A. Bacterial Diseases	
1. Anthrax	a) Four blood smears Flame fix the smears.
	b) Lesion smears from subcutaneous swelling (Swine, Dog and Horse) Flame fix the smear.
	c) Swab of blood from ear vein in sterile container over frozen cool pack (FCP).
	d) A Small piece of ear tip in saline on frozen cool pack.
	e) In case of horses and swine because the organism may not be present in blood, swab should be taken from exudates and cut surface of haemorrhagic lymphnodes
2. Actinomycosis and Actinobacillosis	a) Smears from pus lesions. b) Pus in sterile container over ice.
	c) Affected tissue specimen preserved in 10 formalin.
3. Black uarter (leg)	a) Impression smears from affected muscle tissue (fixed and unfixed).
	b) Exudates from lesions.
	c) Pieces of affected tissue on FCP. Fresh affected tissue are specially important because clostridia rapidly invade tissues after death.
4. Brucellosis	a) Paired serum samples.
(Campylobacteriosis, Abortion)	b) Milk for MRT.
	c)Placenta with 2-3 cotyledons over ice.
	d) Vaginal swabs in PBS.
	e) Impression smears from placenta, lung and cotyledons.
	f) Foetal stomach contents in a vial over ice.
	g) Whole foetus on ice or tissues from all the internal organs on ice and in 10 formalin.
	h) Preputial washing on ice.
5. Enterotoxaemia (Braxy, lamb dysentery	a) Several ounces of fresh contents of small intestine in a jar or plastic bag with and without chloroform over ice or a section of affected intestine tied off at both ends and submission as soon as possible.
	b) idney over ice and in 10 formalin.
	c) Urine sample in sterile container over ice.

6. Glanders	a) Exudate from skin and lung lesion on frozen cool packs. b) Flame fixed impression smears from lesions/ exudates.
7. Haemorrhagic septicaemia	a) Smears from blood and oedema fluid from clinical cases. b) Smears from heart blood, throat swelling and liver. c) Heart blood in a sterile container over ice. d) Tissue from lymphnode and spleen on FCP.
8. Johne s disease (Paratuberculosis)	a) Rectal pinch smears from clinical cases. b) Bowl washing (10.0 gm) preserved in 10 formalin from clinical cases. c) Terminal portion of ileum with ileocaecal valve flushed free of contents mesenteric lymphnode of this region in 10 formalin.
9. Leptospirosis	a) Paired serum samples. b) Milk or urine samples on ice (formalin can be added @ 1drop per 20.0 ml. c) Pieces of liver and kidney on FCP and also in 10 formalin.
10. Listeriosis	a) Aborted foetus and placenta on FCP all internal organs / tissues including brain in 10 formalin and on FCP
11. Mycoplasmosis / contagious bovine pleuropneumonia / contagious caprine pleuropneumonia	a) Nasal and Vaginal swabs in PBS on FCP. b) Swabs from other lesions in PBS on FCP Tissue pieces from lung and mediastinal (regional) lymph nodes in 10 formalin. c) Pleural exudate with the help of a sterile syringe into a sterile container add a few drop of 1:10000 thallium acetate. d) Paired serum samples.
12. Salmonellosis	a) Intestinal swabs, heart blood and bile in sterile containers on FCP
13. Chlamydia infection	a) Nasal swabs in transport medium on FCP. b) Flame fixed impression smears from liver lung, and fetal organs. c) Tissues specimens from lung and liver in sterile container on FCP and duplicate parts in 10.0 formalin. d) Paired serum samples

14. Dermal diseases	a) Skin scrapings for identification of ectoparasites and fungus.
B. iral Disease	
1. African Horse Sickness	a) About 10.0 ml blood at the height of pyrexia in heparin or EDTA on FCP b) Paired sera in sterile container added with antibiotics sent on FCP c) At autopsy, pieces of spleen, lymph nodes and other internal organs in duplicate-one set on frozen cool pack and another in 10 formalin.
2. Blue Tongue	As above for African Horse Sickness
3. Bovine Virus Diarrhoea	a) Blood samples for pyrexic cases in anticoagulant (EDTA/Heparin). b) Swabs from eye, oral cavity and rectumIn PBS on frozen cool packs c) Prescapular and mesenteric lymph nodes and spleen tissue on FCP d) Pieces of all the internal organs including tonsils and intestine in 10 formalin. e) Pieces of intestine on FCP f) Paired serum samples.
4. Bovine Herpes Viral Disease (IBR/IPV/Bovine Mammilitis)	a) Swabs (gauge swab) from nasal and vaginal lesions in transport medium on FCP. b) Pieces of trachea, lung in transport medium on FCP. c) Pieces of trachea, liver, lung and turbine bone in 10 formalin or Bouin s fixatived. Paired serum samples.
5. Caprine Arthritis/ Encephalitis	a) Joint capsules, lung and brain tissue on FCP. b) Joint capsules, lung and brain tissue in 10.0 formalinc. Paired serum samples
6. Canine Distemper	a) Impression smears from urinary bladder and liver b) Tissue specimens from liver and spleen on FCP c) Tissue specimens from liver, spleen, kidney, lungs, lymph node, urinary bladder, trachea, stomach and brain in 10 formalin

7. Canine Parvovirus	a) Heparinized blood samples on FCP b) Rectal swab in PBS on FCP c) Tissue samples from intestine and heart on FCP d) Tissue samples from all the internal organs in 10 formalin e) Paired serum samples
8. Canine Hepatitis (infectious)	a) Nasal, oral and rectal swabs in PBS on FCP. b) Impression smears from liver fixed in methanol. c) Tissue specimens from liver, spleen and tonsils on FCP d) Tissue specimens from liver, spleen, gall bladder and kidney in 10 formalin. i.e. Paired serum samples.
9. Equine Influenza	a) Nasal swabs in PBS or Hank s b) Balanced salt solution or nasal passage washing with sterile PBS on FCP.
10. Equine Infectious Anaenmia	a) Blood with anticoagulant on FCP b) Tissue specimen from spleen, liver, lymph nodes in 10 formalin. c) Paired serum samples.
11. Foot and Mouth disease (Vesicular disease)	a) Blood samples for pyrexic cases in anticoagulant (EDTA/Heparin) on FCP. b) Vesicular fluid from vesicular lesion in 50 buffered glycerine preferably on FCP. c) Oesophago-pharyngeal fluid in 50 phosphate buffered glycerine on FCP. d) Pieces of myocardium in buffered glycerin and duplicate specimens in 10 formalin also. e) Paired serum samples.
12. Peste des petit ruminants (PPR)	Refer to Bovine virus diarrhoea.
13. Rabies	a) Half portion of the brain in 50 buffered glycerin or glycerin saline and other half in Zenker s fluid b) Tissue from sub-maxillary salivary glands in 50 phosphate buffered glycerin.

	c) Alternatively, small pieces from Hippocampus (Ammon s horn), Cerebellum, cerebrum and spinal cord in 50 buffered glycerin and duplilcate samples in Zenker s fluid in separate containers.
	d) Three or four impression smears prepared from cut surfaces of ammon s horn, air dried and fixed in methyl alcohol (acetone free).Caution: All the materials should be securely put in bottles placed in thick polypacks and packed in water tight hard box with sufficient saw dust/ absorbent cotton, sealed and labeled as Suspected for Rabies /
14. Rinderpest	Refer to Bovine virus diarrhoea.
15. Sheep, Goat, Cow, Buffalo Pox	a) Skin lesions scab/papules in sterile vial on FCP
	b) Skin lesions scab/papules in 50
	c) Dermal and lung lesion in 10 formalin.
16. Swine Fever (Hogcholera)	a) Blood (20ml) added with heparin collected from a clinical cases in a sterile vial on FCP.
	b) Pieces of spleen, lymph nodes and Pancreas in 50 buffered glycerin together with heart blood in a separate vial all on FCP.
	c) Tissue from lung, intestine, ileocaecal region, kidney and brain in 10 formalin.
Parasitic Diseases	
1. Anaplasmosis and Babesiosis	Blood smears from ear vain, air dried and fixed with methanol.
2. Surra (Trypanosomiasis)	a) Blood smears from ear vain, air dried and fixed with methanol
	b) Blood samples in anticoagulant on FCP
3. Theileriosis	a) Blood smears from ear vein, air dried and fixed in methanol or alcohol.
	b) Biopsy smears from swollen lymph nodes fixed in methanol.
General Diseases	
1. Abortion	a) Whole fetus on ice or all the internal organs of the foetus on ice.
	b) Vaginal swabs in PBS/Hank s on FCP
	c) Pieces of placenta/cotyledons in sterile containers on FCP

	d) Above mentioned tissues in 10 formaline. Paired serum samples from aborted animals.
2. Entertis	20 gm of feces each from atleast 5 affected untreated animals and from 5 clinically normal, age matched animals in sterile containers in transport medium on FCP.
3. Infertility and Sterility	a) Sterile semen and prepucial swabs on FCP
	b) Paired serum samples
4. Mastitis	c) Milk samples in sterile containers on FCP
5. Pyrexia	a) Blood smears from ear vain, air dried and fixed with methanol
	b) Blood samples in EDTA on FCP
	c) Paired serum samples
6. Septicaemia	a) Blood samples mixed with anticoagulant on FCP
	b) Tissue pieces from spleen, liver, lung, brain, small intestine and mesenteric lymph node in separate sterile containers on FCP.
	c) Heart Blood smears, air-dried.

N Differential diagnoses of Brucellosis → Abortions in Brucellosis- during third trimester of pregnancy, in Campylobacteriosis- early pregnancy, in Listeriosis- 8-9th month, in Trichomoniasis- first half of pregnancy, in IBR- in between 5-9 months (No placentitis), in Leptospirosis- in between 6-7 months

4. Appropriate information sent with samples

i) Name and address of owner/occupier and geolocation (latitude and longitude, if available) where disease occurred, with telephone and fax numbers.

ii) Name, postal and e-mail address, telephone and fax numbers of the sender.

iii) The species, breed, sex, age and identity of the animals sampled along with date of collection.

iv) List of samples submitted with transport media used.

v) Diseases suspected and tests requested from the laboratory.

vi) A complete history would be beneficial for the laboratory and should be included, if possible. Some of the components of the history are:

a) A list and description of the animals examined and the findings of the post-mortem examination along with the length of time sick animals have been on the farm if they are recent arrivals, from where did they originate.

b) The date of the first cases and of subsequent cases or losses.

c) The total number of animals on the farm, the number of dead animals, the number of animals showing clinical signs, and their age, sex and breed.

d) The clinical signs and their duration including the temperature of sick animals, condition of mouth, eyes and feet, and milk or egg production data.

e) The type and standard of husbandry, including the type of feed available, possible contact with poison or poisonous plants including history of foreign travel by owner or of introduction of animals from other countries or regions.

f) Any medication or vaccination given to the animals along with time.

Transportation of samples

General guidelines for transport of specimen

Regulations require that diagnostic specimens transported in interstate or inter country traffic must be packaged and labelled properly. Improper packaging and labelling of diagnostic specimens and other hazardous material can result in unnecessary exposure to postal, shipping, laboratory personnel, etc.

1. The first and foremost thing is that the specimens should be forwarded to the laboratory by the fastest available method and it should reach to laboratory within 48 hours.
2. Transport medium may be used to preserve microorganisms during transportation as charcoal medium improves the isolation of bacteria by neutralizing toxic substances, such as naturally occurring fatty acids found on the skin.
3. The viral transport medium should be used as many viruses, which do not survive well outside the body and the expiry date of transport medium should always checked.
4. Samples submitted for bacterial polymerase chain reaction (PCR) should not be transport in any medium.

5. The specimens must be in securely closed as screw cap container or sealed vial in waterproof manner.
6. Each primary container should be wrapped in sufficient dry absorbent cotton or paper towels to absorb the material, in case of breakage the external surfaces of the primary containers make contaminants free before shipment. In extra precautions, the primary container should be padded with more cotton or paper to prevent jarring.
7. The secondary containers used to keep the primary container should be a half gallon sized or approximate one liter capacity, and the paint cans having friction type lids are totally water proof, should used for this purpose.
8. A tertiary container should used in transport, if a highly infectious disease or zoonotic disease is suspected. Tertiary containers are bigger in size than the secondary container.
9. Finally the sealed secondary of tertiary container should be placed in a shipping container, which is an insulated box with a lid that can be taped shut and it is again packed with packing material like paper. A corrugated shipping box, affixed with the proper labels and shipper s certification, is the final enclosure and contains all other containers.
10. The samples should be sent in refrigerated conditions and if dry ice is used for refrigeration, then the additional packaging requirements must be need.
11. Regular mail or airmail shipment should not be used, when a exotic infectious animal disease is suspected. Courier service is the appropriate method of shipment.
12. Care must be taken to ensure that a exotic infectious animal disease suspicious package is only opened within the confines of a biosecure facility.

The proper specimen collection is the pre-requisite of lab diagnosis. The accurate sampling is the way to reach the correct diagnosis of an issue and make the inferences from the results.

R

1. Veterinary laboratories agency (2003). Submission of Samples to the Veterinary Laboratories Agency. Veterinary Laboratories Agency, New Haw, Addleston, Surrey, United ingdom, 27 pp. www.vla.gov.uk/servtovet/documents/Submissions.pdf

2. Veterinary services (of the united states department of agriculture (2005). Regulations for Classifying Infectious Substances and Diagnostic Specimens, USDA Veterinary Services Notice No. 06-02.

3. World health organization (2005). Guidance on regulations for the transport of infectious substances. http://www.who.int/csr/resources/publications/biosafety/WHO CDS CSR L O 2005 22/en/.

4. World organization for animal health (Oie : Office International Des Epizooties) (2006). Terrestrial Animal Health Code. OIE, Paris, France, www.oie.int

5. Advisory Committee on Dangerous Pathogens (2013) Approved List of Biological Agents. Health and Safety Executive: London.

6. Parsani, H.R and Momin, R.R (2008) Preparation and submission of Specimens for Laboratory Examination. Vet World, Vol. 1(8): 253-255.

7. Collection and shipment of diagnostic specimens (2008) OIE *Terrestrial Manual.*

8. Anon (1993) Removal of blood from laboratory mammals and birds. First Report of the BVA/FRAME/RSPCA/UFAW/Joint Working Group on Refinement. *aboratory Animals*, 27: 1 22.

□□□

Chapter 10

Gross Anatom and Ph siolog of emale Genital Organs in Bovine

Anuj Kumar ikas Sachan and .K. Agra al

Department of Veterinary Gynaecology & Obstetrics, College of Veterinary Science and Animal Husbandry, Uttar Pradesh Pandit Deen Dayal Upadhyaya Pashu Chikitsa Vigyan Vishwavidhyalaya Evam Go Anusandhan Sansthan, Mathura

---

Understanding the anatomy and physiology of the cow s reproductive system is fundamental for good cattle management. Basic knowledge in this area will enable producers to do a better job of getting cows rebred, especially if artificial insemination and estrous synchronization are employed. It will also enable producers to better understand and control reproductive diseases and calving problems. The Female reproductive organs are composed of ovaries, oviduct ,uterus, cervix, vagina and external genitalia.

O

A cow has two oval or almond shaped ovaries located within the abdominal cavity. Size of the ovaries varies with stage of the reproductive cycle and age of the female, but generally are 1.3 to 5cm in length, 1.3 to 3.2cm width and 0.6 to 1.9 cm thick and weighs about 5 to 15 gram.The anterior (cranial) portion of the broad ligament attached to and supports the ovary is called the mosovarium. Mesovarium carries the blood and the lymphatic vessels, which supplies the ovary. The second supportive ligament, the utero-ovarian ligament attaches the ovary to the uterus. The free surface of the ovary is physiologically active, where follicles and corpus luteum develop. The meso- ovarian and utero-ovarian ligament form a bursa like pouch called the ovarian bursa. The ovary is covered by the outer most single layer of cuboidal cells called the germinal epithelium. Beneath the germinal epithelium there is the tunica albugenia, a connective tissue composed of fewer cells and closely packed fibres. Beneath the tunica, albugenia there is the ovarian cortex which contains the follicles and corpus luteum in various stages of development or regression the central part of the ovary is called the ovarian medulla. The medulla houses the vasculature, nerves and the lymphatics and is composed of dense connective tissue.

Follicles begin within the ovary as one of several thousand **primordial follicles**, which consist of a germ cell surrounded by a layer of flattened cells. This germ cell has the potential to mature into an egg, if the follicle completes the development phase. However, only a small percentage of primary follicles continue through the **secondar** and **tertiar follicular** phases and ultimately undergo ovulation. Primary follicles that never complete development die and are replaced by newly formed primary follicles.The relatively few primary follicles that complete development do so through a series of phases. Many layers of cells are added to the single layer of cells surrounding the egg in the primary follicle and a central cavity forms. The follicle and cavity within the follicle grow larger and the egg becomes attached to a stalk of cells on the side of the follicle opposite the future site of ovulation. As the follicle continues to grow larger, the outer layer of the follicle becomes thinner. This follicle is matures and called a **Graafian follicle**. The outer layer of the follicle ruptures at the appropriate time and the egg and along with the contents of the follicular cavity is released. Follicular development occurs in concert with other reproductive and behavioural functions so that near the time of ovulation, the uterus is prepared to receive both the egg from the female and sperm from the bull.

Following ovulation, the cells that developed within the follicle undergo a differentiation process by action of pituitary hormones. This process is called **luteini ation** and gives rise to the second ovarian structure, the **corpora lutea** (pl. **corpus luteum**). This structure is often referred to simply as the CL and has the important function of secreting the hormone progesterone.The CL goes through a maturation and regression cycle much the same as the follicle. A blood clot-type structure known as a **corpora hemorrhagicum** forms in the cavity left by the ruptured follicle and is transformed into a CL by Day 5 of the cycle (Day 0 estrus). The CL is fully functional from Day 5 to Day 15 of the cycle and then begins to regress, if the female does not become pregnant. The CL regresses and no longer secretes progesterone as the follicle of the next estrous cycle begins to develop. As the CL regresses further, it changes into the **corpus albicans** and remains visible on the ovary for several subsequent cycles.

The , or female gonad, is responsible for two basic functions

- **E ocrine** Production of the female gamete, the egg or ovum
- **Endocrine** Production of two primary reproductive hormones, estrogen and progesterone. The ovary also produces oxytocin, relaxin, inhibin and activin.
- **O tocin** : It is also produced by Corpus luteum besides posterior pituitary. It causes contaction of smooth muscles and regulates luteolysis.
- **Rela in** : A polypeptide hormone secreted by placenta and /or secretory granules of corpus luteum of pregnancy that causes the cervix to dilate and softens the ligaments in pelvic region , thus tending to widen the birth canal during parturition.
- **Inhibin** : A glycoprotein produced by the granulose cells in the female that specifically inhibits the release of FSH from the anterior pituitary.
- **Activin** : Is a protein from the follicular fluid shown to cause release of FSH from pituitary cells in culture. It, therefore, causes the opposite of inhibin in-vitro. (it is not as yet considered a hormone.)

The ovary produces the egg by a process called **oogenesis**. In contrast to spermatogenesis in the bull which is continuous, oogenesis is cyclic. This cycle of egg development in cattle is called the **estrous c cle** and is typically 20 to 21 days in length.Any condition that prolongs the period of time that blood levels of progesterone remain high will have the same effect as pregnancy in stopping the regular 21-days cycle. Occasionally the CL does not regress normally (persistent CL) even though the animal does not become pregnant. This requires diagnosis and treatment by a veterinarian.Abnormally short estrous cycles (7 to 11 days) can occur. This condition appears to be caused by either no corpora lutea being formed, or if one is formed, it is non-functional and progesterone levels remain low. An estrous cycle can be shortened intentionally by injecting a hormone called prostaglandin, which causes the CL to regress. Prostaglandin injection is one method used in estrous synchronization.

Estrus is neither always accompanied by ovulation. Heat without ovulation (anovulatory heat) will not result in pregnancy even though the female is bred. Ovulation without behavioral estrus (silent heat) is not uncommon in cows, especially the first few weeks after calving. Such females will not accept service from a male.

There are wide differences between the species of mammals in the various characteristics of the estrous cycle. Some species have only one heat period each year and are called monoestrus. The cow is in a group that exhibits heat more than one time per year and is called polyestrus. Even though cows will cycle at any time during the year, recent research has shown that day length may have an effect on cow fertility. Slightly lower fertility has resulted during the short day length period of the year.

Ovidut

The oviducts are a pair of tortuous, narrow tubes suspended in the mesosalpinx, a peritoneal fold from the lateral layer of the broad ligament. They are about 20 to 30 cms long and about 3 mm diameter extending from the ovary to the uterine horn. The **oviduct** may be divided into four functional segments-the fringe like **fimbriae** funnel-shaped tube that engulfs the ova. This funnel portion of the oviduct is called the **infundibulum**. The more dilated **ampulla** and the narrow portion of the oviduct connecting the oviduct with the uterine lumen-the **isthmus.** The opening of the infundibulum, ostium tubae abdominale lies in the centre of a fringe of irregular processes, that forms the extremity of the oviduct, the fimbriae. The opening of the isthmus into the uterus is called ostium tubae uterinum. The fimbriae greatly increase the surface area of the infundibulum. The infundibulum leads directly into a thick portion of the oviduct called the ampulla. The ampulla occupies one-half or more of the oviductal length and merges with the isthmus of the oviduct. The junction between ampulla and isthmus is called ampullary isthmus junction . isthmus directly connected to the uterus by utero-tubal junction.

The wall of oviduct consists of the mucosa, the muscularis and outer serous coat. The oviductal mucosa is made of primary, secondary and the tertiary folds. The mucosa consists of surface columnar epithelial cells. The epithelium contains ciliated and non-ciliated cells or secretory cells together with peg cells (depleted secretary cells). Ciliated cells are more abundant where the egg is picked up from the ovarian surface, whereas secretary cells are abundant, where luminal fluids are needed as a medium for the interaction of egg and spermatozoa.

The oviduct has following function

1. Captures and transport the ovulated eggs from the ovarian surface to the fertilization site.
2. Conveys the egg and spermatozoa in opposite direction, almost simultaneously.
3. Sperm capacitaton, fertilization and embryo cleavage occur in the oviduct.
4. Transport of the early embryo to the uterus.
5. The oviduct provides an optimal environment that is both nutritive and protective for the sperm, oocyte and early embryo.

When ovulation occurs, the ovum is picked up by the **infundibulum** and channeled into the oviduct (also known as the **allopian tube**), where fertilization takes place, if viable sperm are present. Here, the ovum remains capable of fertilization for only a short time. Thus, it is essential that sperm be present in the oviduct near the time of ovulation. The ovum moves through the oviduct into the uterine horn within the next 3 to 4 days. If the ovum is fertilized, it then begins embryological development if not, it degenerates and disappears and the next estrous cycle ensues.

Uterus

The body of the **uterus** of the cow is short and poorly developed, while the **uterine horns** are relatively long and well-developed (Bicornuate type). The uterine body is having length of about 2 to 4 cm and length of uterine horn is 35 to 40 cm.The horns are joined by the dorsal and ventral intercornual ligaments. The uterus is located either on the floor of the pelvis, on the pelvic brim or in parous cows mostly on the caudal floor of the abdominal cavity. The uterus is attached dorso laterally by the broad ligament and the meso-metrium. Internally the inner surface of the uterus in ruminants contain non glandular convex shaped projections called the caruncles which are arranged in four rows. They are 70 to 120 in number and during pregnancy they increase in size from 15 mm to 10 cm.

The uterus consists of thin outer layer, the perimetrium, a thick myometrium composed of inner circular and outer longitudinal muscle layers and an inner layer, the endometrium. The outer perimetrium is the serous layer, which is part of the peritoneum. During pregnancy the amount of muscle tissue in the uterine wall increases, both by cell enlargement and cell number. The epithelial lining of the lumen of endometrium is of columnar type that undergo structural change during pregnancy to facilitate the attachment of the blastocyst . the endometrium is characterized by numerous openings of the endometrial glands. The glands possess a lamellar connective tissue and are lined by simple or ciliated columnar epithelium. These glands are scattered throughout the endometrium with the exception of the caruncles. These uterine glands reach full secretary capacity under the influence of progesterone. These secretions called uterine milk or histrotroph are important to the survival and function of the preimplantation embryo. The function, thickness and the vascularity of the structures of the endometrium are regulated by the changes in ovarian hormones throughout the estrous cycle and pregnancy. the contraction of the myometrium is essential for the transport of spermatozoa from the site of ejaculation to the site of fertilization. The uterus produce the $PGF_{2\alpha}$ that lysis the corpus luteum and thereby controls the oestrus cyclicity. Endometrial glands secretes the uterine milk, which nourishes the free living zygote preceding implantation. Uterus gives attachment to the placenta and plays a role in the nutrition, excretion and exchange of the carbon dioxide and oxygen. At the time of parturition, the strong muscular contractions of the uterus helps to expel the foetus and placenta.

The fertilized embryo moves from the oviduct into the uterine horn, where fetal and maternal membrane development begins. This newly developing fetus grows within a layer of membranes called the placenta, through which nourishment from the dam diffuses. There is no direct blood connection between the fetus and the dam, but rather a complex system that selectively allows certain molecules to pass from the maternal side of the placenta to the fetal side and vice versa. It also provides nutrients and carries waste products from the fetus.

Cervix

The cervix is a thick walled organ between the vagina and uterus with a constricted lumen. Length of the cervix is 8 to 10 cm, diameter 3 to 4 cm .It has thick walls and a small opening, which softens and relaxes to allow a passage way for sperm at mating and expulsion of the fetus at the time of birth. It serves as a point of orientation during the clinical examination in bovine. The canal of the cervix opens into the anterior vagina through the external os and into the uterus through the internal os. The cervical canal is characterized by various prominences. In ruminants, these prominences are in the form of transverse or spirally inter-locking ridges known as annular rings. They are prominent in cows where they fit into each other to close the cervix securely. In cow, the numbers of annular rings are 3-5 in number. The junction of cervix and vagina is a blind pouch called Fornix. The cervical wall is made up of fibroelastic collageneous tissue and muscular tissue. The collagen is responsible for the high tensile strength of the cervix. During pregnancy, the cervix is filled with a thick mucus secretion known as the **cervical plug**, which protects the uterus from infections entering from the vagina. The cervical plug is expelled and the cervical opening begins to dilate in the days prior to calving.

Vagina

The **vagina** serves as a receptacle for the male s penis during service. The length of vagina is 25 to 30 cm. The mucosal epithelium varies depending on the region of vagina. At the region near the cervix, the epithelium is columnar and highly secretary in nature. Towards the posterior vagina, the epithelium is of stratified squamous type, which thickens dramatically at the time of estrus. In the cow, the semen is deposited in the vagina near the cervix during natural mating with the bull. When artificial insemination is used, an insemination instrument is threaded through the vagina and cervix and semen is deposited at the uterine side of the cervix. Urine is discharged from the urinary bladder through the urethra, which opens into the base of the vagina. The region behind the urethral opening is called the vestibule and is a common passageway for both the urinary and reproductive systems. The cervical canal as well as the biochemical and microbiological milieu of the vagina protected the upper reproductive tract from invading micro-organisms. The external opening of the vagina is called the **vulva**.

Vestibule

Portion of vagina that is common to the urinary system and the reproductive system, Extends from urethral orifice to the labia of vulva. At the floor of the vestibule are the gartners ducts- blind sacs, which are remnants of wolffian duct. Ventral to the urethral opening there is the sub-urethral diverticulum in sow and cow. It is a blind pouch.

Vulva

External part of the female reproductive tract. Consist of labia majora and labia minora. The skin of the labia have numerous sebaceous and sweat glands. The labia consists of adipose tissue into which are embedded small bundles of smooth muscles, which are called constrictor vulvae muscles.

Clitoris

IT is located in the caudal portion of the ventral commisure and is homologues to the penis. It is 5-10 cm long. Most of it is hidden in the tissue between vulva and the ischiatic arch. Clitorial massage at the time of insemination facilitat the sperm transport in female genital tract.

□□□

Chapter 11

Management of Repeat Breeding in Dair Animals

Anuj Kumar ikas Sachan and .K. Agra al

Department of Veterinary Gynaecology & Obstetrics, College of Veterinary Science and Animal Husbandry, Uttar Pradesh Pandit Deen Dayal Upadhyaya Pashu Chikitsa Vigyan Vishwavidhyalaya Evam Go Anusandhan Sansthan, Mathura

I

Repeat breeding is a major reproductive disorder in dairy cattle and its incidence varies among different management systems, environmentals conditions and regions. A repeat breeder cow is a cow that looks apparently healthy with no palpable abnormalities of reproductive tract, apparently normal estrual discharge and has regular oestrous cycle. However, it does not conceive, when bred at least three times continuously, either with a bull of well-known fertility or inseminated artificially with excellent quality semen. Repeat breeding is one of the major infertility problems of herds. The incidence of repeat breeding in dairy cows, worldwide, ranges from 5 to 35 .

Causes of Repeat Breeding in Dairy Animal

The various etiological factors responsible for repeat breeding are-

1. Genetical factors : include numerical chromosomal abnormalities of gametes and other defect of gametes at gene level.
2. Subclinical uterine infection : include various bacterial, viral, protozoal and fungal infections which resulted into sub-clinical infection of uterus.
3. Hormonal factors: includes ovulatory defects, it may be delayed ovulation and/or anovulatory estrus. Ovulatory defects are mainly because of faulty LH secretion, prolong duration of estrus or improper steroid genesis, which resulted into either failure of fertilization or early embryonic death.

4. Managemental factors : includes poor heat detection, wrong time of insemination, unskilled artificial inseminator, parasitic infestation and nutritional deficiency etc. Nutrional deficiency include lack of energy, excess dietry protein and deficiencies of micronutrients etc.
5. Immunological factors : immunological incompatibility of sperm and oocyte because of production of anti-sperm antibodies has also been documented to be a reason for failure of fertilization resulted into repeat breeding.

The fertilization failure and early embryonic death are the two mechanisms resulted in repeat breeding in dairy animals. Both fertilization failure and embryonic mortality occur at a much higher rate than in normal cows to 6 weeks post insemination.

Approximately 50 of embryonic losses occurs during the first 3 weeks embryonic losses of pregnancy in repeat breeder. The incidence of repeat breeding is higher in dairy herds using artificial insemination rather than natural service. Errors in estrus detection may also contribute to repeat returns to service in dairy cows. The higher incidence of embryonic mortality in old cows may be due to a defective uterine environment. When evaluating females for RB, the causes for fertilization failures in part or in complete that would result from because of abnormal male gametes or it s por function must be first eliminated. The possibility of failures caused by semen abnormality appears to be ruled out, when artificial insemination using semen of high fertility is used.

Diagnosis of Repeat Breeder Animal

First of all, a complete clinical history should be obtained at herd and individual level. Age, parity, milk yield, previous diseases, reproductive indexes, estrous cycle characteristics, insemination schedule, bulls, estrus detection, hormones, food and farm hygiene should be registered. Then anatomy, morphology and function of different body systems of the cows should be inspected. The reproductive status of animals must be be evaluated to detect disorders, as muscle or claw lameness. Vulva, vagina, cervix, uterus fallopian tubes and ovaries must be evaluated to diagnoses reproductive defects In general, there are six major diagnostic approaches as follows:

1. External inspection and vaginal evaluation

2. Rectal Palpation
3. Ultrasonography
4. Hormonal function tests
5. Oviductal patency
6. Endometrial cytology and uterine bacterial culture

1. External Inspection and Vaginal Evaluation

External inspection can identify congenital or acquired anatomical defects as pneumovagina, vulvar defects, tumors or injuries etc. The anatomy of the perineal area, secretions around vulva or tail and vulvar and vaginal mucus membrane colouration should be evaluated. It should also be asessed for the presence of adhesions, abnormal structures and cervical defects.

2. Rectal Palpation

Rectal palpation is a widely used diagnostic method in cattle with high accuracy, easy to be implemented and at low cost in comparison with other sophisticated techniques. Palpation helps to diagnose the anomalies, in literus oviduct and ovaries. Animals with poor uterine tone at insemination often have poor conception. Moreover, evaluation is subjective and evaluated differently by different clinician. Ovarobursal adhesions can be diagnosed by rectal palpation of genital organs etc.

3. Ultrasonography (USG)

Transrectal ultrasound diagnosis has improved our ability to assess the reproductive organs in cattle and to follow the dynamic interactions between ovarian follicular cohorts. USG practical uses include routine assessment of follicular and luteal development and differential diagnosis of cystic ovaries, ovarian abscesses and tumors, which can be considered as the factors associated with repeat breeding cow syndrome. At the time of estrus size of graffian, follicle can be monitored by USG. Ovulation of graffian follicle can also be assessed by ultrasonography with more accuracy than manual per-rectal examination.

USG helps to evaluate the uterus by detecting changes in shape and echotexture related with circulating hormonal concentrations during the estrous cycle.

4. Hormonal Function Tests

Progesterone can be considered as a sensor of the reproductive capacity, both for its information about the estrous cycle and for its easy determination. Progesterone assay is an objective and accurate test to evaluate the ovarian function and to diagnose certain abnormalities that otherwise could not be correctly determined, such as delayed ovulation, persistent luteal activity, ovarian cysts or supra basal progesterone levels. A delay or deviation in secretion of LH surge can affect ovulation and development of corpus luteum. Post ovulatory progesterone secretion is also crucial for embryo viability. Late post ovulatory progesterone rise associated with poor embryo development and production of insufficient interferon tau which may lead to embryonic death.

5. Oviductal Patency

The determination of oviductal patency is interesting, although it is difficult to carry out. It is an injection of 500 ml of sterile solution containing 30 gram of starch which is intra-peritoneally injected-starch reaches the oviduct and descends to the cervical mucus, if the fallopian tubes are patent. It takes about 12 hours to arrive at the cervical mucus, where it will remain between 2 and 4 days. A sample of mucus is collected, stained with 2) and observed under the microscope. Another test for patency of fallopian tube is PSP dye test by using a two-way catheter into uterine horn and detection of dye in urine. In case of patent fallopian tube dye is present in urine within 30 minutes. This test may give false positive results in case of any injury in female genital tract.

6. Endometrial Cytology and Uterine Bacterial Culture

Infectious diseases could provoke vulvitis, vaginitis, cervicitis or endometritis and it is interesting to diagnose these disorders. Usually, uterine inflammatory disorders begin with bacterial contamination into the uterine lumen and continue with adhesion of pathogens to the mucosa colonization or penetration of the epithelium and/or release of endotoxins.

In cattle, especially due to the cervical anatomy, samples can be taken using a catheter connected to a syringe containing 30-60 ml of sterile saline. It is deposited into the uterus and then, it is removed and cultured. Diagnostic tests to evaluate such subclinical uterine infections have been developed to a limited extent, but suffer from incorporation of suboptimal uterine secretion collection methods and accuracy of diagnosis. One such test, the white side test , uses cervical mucus of suspected cows (with metritis/ endometritis), which is heated with sodium hydroxide solution upto boiling point. The test is considered positive, if the colour turns yellow. A correlation between the number of leucocytes present in the mucus and the intensity of yellow colour is the basis of this test. Cytological examination of the reproductive tract is often used to evaluate possible reproductive lesions in domestic animals. Endometrial cytological examination in mares and cows are accepted as a good diagnostic techniques. Neutrophils constitute the first defensive barrier against invading pathogenic organisms postpartum, resulting in an increase in the polymorphonuclear neutrophils population within the uterine lumen.

Management of Repeat Breeding

To reduce the negative effects of repeat breeding on the farm profitability, an effective therapy must be established after a proper diagnosis. The choice of a therapeutic regimen depends on the possible cause of repeat breeding:

1. Nutritional supplements have been used to restore certain imbalances at herd level. Diets containing higher concentration of inorganic iodine from 8-12 days before estrus improve the stimulation of the pituitary gland, reducing at the same time the repeat breeding cow (RBC) rate. Herds with problems of repeated estrus were supplemented with copper and magnesium improving fertility problems. Deficiencies of these minerals have been associated with infertility, anaemia or immune suppression.
2. Prophylactic practices have been used, as the intrauterine administration of antiseptic solutions (lugol) 24 h. after mating/ AI, although fertility results are poor. Studies on bacteriology and histology of the uterus concluded that the non-specific genital infection is one of the main causes of repeat breeding cow (RBC) and it is suggested that antimicrobial treatments (chloramphenicol, gentamicin, enrofloxacin, tetracycline, or nitrofurantine) could improve the reproductive indexes.
3. It is also essential to improve all aspects related to heat detection, since it has been demonstrated that estrus detection mistakes involve very significant losses in reproduction and production of cattle.

4. Treatments are being used recently for fixed-timed artificial insemination, without heat detection. These protocols allow the treatment of cows with silent heats or ovulation problems by administration of PGF alpha and GnRH to schedule the insemination time.

5. For the treatment of hormonal (functional) causes of repeat breeding in dairy cattle various hormonal protocols have been developed. In prolonged estrus exhibiting repeat breeder cattle, the use of single insemination along with administration of buserelin acetate, a GnRH analogue, is sufficient, however, in the absence of hormonal treatment, the use of double insemination at 24 h interval also gives optimal results. The administration of GnRH in these animals leads to induction of ovulation. In repeat breeder cattle, GnRH administration at estrus or during luteal phase (between day 11-14 post-insemination) increases plasma progesterone and delays luteolytic response, thus enhancing the embryo survival rate. In fact, the treatment of repeat breeder cattle with 10.5 g GnRH analogue or hCG on day 12 post AI lead to an improvement in conception rate. Another option for improving the conception rate in dairy cattle with functional form of infertility is the use of ovulation induction protocol. The use of ovsynch protocol improved the conception rate, however, there was impact of other protocols like doublesynch and heatsynch on fertility improvement. Pre-synchronization with prostaglandin F2 (PGF2) followed by administration of GnRH analogue along with AI at 60 h post-PGF2 improved conception rate in repeat breeder cattle.

   Parenteral administration of progesterone as a tool to increase conception rate in normal breeding dairy cattle presented for insemination is a fast growing malpractice amongst field veterinary staff in different parts of the state. In fact, the results suggested low conception rate in normal breeding dairy cattle receiving progesterone simultaneous to insemination. Progetserone can be supplemeted as a single intra-muscular injection 1000 mg on 5th day post insemination.

6. In the recent past, several therapies alternative to the use of antibiotics have been suggested for the therapy of endometritis. The intra-uterine infusion of immunomodulators, such as E. coli lipopolysaccarides (endotoxin), oyster glycogen, infusion of

serum, plasma or hyperimmune serum or leukotriene B4 has been reported widely. Besides the use of immunomodulators, some other therapies suggested for resolving endometritis include the use of enzymes and antioxidants. Enzymes like trypsin, chymotrypsin and papain can be infused into uterus to cure uterine inection. Antioxidants, such as vitamins C and E are known to modulate the oxidative stress and reduce the endometrial damage both at the biochemical and histological levels.

❑❑❑

Chapter 12

Procedure for Conducting Artificial Inseminaton in Bovines

Atul Sa ena

Department of Veterinary Gynaecology & Obstetrics, College of Veterinary Science and Animal Husbandry, Uttar Pradesh Pandit Deen Dayal Upadhyaya Pashu Chikitsa Vigyan Vishwavidhyalaya Evam Go Anusandhan Sansthan, Mathura

The primary objective of artificial insemination is to speed up the rate of genetic improvement. The task can be accomplished by greatly increasing the selection differential, wherein one highly selected sire is mated with thousands of females. The commercial use of artificial insemination started in the year 1937, however, the sequence of events leading to AI started way back in the 17th century, when Leeuwenhock saw spermatozoa through the newly discovered microscope and Spallanzani (1780) of Italy discovered that a dog could be impregnated with the cellular portion of semen. In 1933, Professor Ivanov had developed methods for collecting semen and inseminating horses, cattle, sheep and swine. Approximately 60 of the dairy cows in the U.S. are artificially inseminated. This is well below the use of AI in European dairy areas, such as Denmark, Holland and England, where over 90 are artificially inseminated. In India the AI coverage is reported to be 35 40 per cent.

One of the major challenges, which our country faces at present, is low productivity of Cattle and buffaloes. Major reasons attributed are insufficient coverage of animals under Artificial Insemination (AI), low conception rates, non-availability of quality bulls for breeding, poor management practices, high mortality & morbidity losses due to diseases, etc. Government from time to time has addressed these issue which has resulted in accreditation of AI lab with use of semen from these labs only and as per the breeding mandate. Moreover, the AI technicians and paravets are to be tranined from accredited training institute.

A S I

Use of traditional a.m-p.m rule may reduce the conception rates, since cow probably will be bred several hours after the onset of estrus, therefore, the chances of successful fertilization may be missed. The exact onset of estrus is usually unknown for e.g. a cow beginning estrus at 1 a.m. and observed in estrus at 6 a.m. the following morning would be bred approximately 17-18 hr after the onset of estrus. Breeding animals at this time would reduce the number of pregnancies. Hence, a herd should be observed for estrus twice daily adopting at least 30 minutes each time to identify a majority of animals in estrus. It is usually recommended that animals should be inseminated within 4 to 16 hr of observed estrus, when the precise onset of estrus is unknown (for twice daily observation).

Why detection of estrus is important

Among the many components of the reproduction management, heat detection is one of the crucial, as it contributes towards the ultimate pregnancy rate and the survival of the embryo. Improper heat detection and insemination of such animals incurs heavy loss in terms of wasteful expenditure of quality male germplasm, production loss and increase risk of introducing genital infections in the female. In this regard attaining higher heat detection efficiency and accuracy is important key to improve individual animal as well as overall herd fertility. The selection of proper heat detection method for a particular dairy farm is dependent on several factors like scale of operation, availability of manpower type of animals, etc. and a single aid cannot be used invariably.

Behavioural changes during heat

Cows

The usual signs shown at the time of estrus in cows are summarised in the table. Comparison with before and after estrus should always be kept in mind.

Before heat - hr before	**Standing heat hr**	**After heat hr after**	**Metestrous bleeding**
Altered vocalization Smell other cows Attempts to ride other cows Vulva moist , swollen reddening of mucus membrane	Stands to be mounted Nervous and excitable Bawls frequently Rides other cows Clear mucous -string from vulva Vulva moist , swollen reddening of mucus membrane	Will not stand to be mounted Clear mucus discharge from vulva	Bloody mucous discharge, though always may not be seen.

Buffaloes

Buffaloes are shy breeders and many a times, the signs of heat are not overt to be detected easily (Silent heat). Incidence of silent heat is high in the herds practising artificial insemination rather than natural service. Estrus in buffaloes is expressed between the late evening to early morning, *i.e.* during the darker part of the day, which further reduce the chances of detection. The most conclusive sign of estrus in buffalo is considered as standing to be mounted by a teaser bull or androgenised female. However, this method can only be practised in organized large dairy herd. Other signs of classical heat may also be found in buffaloes but with less intensity. The chances of detection of heat in buffaloes can be increased by observing the buffaloes during late evening and early morning for heat signs. The person who is milking the buffaloes, can detect the heat most efficiently and accurately.

The AI Technique (Recto-vaginal method)

General Procedure

- eep the premises of the AI Centre clean and maintain all equipments and materials properly along with properly tagged canisters with complete description of semen.
- Each and every call for AI should be responded considering the fact that delay in this work will add another 21 days for infertility.

- Always keep the AI it clean and ready. Check that the AI kit has the following items:

  Straw cutter/Sharp Scissors

  Thermometer

  Thawing Tray (idney tray) or thawing unit

  Forceps (plastic type)

  Singly packed AI sheaths/AI sheaths

  Sheath container

  AI Gun with container (Universal Gun)

  Full arm disposable gloves

  Clean towel

  Tissue paper role

  Thermos-flask with hot water

  Apron

  1.5/2 liter cryocan with desired semen straws for doorstep AI work

- Be at the centre on the scheduled day and time of semen and liquid nitrogen delivery.
- Always keep the container with proper quantity of liquid nitrogen

Detection of Animal for estrus

- Examine the animal externally and ascertain that animal is in heat by presence of clear, transparent, viscous and ropy vaginal discharge. The primary sign of heat is stands to be mounted.
- Check past breeding records and history. Will be helpful in early detection of cyclic non-breeder.
- Wash hands.
- Proceed with preparation of gun only after per rectal examination of genitalia.
- Have plastic gloves, sheath, gun, scissors, forceps, tissue paper, and clean towel ready before thawing semen.

Preparation of thawing unit

- Plug in a thawing unit filled with clean water with AC supply (220 volt) and wait till the red light turned to green or pour hot water from flask in the thawing tray and adjust temperature of water in the tray to 37 degree centigrade by adding cold or hot water.

Removal of semen from the LN2 tank

- Remove semen from the cryocan with forceps and not with hands. While taking out, raise the canister just high enough not above the frost line. Remove the straw within 10 seconds.
- Always keep LN2 cylinder and thawing apparatus side by side to avoid delay in shifting from LN2 to thawing unit.

Thawing of the semen straw

- Shake straw to remove excess nitrogen and quickly plunge it into thawing tray containing warm water at 37 degree centigrade for 40-45 seconds in the horizontal position (kidney tray) or vertical position (thawing unit). In other words, the straw should be completely submerged in the warm water.
- Use plastic container, as they are having poor conductivity and affect of outside temperature can be minimized.

Loading of AI gun

- Ensure that insemination gun and sheath also have temperature around 37 degree centigrade and not extremely hot or cold. In cold weather briskly rub the gun with tissue paper for maintaining temperature near to thawing temperature.
- Take out straw from tray and wipe the straw with tissue paper. After thawing A.I. should be performed as early as possible (maximum within 20 minutes)
- Before loading the straw in the gun, ascertain that air space in the straw is at the laboratory seal end.
- Load the straw into the gun and make a clean cut at a right angle with a straight and sharp scissors or straw cutter just below the laboratory seal.

- Take out the sheath by holding bottom of the sheath corner of the sheath packet and place the sheath on the gun and secure the sheath firmly with o-ring lock or else, fix it as in universal type gun.

Insemination technique

- Wear shoulder length plastic glove, preferably on left hand and hold the gun with right hand (or as per convenience).
- Ask owner to restrain the animal and hold the tail properly. Speak to the animal and make her calm down.
- Lubricate the gloves with liquid paraffin or any other suitable lubricant (bathing soap) before proceeding to rectum.
- Gently put the gloved hand into the rectum by forming a cone with fingers.
- Clean the rectum by removing the faecal material without ballooning.
- Clean vulva with water and wipe with tissue paper.
- Ask owner to help spread the vulva.
- Never allow gun s tip to touch external coat or anus/ vulva of the animal.
- Insert insemination gun at approximately 30-degree angle till the gun reaches the fornix vagina to avoid entry of gun into the urethral opening/urinary bladder.
- Hold the cervix firmly through rectum and slightly stretch it forward to unfold the vaginal folds.
- Gently and smoothly pass the gun through the vagina to the opening of the cervical canal.
- Hold the external os of the cervix ahead of the gun s tip and negotiate vaginal folds and cervical rings to pass the gun through the cervix till the gun s tip reaches at internal os.
- Feel the tip of the gun at internal os by gently moving the gun tip forward to ensure that the gun is in correct place (just at the internal os i.e. body of uterus). Be certain the gun tip is not caught in a thin area between cervical rings or vaginal folds.

- If the animal moves, STOP. Wait till the movement stops.
- Hold the shoulder of the gun between your ring and middle fingers and push the gun piston with your thumb slowly (5 seconds) to deposit the semen just outside the internal os to allow semen to drain into the body of uterus. Gently remove the gun and check for abnormal discharge and a complete semen deposit.
- Recheck semen ID bull and batch number.
- Properly dispose off the sheath, gloves and tissue papers. Clean gun, if needed.
- Record breeding information in the specified Artificial Insemination cow/Artificial Insemination buffalo register provided by SIA.
- Blood on the gun tip and on the gloves indicate that too much force was used to pass the gun be gentle and patient with the animal.
- Ask farmer to release the animal and let her calm down.

Post Insemination Advice to owner

- Ask owner to keep the animal under observation for next 12-24 hrs.
- Inform the owner to save the animal from scrub bulls during the remaining part of present heat.
- If signs of heat persist even after 18-24 hr call for repeat AI, otherwise observe for heat symptoms after 18-21 days and also after 36-42 days.
- If animal does not repeat heat at 18-21 days intervals, then go for early diagnosis of pregnancy.

Post insemination follow-up

- Follow each and every animal inseminated after around 21 days to find out whether it has repeated.
- Follow each and every animal inseminated for pregnancy diagnosis and record the date and result of pregnancy diagnosis in the register.
- Follow each and every pregnant animal and record calving details of the animals.

- Maintain all records related to artificial insemination, pregnancy diagnosis, and calving.
- Advise farmers on proper heat detection, feeding, management and healthcare of animals.

General Instructions for proper upkeep of AI centres

- eep the liquid Nitrogen container in a location that allows seeing into the neck tube of the container, and ease in withdrawing & replenishment of semen and liquid nitrogen. The surrounding should be well-ventilated, dry and dust free.
- Clean AI gun, scissors and other accessories, whenever they get soiled or at least once a week with hot water and air dry them. Sanitize the AI gun and the scissor with Isopropyl alcohol after drying. The AI Gun piston and the scissors should be wiped clean with water after each insemination. Surgical spirit and soaps are lethal to semen, hence should not be used to clean equipments.
- Maintain the liquid nitrogen level above the straw level in 1.5/ 2/ 3 litre capacity containers.
- Measure the liquid nitrogen level of 35 litre containers weekly with the help of measuring scale provided by the SIA. Maintain the record of measurements to monitor its evaporation rate.
- Carry the required semen doses in the liquid nitrogen container to farmer s doorstep. Never carry semen straws in pocket/ thermos-flask / polythene bags filled with water/ice, etc.
- Maintain an accurate semen inventory to lessen the risk of semen exposure.
- Always attach the paper tag provided with each goblet to the requisite canister of the container to identify the type of semen in each canister.

❑❑❑

Chapter 13

Ultrasound A Tool for Increasing Reproductive Efficienc in Bovines

Atul Sa ena

Department of Veterinary Gynaecology & Obstetrics, College of Veterinary Science and Animal Husbandry, Uttar Pradesh Pandit Deen Dayal Upadhyaya Pashu Chikitsa Vigyan Vishwavidhyalaya Evam Go Anusandhan Sansthan, Mathura

Ultrasound (US) has been used a diagnostic tool for reproductive control since 1990s, however it has gain its importance following availability of small portable, affordable scanners, with a good quality image. Since its wide use, people have shifted in their earlier concept of the use of ultrasound in early pregnancy diagnosis and has started comparing its accuracy with that of rectal palpation.

In developed countries, a significant decrease in fertility was observed in dairy cattle during the last two decades after starting and realizing the use of US in quick identification of the problems and its efficiency in solving it. Traditionally, the main diagnostic methods used for reproductive control in cattle included rectal palpation, inspection of vaginal discharge and vaginoscopy. According to Ginther (1995), the information-gathering capabilities of ultrasonic imaging is far exceed those of rectal palpation. Ultrasound improves accuracy in the diagnoses of stages of the oestrous cycle, ovarian and uterine pathologies, and pregnancy diagnosis. In addition, it facilitates the diagnosis of alterations during pregnancy (embryo mortality, foetal malformations, etc.) and helps determining foetal sex from day 55 of pregnancy.

T U

In general, linear-array, real-time, B-mode ultrasound scanners are best suited for veterinary applications involving cattle reproduction. Ultrasound machines consist of a console unit that contains the electronics, controls, and a screen upon which the ultrasound image is visualized by the operator, and a transducer, which emits and receives high-frequency ultrasound waves. Linear-array transducers consist of a series of piezo electric crystals arranged in a row. These crystals emit high frequency sound waves upon being energized. The linear-array transducer results in a rectangular image. In bovine, reproductive organs are most commonly scanned per rectum using a linear-array transducer specifically manufactured for transrectal use. Linear-array transducers of 5.0 and 7.5 MHz frequency ranges are most commonly used in cattle, and most veterinary ultrasound scanners are compatible with probes of different frequencies. Depth of tissue penetration of sound waves and image resolution is dependent upon and inversely related to the frequency of the transducer. Thus, a 5.0 MHz transducer results in greater tissue penetration and lesser image detail, whereas a 7.5 MHz transducer results in lesser tissue penetration and greater image detail. An ultrasound scanner equipped with a 5.0 MHz transducer is most useful for conducting routine reproductive examinations, however, small ovarian structures, such as developing follicles are best imaged with a 7.5 MHz transducer.

I I

The ultrasound waves (pulses of sound) are sent from the transducer, propagate through different tissues, and then return to the transducer as reflected echoes. The returned echoes are converted back into electrical impulses by the transducer crystals and are further processed to form the ultrasound image presented on the screen.

Ultrasound waves are reflected at the surfaces between the tissues of different density, the reflection being proportional to the difference in impedance. If the difference in density is increased, the proportion of reflected sound is increased, and the proportion of transmitted sound is proportionately decreased.

If the difference in tissue density is very different, then the sound is completely reflected, resulting in total acoustic shadowing. Acoustic shadowing is present behind bones, calculi (stones in kidneys, gallbladder, etc.) and air (intestinal gas).

Echoes are not produced, if there is no difference in a tissue or between tissues. Homogenous fluids like blood, bile, urine, contents of simple cysts, ascites and pleural effusion are seen as echo-free structures. Normal B (Brightness) mode Ultrasonography displays an image at grey scales from bright to black according to the tissue characters and nature of sound wave transmission.

T E

When an echo returns to the transducer, its amplitude is represented by the degree of brightness (i.e. echogenicity) of a dot on the display. Combination of all the dots form the final image. Strong specular reflections give rise to bright dots (hyperechoic) e.g., diaphragm, gallstone, bone, pericardium. Weaker diffuse reflections produce grey dots (hypoechoic) e.g., solid organs. No reflection produces dark dots (anechoic) e.g., fluid and blood filled structures because the beam passes easily through these structures without significant reflection. Also, deep structures often appear hypoechoic because attenuation limits beam transmission to reach the structures, resulting in a weak returning echo.

S N

Scanning of non-pregnant uterus is aimed to either determine the stage of the oestrous cycle or diagnose pathologic conditions of the uterus. The histology of the uterus determines its ecographic appearance, as the submucosa can be visualized as an anechoic layer beneath the endometrium. During the follicular phase, under the influence of oestrogens, the blood vessels in the submucosa become hyperaemic, the endometrium becomes oedematous, increasing its thickness, and the anechoic vascular zone is more easily visualized (Griffin and Ginther, 1992). The content of the uterine lumen may also vary during the oestrous cycle, being typically absent during the luteal phase, whereas a small amount of fluid may be present during the follicular phase (Barlund *et al.*, 2008). However, to further clarify the stage of the oestrous cycle, observation of the ovaries is required.

Ultrasound examination of the uterus may help to identify pathological conditions. The frequently encountered alterations that cause substantial economic losses is uterine inflammation. Studies reported prevalence of 53 cases of endometritis in USA dairy herds (Gilbert *et al.*, 2005). Using US and uterine cytology uintela *et al.*

(2010) reported incidences of 45.7 endometiritis in north-west Spain dairy animals.

As per Sheldon *et al.* (2009), metritis, (first 21 days after parturition) and endometritis (beyond 21 days postpartum) can be detected through direct exploration of the external genital organs or by rectal palpation and/or vaginoscopy. Ultrasonography is useful in the diagnosis of uterine diseases (Barlund *et al.*, 2008).

To determine the real usefulness of US for diagnosing uterine infections, we are going to recall the common methods used for an endometritis diagnosis. In several studies (asimanickan *et al.*, 2004 McDougall *et al.*, 2007 Barlund *et al.*, 2008) the results obtained when using vaginoscopy, rectal palpation, US or a metricheck have been compared with those obtained by uterine cytology (considered the gold standard test for diagnosing endometritis). All of them concluded that cytology allows us to detect some endometritis that could not be detected by any of the other methods, and that US should be the second method of choice. Rectal palpation and animal inspection is subjective, often fails to account for normal events and variability in uterine involution (Lewis, 1997) and is not useful for identifying subclinical processes. Rectal palpation or the casual observation of a genital flow is not sensitive enough for diagnosing endometritis (Miller *et al.*,1980 De ruif *et al.*, 1982). Vaginoscopy and Metricheck are not very useful for diagnosing endometritis, as the absence of a purulent vaginal discharge does not exclude the problem, and it might lead to an erroneous diagnosis of endometritis instead of vaginitis also.

They concluded that diagnoses based on rectal palpation were not related to cow fertility, whereas those based on the use of US or cytology showed a high correlation. The proportion of endometritis not diagnosed by US varied between 10 and 20 , depending on the use of a 5 or 10 cut-off point for PMN in the cytology (uintela *et al.*, 2010).

Other uterine conditions that can be detected by US include mucometra, pyometra, abscess of the uterine wall. The ecographical difference between mucometra and pyometra is the ecogenicity of the uterine content. Whereas, the sterile mucus has an anechoic appearance, the purulent content shows a certain degree of ecogenicity, depending on the amount of purulent material in the mucus (uintela *et al.*, 2006). Abscesses in the uterine wall will appear to have a hyperechoic content surrounded by a wall of certain ecogenicity (uintela *et al.*, 2009).

S

The structure that can be visualized through US of a normal cyclic ovary is follicle and corpus luteum. The follicle is anechoic spherical structure and can be found in variable numbers and size (Griffin and Ginther, 1992). The advantage of US compared with rectal palpation is that the subjectivity inherent in the estimation of size and content can be eliminated, as the follicular fluid can be visualized and the diameter can be measured. This makes it possible to detect the presence of a cohort of follicles, dominant follicles or pre-ovulatory follicles. To determine the stage of the oestrous cycle of a cow visualization of CL, an estimation of its stage is important. Ultrasound is believed to be the most accurate method for detecting the presence of a CL in a bovine ovary. Many of the CL, which is embedded in the ovary, could not be palpated by rectal examination and hence, use of US facilitate such detection and increase efficiency of detection of CL. Moreover, haemorrhagic and cavitary CL (cystic CL) with a soft consistency may be confused with follicles (Hanzen *et al.*, 2000 uintela *et al.*, 2006) and US helps in detection of the same. The incidence of cavitary CL ranges from 25.2 to 78.8 during dioestrus and decreases with the progression of the oestrous cycle (ahn, 2010). In a study carried out on 28 cows, Perez-Mar n (2009) found that 28.6 of the CL were cavitary 4 days post-ovulation and 50 of the CL were cavitary 8 days post-ovulation, this proportion decrease after that period. Gnemmi (2004) also indicated that about 50 of the corpora lutea are cavitary during the first 10 days of the oestrous cycle, about 30 maintain the cavity between 10 and 13 days post-ovulation, and only a small percentage of the CL are cavitary during pregnancy. It can, therefore, be assumed that when a CL has a cavity, it is likely to be in the first half of the oestrous cycle, and if there is no cavity, the CL is more likely to be in the second half.

The size of the CL may also be used to estimate its age. Perez-Mar n (2009) indicated that the CL increases in size until about day 8 post-ovulation, maintains a constant size until about day 16 post-ovulation and decreases after this period.

nowledge about the ovarian cycle and follicular dynamics together with US examination of the uterus and ovarian structures (number and size of follicles, existence of a cavity and size of CL) allows us to estimate the stage of the oestrous cycle of a cow. At this point, new technologies, such as colour Doppler available in many portable US scanners, may provide new and interesting information. By studying the blood flow to follicles and CL, it is possible to determine with a certain degree of accuracy the time of ovulation and of CL regression (Herzog and Bollwein, 2007).

S

The first studies using ultrasound revealed that follicular growth occurs in waves, each wave culminating with formation of a large follicle. A follicular wave begins with emergence of a group or cohort of small antral follicles just before the day of ovulation. During the next several days, one of the follicles in this cohort continues to grow and becomes dominant, thereby suppressing subordinate follicles within the wave, from which it originated as well as emergence of follicles in an ensuing follicular wave. As the dominant follicle continues to grow, growth of the remaining follicles in the cohort ceases or slows, and these subordinate follicles eventually undergo atresia. A second wave of growth emerges on approximately Day 10 after ovulation and, for three-wave cycles, an additional wave emerges at Day 16 after ovulation. For both two and three-wave cycles, the ovulatory follicle arises from the final wave (Ginther *et al.*, 1996).

Cystic ovarian follicles (COF) are an important cause of subfertility in dairy animals. COF are follicles with a diameter of at least 2 cm that are present on one or both ovaries in the absence of any active luteal tissue and that clearly interfere with normal ovarian cyclicity (Vanholder *et al.*, 2006). There are two types of COF depending on the wall thickness: follicular cysts have a wall thickness 3 mm and luteinized cysts have a wall thickness 3 mm (Tebble *et al.*, 2001 Vanholder *et al.*, 2006).

Ultrasound examination of ovarian cysts allow us to distinguish follicular and luteinized cysts much more efficiently than rectal palpation (Douthwaite and Dobson, 2000).

In a study on 584 cows (Stevenson, 2006), 51 were diagnosed with ovarian cysts. Following a more detailed follow-up, they concluded that only six were really having ovarian cysts. In 19 cows, the cyst co-existed with a CL, in 12 animals the cyst was suspected to be a pre-ovulatory follicle, as it responded to GnRH treatment, and in 14 cows the cyst was suspected to be a cavitary CL. Ultrasonography allows us to reduce some of the confusing factors: the presence of a CL can be easily detected, the exploration of the uterus may show an oedematous endometrium typical of cows with a pre-ovulatory follicle, but not normally seen in cows with ovarian cysts (Bartolome *et al.*, 2005 Archbald *et al.*, 2009), and the size of the follicular structure can be objectively determined.

Granulose-theca cell tumours are the most common ovarian tumours in cattle (incidences 0.5). This type of tumour arises from the sex cord stromal tissue within the ovary and may be relatively small, solid, and yellow to white, or large, filled with cysts of varying sizes and weight upto 11.9 12.3 kg (Roberts, 1986). The ultrasonographic appearance will vary depending on the tumour aspect. An image resembling a honeycomb is often seen because of the presence of fluid-filled cavitary lesions inside the tumour (uintela *et al.*, 2006).

P

Many non-pregnant animals do not show heat, or their heat is not detected which significantly increases the days open (Roelofs *et al.*, 2010). An early pregnancy diagnosis facilitates the detection of non-pregnant cows and enables them to be treated for a new insemination (Romano *et al.*, 2006).

For early pregnancy diagnosis, the entire uterus should be systematically explored as during early pregnancy, the majority of the endometrial surface is not different from that seen in a non-pregnant cow, moreover, its appearance can be confused with that of a uterus during oestrus or endometritis.

The embryonic vesicle can be seen as an anechoic zone with slightly dilated uterine horn. Inside the embryonic vesicle, the embryonic mass can be located (Griffin and Ginther, 1992 uintela *et al.*, 2006). Once the embryo is visualized, its viability can be confirmed by checking the heartbeat frequency. Accuracy of early pregnancy detection depends upon the methodical examination of uterus and the gestation stage. Before 26 27 days of pregnancy, using 5 MHz probes, about 40 50 of the embryos cannot be visualized (Gnemmi, 2004), as they are adhered to the uterine wall at this time, and consequently, the diagnosis cannot be accurate. After 27 days of pregnancy, the reliability of the diagnosis is high (uintela *et al.*, 2006 Romano *et al.*, 2006). The accuracy of the diagnosis is higher in negative than positive cases, as embryonic loss usually occurs in the second month of gestation and hence, certain degree of false positive occurs. US examination also helps in the detection of twins. The presence of a higher amount of fluid in the uterine lumen, more alantoid membranes than expected for the gestational age, together with the visualization of a hyperechoic zone, which would correspond to the anastomosis of alantoid membranes, and of two CL, suggest the presence of a twin pregnancy (uintela *et al.*, 2009). The diagnosis of twins is important for dairy farms as the risks of pregnancy losses, free martinism or dystocia are higher than in single pregnancies (Eddy *et al.*, 1991 Silva del Rio *et al.*, 2009).

One of the most frequent alterations in pregnancy is embryonic or foetal mortality. An embryo resorption can be ultrasonographically recognized by the following characteristics: the amount of alantoid fluid is lower than expected for the gestational age there is a presence of membrane fragments freely floating in a cloudy fluid, an absence of embryo/foetus, an absence of heartbeat. The existence of one or several of these signs are indicative of gestation loss (Gnemmi, 2004 uintela *et al.*, 2006).

Foetal malformations can be detected after approximately 55 60 days of pregnancy. Most large organs of the head, thorax, abdomen and pelvis were visible with ultrasound during the first 4 months (Rajamahendran *et al.*, 1994). Alterations of the normal anatomy, as for example, ascites, umbilical cord alterations, etc., are indicative of reduced foetal viability, so it may be appropriate to induce abortus to avoid increasing the days open.

Diagnosis of foetal sex could increase the price of a pregnant cow, in which case it would be profitable. It will also help dairy farmers in deciding whether or not to retain pregnant cows already earmarked for culling, depending on the sex of the foetus. The sexing of twins is also advantageous, as it allows selective termination of unwanted pregnancies, such as those involving a male and female foetus, which would otherwise bear a freemartin (Rajamahendran *et al.*, 1994).

The external genitalia are initially formed on the caudoventral surface of the abdominal wall, between the hind limbs (Des C teaux *et al.*, 2010). These primordial structures are seen as poorly defined elevations and constitute the genital tubercle (GT), the urogenital fold and the genital swellings, which are developed in the male or female embryos.

In males, the GT becomes elongated to form the penis, the urogenital fold encloses the penis to form the prepuce and the genital swellings become enlarged to develop into the scrotum. In females, the GT forms the clitoris, the genital swellings completely disappear and the urogenital folds develop to enclose the GT, forming the labia (Noden and De la Hunta, 1985 Des C teaux *et al.*, 2010).

The GT is a reliable indicator for bovine foetal gender determination between days 55 and 60 of gestation (Curran *et al.*, 1989 Shunichi *et al.*, 1994). When the GT is located immediately caudal to the abdominal attachment of the umbilical cord, the foetus is male. On the contrary, when the GT is located towards the base of the tail, the foetus is female (Ali, 2004). According to Ali (2004), the best time for foetal gender determination is between days 56 and 98 of gestation. The period of GT migration is a vital parameter and must be verified to avoid male foetuses being incorrectly classified as females because of GT migration after examination (Santos *et al.*, 2005).The possibility of gender determination decreases as pregnancy progresses after the first trimester.

U

The black and white US is helpful to understand the reproductive physiology and hence, the development of reproduction management systems in the cow. To gain more precise information on the physiological status of the ovaries, the local blood flow in individual ovarian follicles and CLs can be observed using colour Doppler US (Herzog and Bollwein, 2007). The technique is based on the Doppler Effect that establishes that when an US bunch with a given frequency finds a flow of erythrocytes, part of the US bunch is reflected towards the probe with modified frequency, higher, if the interface is approaching to the probe and lower, if it is moving away. Therefore, by measuring the apparent change of frequencies between emitter and receiver, the blood flow velocity can be determined (Herzog and Bollwein, 2007).

A colour Doppler image shows the area where a blood flow is detected, so the amount of colour represents the volume of blood present in the examined structures rather than its flow rate. Blood flow changes in the ovaries.

The growth, atresia and ovulation of the follicle and CL functionality can be assessed by colour Doppler US.

- Follicular growth: Before deviation the blood flow in the recruited follicles are same, however, after deviation the flow is maximum in the dominant follicle and reduced in the subordinate follicles with simultaneious reduction in size (Acosta *et al.*, 2005). The atretic follicle was characterized by a lack of detectable blood flow and a progressive decrease in diameter (Acosta *et al.*, 2003). These data suggest that follicular growth, selection and atresia are closely associated with changes in blood supply to an individual follicle.
- Ovulation: There is an increase in the blood flow in the mature follicle following LH surge that reflect the process of ovulation (Acosta *et al.*, 2003).
- Corpus luteum: The CL is one of the most highly vascularized organs and receives the greatest rate of blood flow per unit of tissue of any organ in the body (Wiltbank *et al.*, 1988). During its initial development (48 120 h), a gradual increase in the blood flow around the CL matches with an increase in its volume and in the serum progesterone concentration (Acosta *et al.*, 2003), which suggests that local blood flow in the CL is related to its potential to produce and release progesterone.

In the process of spontaneous luteolysis, blood flow in the CL was observed to increase during the days 16 17 of the oestrous cycle, concomitant with an increase in plasma levels of 14-dihydro-15-keto-prostaglandin F2α (PGFM) and was followed by a decrease in plasma progesterone concentration 1 day after (Miyamoto *et al.*, 2005 Shirasuna *et al.*, 2008 Shirasuna, 2010).

Applications of Doppler Colour to Reproduction in Cattle

- Functionality of the Corpus Luteum: Luteal blood flow (LBF) is more informative about luteal function during the bovine oestrous cycle than is the assessment of luteal size (LS) (Herzog and Bollwein, 2007). In the luteal growth phase LBF, LS and

P_4 increase simultaneously during the luteal static phase, the three parameters are high, however, during the regression phase LBF and P_4decrease parallel, whereas LS decreases later (Herzog *et al.*, 2011). During the static phase of the oestrous cycle and at the onset of CL regression, the luteal size is similar and using only this parameter may cause diagnosing errors.

- Pregnancy diagnosis : By using colour Doppler US, pregnancy diagnosis can be carried out earlier by evaluating the LBF, as non-pregnant animals can be identified based on the decrease in CL blood flow associated with luteolysis. In pregnant cattle, active blood flow surrounding the CL was continuously observed during the late luteal stage (16 23 days after ovulation). However, in non-pregnant cattle LBF clearly decreased at 19 days after ovulation (Matsui and Miyamoto, 2009 Utt *et al.*, 2009).
- Ovarian cysts : The use of colour Doppler US helps to confirm the structure of the follicular wall, as it shows the location of blood vessels in the wall thickness. Follicular cysts show the presence of blood flow inside the wall, whereas luteinized cysts show blood vessels surrounding the wall (Matsui and Miyamoto, 2009).
- Embryo and foetal losses : An evaluation of the status of CL blood flow could be used not only to diagnose the pregnancy, but also early embryonic death. Corpus luteum regression precedes embryo death, when it occurs before day 25, but if embryo mortality occurs between days 25 and 40 of pregnancy, the CL regression may delay upto 3 days (astelic *et al.*, 1991). Thus, detection of a reduced LBF may predict or confirm embryo mortality.

R

Acosta TJ, Hayashi G, Matsui M, Miyamoto A, 2005: Changes in follicular vascularity during the first follicular wave in lactating cows. J Reprod Dev 51: 273 280.

Acosta TJ, Hayashi G, Ohtani M, Miyamoto A, 2003: Local changes in blood flow within the pre-ovulatory follicle wall and early corpus luteum in cows. Reproduction 125: 759 767.

Ali A, 2004: Effect of gestational age and fetal position on the possibility and accuracy of ultrasonographic fetal gender determination in dairy cattle. Reprod Dom Anim 39: 190 194.

Archbald LF, Bartolome JA, Thatcher WW, 2009: Nuevas estrategias en el diagnostico y tratamiento de los quistes ov ricos en la vaca de leche. IV Congreso Internacional de Medicina Bovina, A Coru a, 141 145.

Barlund CS, Carruthers TD, Waldner CL, Palmer CW, 2008: A comparison of diagnostic techniques for postpartum endometritis in dairy cattle. Theriogenology 69: 714 723.

Bartolome JA, Thatcher WW, Melendez P, Risco CA, Archbald LF, 2005: Strategies for the diagnosis and treatment of ovarian cysts in dairy cattle. J Am Vet Med Assoc 277: 1409 1414.

Curran S, astelic JP, Ginther OJ, 1989: Determining sex of the bovine fetus by ultrasonic assessment of the relative location of the genital tubercle. Anim Reprod Sci 19: 217 227.

De ruif A, Gunnink JW, De Bois CH, 1982: Diagnosis and treatment of postpartum endometritis in cattle. Tijdschr Diergeneesk 107: 717 725.

Des C teaux L, Colloton J, Gayrard V, Picard-Hagen N, 2010: Bovine pregnancy. *In:* DesC teaux L, Gnemmi G, Colloton J. (eds), Practical Atlas of Ruminant and Camelid Reproductive Ultrasonography. Blackwell Publishing, Iowa, pp. 81 100.

Douthwaite R, Dobson H, 2000: Comparison of different methods of diagnosis of cystic ovarian disease in cattle and assessment of its treatment with a progesterone-releasing intra-vaginal device. Vet Rec 23: 355 359.

Eddy R, Davies O, David C, 1991: An economic assessment of twin births in British dairy herds. Vet Rec 129: 526 529.

Ginther OJ, Wiltbank MC, Fricke PM, Gibbons JR, ot , 1996. Minireview. Selection of the dominant follicle in cattle. Biol Reprod 55: 1187-1194.

Ginther OJ. 1995. Ultrasonic imaging and animal reproduction. Equiservices Publishing, Cross Plains, WI.

Gnemmi G. 2004: Atlante di ultrasonografia ginecol gica buiatrica. Ed. Le Point Veternaire, Milano, Italy, Pp 127.

Griffin PG, Ginther OJ, 1992: Research applications of ultrasonic imaging in reproductive biology. J Anim Sci 70: 953 972.

Hanzen CH, Pieterse M, Scenzi O, Drost M, 2000: Relative accuracy of the identification of ovarian structures in the cow by ultrasonography and palpation per rectum. Vet J 159, 161 170.

Herzog , Bollwein H, 2007: Application of doppler ultrasonography in cattle reproduction. Reprod Dom Anim 42: 51 58.

Herzog , Vossa C, astelic JP, Beindorff N, Paul V, Niemann H, Bollwein H, 2011: Luteal blood flow increases during the first three weeks of pregnancy in lactating dairy cows. Theriogenology 75: 549 554.

ahn CM, 2010: Cystic ovary disease. *In:* Scott Line (ed.), The Merck Veterinary Manual, 10th edn. Whitehouse Station, NJ: Merck, pp. 1243 1247.

asimanickan R, Duffielda TF, Fosterb RA, Gartleya CJ, Lesliea E, Waltonc JS, Johnsona WH, 2004: Endometrial cytology and ultrasonography for the detection of subclinical endometritis in postpartum dairy cows. Theriogenology 62: 9 23.

astelic JP, Bergfelt DR, Ginther OJ, 1991: Ultrasonic detection of the conceptus and characterization of intrauterine fluid on days 10 to 22 in heifers. Theriogenology 35: 569 581.

Lewis GS, 1997: Health problems of the postpartum cow, uterine health and disorders. J Dairy Sci 80: 984 994.

Matsui M, Miyamoto A, 2009: Evaluation of ovarian blood flow by colour Doppler ultrasound: practical use for reproductive management in the cow. Vet J 181: 232 240.

McDougall S, Macaulay R, Compton C, 2007: Association between endometritis diagnosis using a novel intra-vaginal device and reproductive performance in dairy cattle. Anim Reprod Sci 99: 9 23.

Miller HV, imsey PB, endrick JW, 1980: Endometritis of dairy cattle: diagnosis, treatment, and fertility. Bovine Pract 15: 13 23.

Miyamoto A, Shirasuna , Wijayagunawardane MP, Watanabe S, Hayashi M, amamoto D, Matsui M, Acosta TJ, 2005: Blood flow: a key regulatory component of corpus luteum function in the cow. Domest Anim Endocrinol 29: 329 339.

Noden DM, De la Hunta A, 1985: The Embriology of Domestic Animals. Development Mechanisms and Malformation. Williams and Wilkins, Baltimore, MD, pp. 330 335.

Perez-Mar n C, 2009: Formation of corpora lutea and central luteal cavities and their relationship with plasma progesterone levels and other metabolic parameters in dairy cattle. Reprod Dom Anim 44: 384 389.

uintela LA, Becerra JJ, Cainzos J, Prieto A, D az C, Mourazos N, Fern ndez FI, Mart nez D, Barrio M, Herrad n PG, 2010: La citolog a endometrial en la vaca. Boletin de Anembe, Journal of the National Association of Spanish Specialists in Bovine Medicine, pp. 16 32.

uintela LA, Becerra JJ, P rez-Mar n CC, Barrio M, Cainzos J, Prieto A, D az C, Herrad n PG, 2011: Fetal gender determination by first-trimester ultrasound in dairy cows under routine herd management in North-west Spain. Anim Reprod Sci 125: 13 19.

uintela LA, D az C, Becerra JJ, Herrad n PG, 2009: Atlas de ecograf a en la vaca. Ed. uintela L.A., Spain, Pp. 205.

uintela LA, D az C, Herrad n PG, Pe a AI, Becerra JJ, 2006: Ecograf a y reproducci n en la vaca. Ed. Servicio de publicaciones e intercambio cient fico of the University of Santiago de Compostela, Santiago de Compostela, Spain, Pp 92.

Rajamahendran R, Ambrose DJ, Burton B, 1994: Clinical and research applications of real-time ultrasonography in bovine reproduction: a review. Can Vet J 35: 563 572.

Roberts SJ, 1986: Veterinary Obstetrics and Genital Diseases Theriogenology. Woodstock, Vermont, Vol. 12: 533 535.

Roelofs J, L pez-Gatius F, Hunter RHF, van Eerdenburg FJCM, Hanzen CH, 2010: When is a cow in estrus Clinical and practical aspects Theriogenology 74: 327 344.

Romano JE, Thompson JA, Forrest DW, Westhusin ME, Tomaszweski MA, raemer DC, 2006: Early pregnancy diagnosis by transrectal ultrasonography in dairy cattle. Theriogenology 66: 1034 1041.

Santos MHB, Chiamenti A, Aguiar Filho CR, Moraes EPB , Cavalcanti Neto CC, Lima PF, Oliveira MAL, 2005: Utiliza o da ultra-sonografia na sexagem de fetos de ra a Anglo-nubiana pela idenfica αo do tub rculo genital e da genit lia externa. Veterin riae Zootecnia 12: 1 112.

Shirasuna , 2010: Nitric oxide and luteal blood flow in the luteolitic cascade in the cow. J Reprod Dev 56: 9 14.

Shirasuna , amamoto D, Morota , Shimizu T, Matsui M, Miyamoto A, 2008: PGF2 stimulates endothelial nitric oxide synthase depending on the existence of bovine granulose cells: analysis by co-culture system of endothelial cells, smmonth muscle cells and granulose cells. Reprod Dom Anim 43: 592 598.

Shunichi , ondoh S, Enomoto S, Sameshima H, Goto , Hamana , 1994: Ultrasonic diagnosis of bovine fetal sex by relative location of the genital tubercle in early pregnancy. J Reprod Dev 40: 343 347.

Silva del Rio N, Colloton JD, Fricke PM, 2009: Factors affecting pregnancy loss for single and twin pregnancies in a high-producing dairy herd. Theriogenology 71: 1462 1471.

Stevenson J. 2006: What s all the fuss about cysts . Hoard s Dairyman, *ct* 10: 682.

Tebble JE, O Donnell MJ, Dobson H, 2001: Ultrasound diagnosis and treatment outcome of cystic ovaries in cattle. Vet Rec 31: 411 413.

Utt MD, Johnson GL III, Beal WE, 2009: The evaluation of corpus luteum blood flow using colour-flow Doppler ultrasound for early pregnancy diagnosis in bovine embryo recipients. Theriogenology 71: 707 715.

Vanholder T, Opsomer G, De ruif A, 2006: Aetiology and pathogenesis of cystic ovarian follicles in dairy cattle: a review. Reprod Nutr Dev 46: 105 119.

Wiltbank MC, Dysko RC, Gallagher P, eyes PL, 1988: Relationship between blood flow and steroidogenesis in the rabbit corpus luteum. J Reprod Fert, 51: 3 520.

□□□

Chapter 14

Handling Tha ing Procedure of Semen

ikas Sachan Anuj Kumar and itendra K. Agra al

Department of Veterinary Gynaecology and Obstetrics, College of Veterinary Science and Animal Husbandry, Uttar Pradesh Pandit Deen Dayal Upadhyaya Pashu Chikitsa Vigyan Vishwavidhyalaya Evam Go Anusandhan Sansthan, Mathura

---

Artificial insemination (AI) is first generation reproductive biotechnology which has revolutionized the animal production. AI can be done with the fresh semen, semen preserved at room temperature, refrigerated semen as well as with the cryopreserved semen. Last one is the most popular and successful method of AI in bovines at field level throughout the country to achieve the fast genetic progress regarding livestock production. There are a lot of technical and non-technical aspects related to AI, among which handling of semen as well as liquid nitrogen (LN_2) cylinder management has its own importance.

Frozen semen straws are always preserved in liquid nitrogen (BP -196^{0}C and FP -212^{0}C) in special container called as LN_2 cylinder or cryocan. In general, it is a double-walled metal/aluminium vacuum vessel with an efficient insulation. There is an inner chamber and an outer chamber with a bad conductor of heat as non-metalic neck. Space between inner and outer chamber is filled with high quality insulator material (No heat exchange) with vacuum system. Failure of this system will lead to loss of the filled gas rapidly. Frost line at the top of container is sign of increased evaporation due to damaged container. Weight of LN_2 in the container is supported by neck tube. The neck of the most cryocan is delicate and easily get damaged on mishandling because of poor knowledge about structure and function. Thus, some points should be kept in mind in order to increasing efficiency of cryocan.

LN_2 cylinder should be kept on rubber, jute or wooden carpet in order to avoid the direct contact with hard floor. Wet floor, hard cement or chemicals may cause corrosion to the cylinder with due course of time and may lead to loss of vacuum system. LN_2 cylinder should be kept always in vertical position. It should never be tilted or rolled to avoid any damage or dent. eeping one cylinder on other should not be practised. Platform base trolley should be used during shifting from one to another place. Placing of cryocan should be done in cool place and avoid direct sunlight exposure to increase the LN_2 holding capacity. There should be an alternate arrangement of cryocan in case of appearance of frost line or condensed moisture on outer shell. Handling should be careful to avoid damage to vacuum knob of the cylinder to avoid vacuum loss. Handling of cryocan should be gentle as any jerk or shock/vibration during lifting, putting or carrying may cause damage to the neck tube and loss of vacuum system. Punching or drilling on the container wall is prohibited. Neck plug or lid of cryocan should be opened only during filling of gas, measuring of LN_2 gas level or taking straw out. Neck should be kept dry with use of cloth or tissue paper to avoid jamming of the neck plug. The lid should always be kept in vertical position to avoid damage. Lids or canisters are never be recommended to exchange, as they are specific for individual models of cryocan otherwise there may be damage due to tight fitting or frost formation with LN_2 loss due to loose fitting. Frequent opening, closing or shifting of the cryocan should be avoided to keep evaporation rate minimum. For proper charging and filling of the container, the gas should be filled slowly and non-splashing. Funnel should be used to transfer the gas from one to another cryocan and avoid overfilling of gas. LN_2 cylinder can be secured with rubber band rings during transportation as shock absorbent and damage proof. One should always be careful while transporting filled cryocans in bus or train or in gathering, as sudden evaporation may cause any unwanted or panic situation among people. Regular checking for frost formation, leakage and also the LN_2 level in the container should be practised and replace immediately, if there is increased evaporation rate or any damage diagnosed. Metal or wooden dipstick should be used to measure the LN_2 level in cryocan. Plastic or any hollow rod is not recommended for the purpose. Always use forceps to take semen straw out.

On filling new container with LN_2 gas, one should wait for 24 hr for charging and cooling of the can, then it should be refilled to its full capacity. It is found that first filling lead to excess evaporation due to charging so, one should not worry about any damage to container. Also there be is frost appearance on first filling but it vanishes by its own within two hours. First noting of the LN_2 level should be done after 10 days of first filling, as it is the normal time taken for thermal balance by the new container.

Use of protective clothing and eye glasses is recommended to avoid any direct contact of the LN_2 to body surface. Although LN_2 is a non-toxic and non-inflammable gas but if there is any direct exposure of the gas to body tissue, it may cause tissue damage or frost bite. In this situation, water should be used immediately to wash off the affected part. In poorly ventilated room, it may cause suffocation and lead to unconsciousness and dizziness, so quick movement to fresh ventilated area is needed.

S

It is another important aspect in order to get better success rate of artificial insemination. Semen straws should be kept in the goblets in canisters with proper identification marking like date of freezing, animal species, sire information, goblet no., canister no. and no. of straws, etc. on locator strips tagged with canister. Maintenance of the proper inventory of stored semen must be done by preparing the Inventory map of storage container with above information. The seminal quality should be checked regularly after every 7 days to ensure the quality of stored semen for long period. Also the LN_2 level should be checked regularly to ensure the proper exposure of straw canisters to the gas inside. If the cold chain is disturbed once, whole of the semen stored in particular cryocan will get spoiled because of the thermal shock. LN_2 should be replenished regularly according to the level and evaporation rate of gas in order to maintain the level of LN_2 more than about 8 cm in cryocan having straws. It should also be taken care of that semen straws should not be exposed above LN_2 level more than 10 seconds, otherwise sperm will be thermally damaged. During transferring the straws from one container to another, keep the containers side by side in close proximity with filled LN_2 and each transferring procedure should be fast enough to complete within 5 seconds. It is not recommended to touch the straws with bare hands.

The process of converting frozen semen into the liquid state with retention of maximum semen fertilizing capacity is called thawing. It is very important procedure during AI with frozen semen, as there are maximum chances of sperm damage during freezing and thawing (Approx 50). Thawing can be done with rapid thawing or slow thawing process depending on the extender used and freezing process adopted. Rapid freezing required rapid thawing process. The process from withdraw of the semen straw from canister and loading to the AI gun after thawing should be emphasized with minimum damage to quality of the sperm. Standard procedure of thawing should be followed as:

1. Wear gloves, eye glasses and apron in order to avoid any tissue damage by LN_2 gas.
2. eep ready the thawing machine or thermos flask with the water capacity of 1-2 lit i.e. sufficient for dipping the whole straw maintained at temperature of 37^0C.
3. Calibrate the thermometer on regular basis to avoid any temperature fluctuation during thawing.
4. Remove the lid of cryocan and lift the desired canister upto the neck only (3 inch below the top of the neck i.e. never above the frost line) of cryocan. As it may lead to irreversible thermal damage to the spermatozoa.
5. Pre-cool the straw holding forceps in LN_2 vapors for few seconds and then pick up the straw and shake vigorously in the air for once or twice and wipe it with cotton or tissue paper to dry within few seconds and quickly transfer to warm water (37^0C) in thawing flask for 45 sec.
6. If it takes more than 10 sec. to take the straw out of canister, It should be lower back to tank floor to dip in LN_2 and then, lift it again to complete the task.
7. Never thaw semen by rubbing between palms or in pocket as thawing temperature is not maintained properly and mechanical damages are also there, leads to dead and damaged sperm.
8. After retrieving the straw, immediately lower the canister in tank and close the lid.
9. Take straw out of the water after 45 sec. and dry it with tissue paper, as water is spermicidal and also to avoid the rapid cooling back.

10. Shake straw to create air space at lab end to avoid loss of semen during cutting.

11. Cut the straw from lab end at right angle for proper sealing with AI sheath and to prevent backflow within sheath during insemination.

12. Load the thawed semen straw to the AI gun and perform the artificial insemination within 10-15 minutes.

Proper handling of the LN_2 storage as well as semen straws will always result into the greater success rate of the AI programme. By keeping the points in mind, discussed above for semen straw management and thawing, will lead to better post thaw motility and will give better conception rate which is ultimate requirement of AI for the more production in the form of the livestock population, milk production as well as economic benefits to the animal owner.

L P AI G P I

Recto-vaginal method of insemination is most popular method of artificial insemination (AI) with frozen thawed semen in bovines. Not only the upkeepment of artificial instrumentations, but also for proper loading of the AI gun for insemination has key role for successful insemination in terms of better conception rate. AI gun, AI sheath, forceps, etc. should be clean, dry and sterilized, always be kept in sterilized chamber/box. Clean water, thawing flask, thermometer, paper towel, tissue paper, etc. should be available at time of AI.

Packet of AI sheath should not be opened from the side of their tip in order to avoid the touching with unsterilized hand or surface. After thawing semen straw should be hold with the help of forceps from the laboratory seal end and wipe the water with tissue paper. Holding of the straw should be by the end, to avoid thermal shock to sperm. Shaking of the straw should be done to create air space at the lab seal end to avoid any loss of semen during cutting of the straw. Tip of the AI gun should never be touched with bare hand, dung, perineal region of animal or water and also should not be placed on unsterilized surface. Warming of the AI gun is recommended by rubbing it with paper towel to avoid cold shock to the sperm. This activity should be practised specially in winter season. After pulling back the plunger of the AI gun about $1/4^{th}$ of its length, semen straw should be inserted into the AI gun with manufacturer s end. In some

AI guns, there is an in-built stopper preventing the straw going too far. With clean sharp scissors / straw cutter, semen straw should be cut open at right angle to remove the lab seal end after holding the loaded gun vertically at eye level. It is needed for proper sealing of loaded straw with AI sheath and to prevent backflow of semen within sheath during insemination. Then, fixing of the AI sheath is done over the barrel of the gun to get a perfect fit between extremity of straw and cone of AI sheath. Touching the tip or middle part of the sheath should be avoided to avoid entry of contamination into the female genitalia. Sheath is pulled and twisted through the central hole of the locking ring and over the conical seal of AI gun for locking. Proper seal between straw and sheath is extremely important. Plunger of the AI gun should be pushed until the semen is just visible at the end of the gun. This reduces the stretching of fingers needed during handling of the loaded gun. Now, loaded AI gun is ready to inseminate the bovines.

The loading of the AI gun is strategically scientific process and should not be taken as general. Even if the female is fit for conception, semen used is of good quality, Heat detection is proper but if the handling of AI instruments and process of loading the AI gun is not as per the standard protocol, conception rate will be low. Furthermore, unsterilized and improper insemination may lead to repeat breeding, uterine infection and embryonic death with questionable future fertility of the female animal, ultimately there will be economic loss to the herd or individual animal owner.

❑❑❑

Chapter 15

Advanced Bovine ro en Semen Evaluation Techni ues

Dilip Kumar S ain and Sarvajeet adav

Department of Veterinary Physiology, College of Veterinary Science and Animal Husbandry, Uttar Pradesh Pandit Deen Dayal Upadhyaya Pashu Chikitsa Vigyan Vishwavidhyalaya Evam Go Anusandhan Sansthan, Mathura

---

B O S A R

Frozen semen technology has been the pillar behind artificial insemination and one of the major strengths of assisted reproduction. The discovery of liquid N_2 and different extenders has made it relatively easy for the preservation of liquid semen. Frozen semen technology has been used as a method for dissemination of superior germplasm and also going to cater the increasing demands of meat, milk and other animal product in future. Some of the major advantages of the frozen semen are :

- Long term of storage of superior quality of sperm
- Faster propagation of germplasm
- Prevents the loss of semen in excess
- Increase possibility of inseminations by using semen from a bull
- Ease in transport and avoid country or border as a limitation for best semen
- Animal cloning and stem cell technology are dependent on frozen semen
- Upgradation of local breeds with superior sperm

The mammalian sperm is a deceptively simple, and terminally differentiated cell. Although it seems to have a limited array of functional features, in essence to deliver an intact haploid genome to an oocyte at fertilization. Despite the extensive knowledge on spermatology, a definition of what constitutes a good spermatozoon (i.e. a male gamete with high fertilization potential) remains elusive. Besides the already mentioned species-specific differences, the fact that ejaculates from the same male may vary according to several factors, and that they are always very heterogeneous, containing both functional sperm and defective cells, is the main obstacle for proper analysis. However, there are several aspects of sperm biology that can be monitored, and which can give clear indications on the potential fertility of a given sample. Furthermore, the analysis of sperm structure and function may be adjusted and complemented according to specific needs, be they clinical, teaching or research and several methods can be chosen according to both the purpose of the assay, and the available resources.

Since the advent of AI, researchers have sought laboratory assays that would accurately predict the fertilizing potential of a semen sample. This goal, however, has proven difficult to achieve. This difficulty arises from the complex nature of the problem, dealing with the complexities of the spermatozoon itself, with our ability to evaluate fertility, and with our ability to manage the females to be inseminated. Part of the complexity dealing with the spermatozoa, comes from the fact that each spermatozoon is a multi-compartmental cell that must possess many different attributes to be able to fertilize an oocyte. Each spermatozoon must possess.

- Motility: To carryout transit in the female reproductive tract.
- Active mitochondria to supply the energy necessary for motility and other metabolic functions.
- Intact acrosomal membranes that are capable of undergoing capacitation changes thereby permitting the acrosome reaction to occur, but only at the correct moment that is during fertilization.
- Receptors that permit the cell to bind to the zona pellucida and to the oolemma.
- Plasma membranes that permit fusion with the oolemma.
- A nucleus that is capable of proper decondensation, nuclear re-organization, and genetic performance to maintain zygotic and embryonic development.

Advanced senior evaluation techniques are required for the exact functional evaluation of sperm cells in terms of their fertilising competance. Due to multicompartment structure, sperm cells requre functional evaluation using advanced techniques.

Sperm Compartments and their Functional Significance

A functional sperm is composed of three main regions: the head, the mid-piece, and the tail. The head contains the nucleus, in which sperm-specific DNA binding proteins, called protamines, have replaced histones. The presence of protamines allows for tighter chromatin packaging, and, together with the loss of most of the typical cell organelles and cytoplasm that takes place during spermiogenesis, this is thought to have a role in reducing cell volume and increasing the sperm s aerodynamic properties, thus potentially facilitating fertilization. It should be noted that these characteristics are also widely believed to render the sperm transcriptionally inactive, or at least translationally impaired. Overlaying the nucleus is a large secretory vesicle, the acrosome. This vesicle contains hydrolitic enzymes thought to aid in sperm penetration through oocyte-protecting layers, namely the translucent glycoprotein-based *zona pellucida.*

Release of acrosomal contents, an exocytotic process dubbed the acrosome reaction, must only take place in the vicinity of an oocyte, and the lack of an acrosome in any other circumstance signals that the sperm will likely not be fully functional. However, before the sperm can undergo the acrosome reaction, it must be primed by a series of poorly understood maturation steps involving tightly regulated intra-cellular signalling and protein phosphorylation (characteristically on tyrosine residues), which comprise of what is called sperm capacitation. The sperm tail (or flagellum) is paramount for sperm motility, and is comprised of an axoneme containing a typical 9 2 microtubular arrangement, consisting of nine doublet pairs of peripheral microtubules, arranged in circle around a central pair.

Other protein structures (the outer dense fibers and fibrous sheath) are arranged around the axoneme, adding strength and resistance to the tail. The sperm mid-piece, as its name indicates, apparently connects the head and the tail, although it in fact consists of a variable number of mitochondria wrapped helically around the anterior portion of the flagellum. It has been assumed that the role of these mitochondria might be to provide ATP for sperm movement through oxidative phosphorylation. However, it is also possible that the necessary ATP is produced mostly by glycolitic pathways throughout the flagellum, with mitochondrial ATP required only in specific circumstances. It is also very important to note that there are many species-specific differences, and what holds true for one species may not translate well (or at all) to another.

Acrosome and its Functional Significance in Frozen Semen

In order to fertilize an oocyte, a spermatozoon must first become capacitated and bind to the zona pellucida of the oocyte. Capacitation is a process in which many changes occur within the spermatozoon including but not limited to cholesterol efflux from the plasma membrane, increases in intra-cellular calcium, bicarbonate, potassium, protein phosphorylation, and a decrease in intra-cellular pH. In the best case scenario, a spermatozoon reaches the site of fertilization and completes capacitation at the time the oocyte is present. However, cryopreservation results in a loss of lipids from the sperm membranes and a re-arrangement of lipids and proteins within the membrane, which results in a pre-capacitated spermatozoa, resulting in a reduced fertilizing lifespan for the spermatozoon. Therefore, assays to evaluate sperm capacitation can be used to evaluate the normalcy of spermatozoa after freezing and thawing, as well as to monitor techniques designed to induce sperm capacitation for assisted reproductive technologies.

Since there are many aspects of sperm capacitation, many assays have been developed which monitor one or more parts of the capacitation process. Changes in membrane fluidity can be measured, using the probe merocyanin 540, as capacitation occurs. Similarly, changes in intra-cellular calcium levels using chlortetracycline, Indo-1 AM or fluo-3 AM, changes in protein phosphorylation or the ability of sperm to undergo an acrosome reaction, when challenged with various acrosome reaction-inducing compounds can be assessed as sperm undergo capacitation.

Sperm Mitochondria and its Functional Significance

Several fluorescent probes have been used to evaluate sperm mitochondrial function. Mitochondrial probes are actively transported into actively respiring mitochondria, therefore, the more active the mitochondrial respiration, the more probe is accumulated. Rhodamine 123 was initially used to evaluate sperm mitochondrial function, but can only differentiate between respiring and non-respiring mitochondria. More recently, JC-1 has been used to assess spermatozoal mitochondria function. At low concentrations, JC-1 remains in the monomeric state and fluoresces green. However, at high concentrations, JC-1 forms aggregates that fluorescence orange. Therefore, JC-1 has not only the ability to distinguish functional from non-functional mitochondrial, but permits different levels of mitochondrial function to be determined by intensity of mitochondrial orangeness . In support of sperm motility being a measure of mitochondrial function, the percentages of sperm with functioning mitochondria is highly correlated to sperm motility, regardless of whether rhodamine 123 or JC-1 is used to evaluate mitochondrial function.

Sperm DNA Evaluation and its Functional Significance

The genetic integrity of the spermatozoan is essential for normal embryo development. A high level of DNA fragmentation in sperm cells may represent a cause of male infertility that conventional examinations - sperm concentration, motility analysis, morphology assessment - cannot detect. Results reported in the scientific literature show regardless of the assisted reproductive technology used, elevated levels of DNA fragmentation above the critical threshold will significantly compromise the possibility of a successful pregnancy.

- High sperm DNA fragmentation does not appear to affect fertilisation or the first or second embryo cleavage stages.
- High sperm DNA fragmentation can affect embryo cleavage once the paternal genome is switched on, and subsequent blastocyst development.
- DNA fragmentation levels are closely correlated with IUI, IVF and ICSI miscarriage and pregnancy rates.
- DNA fragmentation is significantly higher in frozen semen.
- Animals with poor semen parameters are more likely to have high DNA fragmentation.
- High sperm DNA fragmentation is also found in animals with normal semen parameters.

Freeze thaw process induces a high amount of oxidative stress to the sperm causing induction of DNA fragmentation. This instead makes the sperm prone to apoptois and thereby a reduction in the sperm quality. That is why, sperm DNA evaluation is a key process in frozen semen analysis. This can be achieved by:

- Comet assay of the sperm
- Sperm chromatin assay
- TUNEL assay of the sperm
- Detection of apoptotic like changes in the sperm through the evaluation of caspases and various death ligands

Major Setback of Cryopreserved Sperm

- Cold stress to the sperm
- Formation of inter and intra-cellular ice crystals
- Free radical generation and oxidative stress to the sperm
- Capacitation like changes in the sperm
- Acrosome damage and loss of functional intact acrosome
- Loss of membrane integrity and thereby osmotic stress to the sperm
- Cholesterol loss from the membrane causing reduction in the fluidity of the sperm membrane
- Chromatin crosslinking, protein denaturation and lipid peroxidation of sperm plasma membrane
- Induction of cell death in sperm leading to apoptosis
- Loss of functional proteins from the sperm and a consequent loss of motility and fertility in the sperm
- Abnormal sperm motility and altered ion channels of the sperm.
- Reduction in seminal attributes after freezing
- Enzyme leakage causing loss of sperm function
- Reduced metabolic activity of the sperm
- Protein tyrosine phosphorylation causing pre-capacitation in the sperm
- Induction of acrosome reaction in the sperm
- Altered ionic equilibrium in the sperm.
- Deprotamination in the sperm and hence, there is a loss in the chromatin compaction.

- Reduction in the viability of the sperm.
- Damage to the sperm at cellular and molecular level causing overall loss of sperm competence for the process of fertilization.

Major of Sperm Dysfunction During Freezing and Thawing

Freezing and thawing of the semen target primarily four structures of the sperm leading to reduction in the sperm quality. These sites are:

- Sperm Plasma membrane and its molecular alteration in terms of ion channels and cholesterol.
- Sperm acrosome inducing precapaciation like changes along with acrosome reaction.
- Sperm nuclear DNA causing or inducing the sperm DNA fragmentation, deprotamination.
- Sperm mitochondria and alterations in the mitochondrial function along with compromised sperm motility.

Logic Behind the Evaluation of Frozen Semen

- Freezing process induces a large number of irreversible changes in the sperm, which make the sperm incapable of fertlisation.
- Generation of free radicals and oxidative stress to the sperm substantially reduce the sperm quality.
- Multiple alterations occur in the sperm both at cellular and molecular level leading to a dramatic loss in post thaw sperm quality.
- Multiple sites of sperm damage are possible during freeze thaw process as a consequence, there will be a reduction in the sperm fertilizing ability.
- Cold stress, stress associated with freezing and alterations in sperm are still not understood at molecular level and hence, a number unknown causes are defined for the reduction in the sperm quality.

Advanced Tests for Semen Evalution-Need of the Hour

Routine laboratory tests cannot evaluate the inherent competence of the sperm to bring out successful fertilization. The increase in trend of molecular abnormalities at cellular and subcellular level again makes it very difficult to predict the male fertility in terms of sperm functional competence. Routine laboratory procedures are also failed to determine the future consequence of embryonic development and hence, it is essential to evaluate the sperm competence by using advanced techniques. The primary advanced techniques are:

1. Use of fluorescent probes to detect intact acrosome, intact plasma membrane and viable sperm population.
2. Targetting sperm flagella by using CASA to monitor sperm motility competence.
3. Targetting sperm mitochondria to evaluate sperm energetic as well as sperm ageing.
4. Targetting sperm DNA and protamine to evaluate the organization of sperm DNA for successful fertilization as well as embryonic development.
5. Sorting of sperm to differentiate between normal and apoptotic sperm so as to enhance semen quality.
6. Evaluation of sperm ion channels, a new venture to understand minute to minute regulation of sperm functions.
7. Evaluation of membrane architecture in terms of cholesterol content as well as functional significance in bringing out acrosome reaction and capacitation.
8. Targetting the residual cytoplasm of sperm to know their functional significance.
9. Targetting sperm sub populations with less activity to understand sperm dynamics.
10. Targetting molecular surface architecture of sperm to understand sperm functions.

Evalution of Frozen Semen and its Significance

Correlations between laboratory results and fertility are inconsistent between studies. Part of the reason for this is that sperm must possess many attributes to fertilize an oocyte, not merely one or two or even three attributes. Secondly, for most attributes, there is not a continuum from a minimum to a maximum that affects fertility, but instead spermatozoa must possess a sufficient amount of each attribute to fertilize an oocyte. Therefore, when evaluating a specific sperm attribute, we can postulate which samples are likely to have poor fertilizing capacity, but are unable to determine, if a particular sample will be fertile.

Over the past 75 years, researchers developed laboratory assays for many of the attributes spermatozoa require to fertilize an oocyte, but there are likely many sperm attributes necessary to fertilize an oocyte that are unknown. There may also be problems inherent in a specific assay that may limit the usefulness of the data obtained using that assay. In addition, because each spermatozoon requires many attributes to fertilize an oocyte, an assay measuring only a single attribute will fail to detect spermatozoa defective in a different attribute, and therefore, overestimate the number of fertile spermatozoa in a semen sample.

Unfortunately, because these assays evaluate a population mean for each attribute measured, combining results from two or three different assays on the same sperm population does little to determine the true number of fertile sperm in a population. To achieve this, we would need to assess all the attributes necessary for fertilization simultaneously on each individual spermatozoon.

Problems also exist in defining and measuring fertility. Fertility can be described as the percentage of females, from which embryos are flushed after insemination, the percentage of females that are pregnant a defined number of days after a single insemination or multiple inseminations during a single heat cycle or several heat cycles, or the percentage of females that deliver a live offspring after insemination (again single or multiple inseminations over one or many heat cycles). Each of these is a very different response and each reflects a different aspect of maternal input that is not likely to be detected in a semen assay. In addition, for fertility data to be useful, it must accurately reflect the true fertilizing potential of the semen used.

Altogether above mentioned events mediate a time dependent irreversible damage to the sperm and as a consequence to this, there is a reduction in sperm quality. The sperm loses the functional competence to bring out fertilization. These cellular and molecular changes are not assayed through the routine semen analysis and hence, require sophisticated assays and imaging to evaluate the sperm functions. Following are some of the assays, which are employed to evaluate the sperm functional competence in terms of sperm fertilization:

- Fluorescent based evaluation of sperm viability by employing PI or EBr.
- Evaluation of sperm acrosomal integrity by employing FITC-PSA staining.
- Evaluation of sperm mitochondrial activity by JC I staining.
- Evaluation of sperm DNA integrity by employing various techniques, namely Comet assay, TUNEL assay, Sperm chromatin structure assay (SCSA).
- Evaluation of sperm motility through CASA.

Optimization of Conception Rates in Bovines in Sepcific Reference to Frozen Semen Evalution

Optimization of conception rates in bovines can be achieved by both, male and female factors. Following are some of the parameters which can be incorporated to enhance the conception rates in the bovines and in specific reference to frozen semen:

- Proper evaluation of semen samples by using multiple automatic and visual methods.
- Evaluation of sperm basic and subcellular parameters.
- Proper evaluation of sperm motility by using CASA.
- Evaluation of sperm DNA integrity/Chromatin structure.
- Employment of highly sensitive fluorescent based staining of sperm components.
- Proper care of the sperm during freezing and thawing.
- Pre-screening of sperm for the process of freezing.
- Selection of best quality of semen alongwith best ejaculates for preservation.

Concluding remarks

No doubt that frozen semen is the best choice for artificial insemination but simultaneously one cannot avoid the abnormalities induced by freeze-thaw process. This ultimately compromises the fertility response, when used and hence, time demands to opt for multiple advanced tests for quality evaluation of sperm samples.

Employment of various staining (fluorescent) will effectively solve the issue for semen evaluation along with incorporation of automation will substantially improve the semen for artificial insemination and the consequence thereof. Relatively few of these assays are conducted on every semen sample, and it is unreasonable that many of these assays should be conducted on every semen sample, due to time and expense. However, these assays might be performed on selected semen samples from males that are exhibiting low fertility to determine more precisely what spermatozoal attributes are compromised. Steps may then be taken to attempt to correct the deficiency, if possible. Unfortunately, it is very unlikely that results from any single laboratory assay will effectively estimate the fertilizing potential of a semen sample. However, laboratory assays are important, as they can help to eliminate poor samples from being used for artificial insemination and to determine what spermatozoal defects are present in samples with poor fertility. Several laboratory assays have been developed that evaluate several spermatozoa attributes simultaneously on the same spermatozoon. Such assays increase the likelihood of more accurately identifying sub-populations of fertile sperm in a sample and are more powerful than conducting single assessments of the same sperm attributes on different sub-samples of the semen sample, which may only still measure two or three attributes. In conclusion, besides employing routine semen analysis tests, one should employ specialized sperm assays to get best quality sperm for fertilization. Along with this, optimization of freezing with the selection of best extenders will enhance the quality of frozen semen, opted for artificial insemination purposes.

□□□

Chapter 16

Use of Approved Ethno- eterinar Products and Practices

Atul Prakash Rajesh Mandil and Satish Kumar Garg

Department of Veterinary Pharmacology and Toxicology, College of Veterinary Science and Animal Husbandry, Uttar Pradesh Pandit Deen Dayal Upadhyaya Pashu Chikitsa Vigyan Vishwavidhyalaya Evam Go Anusandhan Sansthan, Mathura

India has large livestock population and it is the major income source of tribal, rural and semi-urban people. Livestock rearing in rural and tribal areas is quite different than urban areas due to their economical status, at the same time to keep their animals healthy, traditional healing practices have been applied for centuries (Balaji and Chakravarthi, 2010 aur *et al.*, 2015 Hema *et al.*, 2016). According to the World Health Organization, at least 80 of people in developing countries depend largely on indigenous practices for the control and treatment of various diseases, affecting both human beings and their animals. Ethno veterinary medicine (EVM) is the knowledge developed by local livestock holders and contrast the allopathic veterinary medicine taught in veterinary colleges/ universities. The term *thno Veterinary* was coined by MC Corkle (1986). Though, there is no authentic evidence of when and how plants came into usage for curing the domestic animals, the rural people seems to be aware of it through generations. Ethno-veterinary medicine refers to holistic and inter-disciplinary study of traditional knowledge, beliefs, practices, skills and methods pertaining to the health care of animal ailments.

The growing interest in traditional medicine practices have been encouraged by the recognition of some efficacious ethno-veterinary medicinal products. Ethno-veterinary medicine practice started as early as 1800 B.C. at the time of ing Hamurabi of Babylon for treating cattle and donkeys (Schillhorn van Veen, 1996 Selvaraju *et al.*, 2011).

Ethno veterinary practices are often cheap, safe, time tested and based on local resources and strengths. These can provide useful alternatives to conventional animal healthcare (atewa *et al.*, 2000). The ethno veterinary practices all over the world are an integral component of livestock healthcare and management practices. Many medicinal plants grow in India, in plains and hills are most commonly used ingredients in the preparation of ethno-veterinary medicines. In most rural areas, people prefer to treat their animals with indigenous drugs. At present over 35, 000 plants are known to have healing properties. All parts of the plants, including leaves, bark, fruits, flowers, seeds are used in medicinal preparation (Patil and Deshmukh, 2013). Resource-poor livestock farmers all over the world frequently depend on traditional knowledge for the management of animal health problems and to improve their productivity particularly in the areas with inadequate health coverage facilities. However, ethno-veterinary medicine is in danger of extinction with the advancement of the modern veterinary medicine because, it is developed by farmers in field and barns rather than in scientific laboratories and is less systematic, less formalized and usually transferred by word of mouth rather than in writing (Phondani *et al.*, 2010). Therefore, it has not yet been well-documented and much effort is needed in research and integration activities in developing countries particularly India (ineger *et al.*, 2007). Hence, documentation of ethno-veterinary medicine from regions having a rich ethnographic and biodiversity setting would be of great significance. Some studies on ethno veterinary practices from different regions of India have been reported.

E

Rigveda (10:97:2) mentions that this motherly earth has provided us hundreds and thousands of plants, which have got capabilities of keeping us healthy and if required, cure us from various ailments/ diseases. In Atharvaveda (8:7:2), the sun has been mentioned the father of plants and the earth is considered mother of plants. The extracts of these plants, when taken as prescription have potential of penetrating into our muscles, joints and relieve ailments (Rigveda 10:97:12). Further, it has been mentioned that these herbs conquer diseases as fast as swift horses, prove their efficacy for the sick, and make them healthy and happy (Rigveda 10:97:3). The knowledge of identification of these plants and their use was mandatory for the clinicians. To strengthen this point in the Atharvaveda, it has been mentioned that king should punish such clinicians who are unaware of medicinal properties of plants or if they are engaged in production of certain spurious/toxic medicine(Atharvaveda 4:17:4). Atharvaveda (8:7:10) also mentions that the plants which are used as antidote of the poison, should never be destroyed. In Atharvaveda (11:4:16), there are mention of remedies of ailments. According to it, there are four kinds of remedies, which are considered to protect life as well as they help increase lifespan of individual (C. Varshney: www.hillagric.ac.in/edu/covas/vpharma/winter 20school/lectures/33 20 Ethnoveterinary 20 practies 20 of 20 India. pdf.

These include:

- The drug of the angirasas (juice of plant and herbs).
- The drugs of the artharvans (a part of mantra therapy).
- The divine drugs in the form of prayers.
- The drugs of human artifice and contrivance.

Thus, ethno-veterinary medicine is:

- Accessible
- Easy to prepare and administer
- Inexpensive: low cost or even free
- Part of one s own traditional culture

Elements of ethno-veterinary medicine

Ethno-veterinary practices have grown recently because these practices are much less prone to drug resistance and have fewer damaging side-effects on the environment than conventional medicine.

Traditional healing practices make use of three important elements:

- Application of natural products
- Appeal to spiritual forces
- Manipulation and surgery

Natural products used are:

- Medicinal plants and by-products
- Edible earth and minerals
- Parts and products of animals
- Other ingredients

a) Plants

Plants are the most commonly used ingredients in the preparation of ethno-veterinary medicines. All parts of the plants, including leaves, bark, fruits, flowers, seeds are used in medicinal preparations. At present over 35,000 plants are known to have healing properties. At least 1,00,000 species of plants are used by humans for as food, medicine, fibre, fuel, oils, shelter, poisons, intoxicants, ornamentals and other purposes. By virtue of specialized biochemical capabilities, plants synthesize and accumulate a vast array of primary and secondary metabolites/chemicals. For reasons, both cultural and economical, 75 of the world s population depends on medicines from plants. Of the proprietary medicines in the western market, 35 are phytic in origin however, these medicines are derived from less than 0.1 of known plant species. So far, more than 100,000 biologically active secondary plant compounds have been isolated from higher plants, these diverse structures falling into four main chemical classes. The phenolics (phenols, flavonoids, quinones, tannins and lignins), terpenoids (monoterpenes, lactones, diterpenes,saponins and others), sulphur compounds (glucosilates, disulphides and acetylenic thiophenes) and nitrogen compounds (alkaloids, amines, non-protein amino acids and cyanogenetic glycosides). Certain organic acids and polyacetylenes are also known to exist (Cotton, 1996 Balaji and Chakravarthi, 2010).

b) Edible earth and minerals

Edible earth, especially from termite and ant hills, is commonly used in ethno-veterinary preparations. Limestone is a commonly used edible type of earth used in decoctions and concoctions. Other ingredients Honey, vegetable oils and butters, and salt are used for their healing and preservative properties.

c) Parts and products of animals

Parts and products of animals, such as skin and hides, bones, milk, butter and even urine and dung are ingredients of ethno-veterinary medicines.

E B

Ethno-botany is the term used to define the experience of the humans, who observed birds and animals and tested leaves, fruits and tubers for their ability to satisfy hunger or heal wounds. Ethno-botany is now almost universally taken as the total direct relationship between humans and plants. Indian epics, ancient literature and folklore are replete with references to plants (Jain, 2000).

Ethno-Vet Preparations

The most common forms of ethno-vet preparations are powders, poultice, ointment, decoction, infusion, cold ware extract, tincture and fumigation.

T Ethno-veterinary medicine (products) used in different disease conditions in Cattle

Name of disease	Cause	Treatment	Procedure for application of therap
		E e diseases and problems	
Pinkeye (keratoc-onjunctivitis)	Injuries, dust particles and germs bacteria and flies	Milk- 250 ml Salt- 2 tablespoons	Dissolve 2 tablespoons of salt in 1 cup (250ml) of fresh milk. Milk alone can also be used, especially if it is the first milk after birth (parturition).Using a clean syringe (without a needle) wash the affected eye with the milk solution twice a day until the animal recovers.
Worms in the eye (thelazia)	Eye worms are carried into the eye by dust, flies , worms or Ticks Parasites carried by flies, or from one animal to the other	*Pilostigma thonningii* B - 0.25 kg	Pound or chew the fresh fibrous bark of *Pilostigma thonningii*.Squeeze it and collect the liquid. Apply some of the liquid directly to the eye daily, continue for 3-7 days.
Poison in the eye		Fresh milk 3-5 drops	Using a syringe or your own mouth, put 3-5 drops of fresh milk into the eye every 2-3 hours until the pain disappears. The use of the syringe is highly recommended, as the syringe flushes the eye better.
		Skin diseases and problems	
Ectoparasites	Bokkaje (flies), Sufi (mosquitoes), Buubi (tsetse flies)	*Azadirachta indica* SD -2 kgWater - 250 ml	Pound the seeds of *Azadirachta indica* until they turn brown and sticky. Add a little water to make a paste. Squeeze the paste to remove all the oil out of the seeds.Rub the oil on the animals to repel flies and other biting insects.

Lice	Poor hygiene and malnutrition	*Tephrosia vogelii* L - 5 kg Wood ash - 2 kgCow urine - 1 l Water - 3 l	Collect and pound 5 kg *Tephrosia vogelii* leaves. Soak 2 kg wood ash in 3 litres of water and stir thoroughly. Filter and mix the pounded *Tephrosia vogelii* with the wood ash solution. Filter it and add 1 litre of urine. Bathe or spray the affected animal with the solution. Parasites will die within one day.
Ticks		*Adenium obesum* WP 1 plant	Crush *Adenium obesum* and mix it in water. Wash the affected animals with the preparation. (Caution: *Adenium obesum* is potentially very poisonous and must be handled with care. Avoid direct contact by always using gloves or covering your hands with plastic bags, when andling it.)
Ticks and lice	Poor hygiene and malnutrition	*Psorospermum febrifugum* B - 1 kg*Tephrosia vogelii* L - 3 kg*Nicotinia tabacum* L - 2 kg Water - 10 l	Pound the fresh plant parts and soak in 10 litres of hot water while stirring thoroughly until the colour changes. Filter. Spray the affected animals with the mixture. Adjust the quantity of material, according to the number of animals to be sprayed.
		Nicotinia tabacum L - 250 gSoap - 250 gWater - 4 L	Boil 250 grams of *Nicotinia tabacum* leaves in 4 litres of water. Add just enough soap to cause a little foaming. Wash or spray the affected animals with this liquid.
Ringworm	Fungus (Ringworm manifests itself especially in calves. Healthy calves can catch the disease, if they come in direct	*Bridelia ferruginea* B - 2 kgLimestone handfulWater - 3 l	Collect 2 kg of *Bridelia ferruginea* bark. Prepare a decoction by adding the bark to 3 litres of boiling water, which contains one handful of limestone. Boil the mixture for 10 minutes, cool and filter.Drench animal with 0.5 litres twice a day for 1 week.

	contact with infected animals)		
		Phaseolus vulgaris SD - 0.5 kg *emizygia welwitschii* L - 0.5 kgHoney - 0.5 kgWater - 2 l	Collect 0.5 kg of *Phaseolus vulgaris* seeds and *emizygia welwitschii*leaves. Add these plants and 0.5 kg honey to 2 litres of water and boil for 30 minutes cool and filter.Drench each calf with 0.5 litres each morning and evening for 1 week. Animals will recover within 5-7 days.
Streptothricosis dermatophilosis	Germs which are considered to be evil spirits.Bacteria. Factors, such as prolonged wetting by rain, high humidity, high temperatures and various ectoparasites like ticks reduce the natural barriers of the skin and are risk factors in developing streptothricosis.	*Khaya anthoteca* B - 1 kg*Psorospermum febrifugum* B - 1 kg*Ricinus communis* SD - 0.5 kg Limestone handful Butter - 2 kg	Pound 1 kg each of the bark of *Khaya anthoteca* and *Psorospermum febrifugum* and add one handful of limestone powder. Roast 0.5 kg of *Ricinus communis* seeds and grind them to powder. Mix the powders and add butter to make a paste.Remove any hard crusts from the skin of the affected animal. Apply the paste on the affected area daily for 3-7 days, depending on the severity of the infection. New crusts may appear but will fall off. New hair will grow on treated areas in about 2 weeks.
		Solanum aculeastrum F 5 or more fruits, depending on the surface area affected.	Roast the fruits of *Solanum aculeastrum* and slice them into halves. Tether the infected animal and remove the crusts before treatment. Thoroughly scrub the affected area for 1-3 days with the fruits. The crusts will fall off and new hair will start growing on the affected area.

Digestive diseases and problems

Bloat (tympany)	Eating in fresh succulent pastures After eating dry feed and there is no water or when the animal eats very succulent pastures high in nitrogenous compounds. The rumen compartment fills with gas and the animal suffocates from pressure on the chest.	*Khaya anthoteca* B - 0.5 kgWater - 3 l	Boil the fresh bark of *Khaya anthoteca* in 3 litres of water for 30 minutes filter.Drench each animal with 2 litres of the liquid.
		Fresh milk - 4 l	Collect 4 litres of fresh milk.Drench 4 litres for adult cattle and 2 litres for calves. The animals will recover within 1-3 hours.
		eep the bloated animal running until it passes gas.	
		Any type of oil (edible, or even paraffin/kerosene)	Drench the animal with the oil.
Stomach and intestinal worms	Animal get worms from pastures and milk. Animal get infected with worms by eating grass or drinking water, which is contaminated with eggs or larvae of worms.	*Vernonia amygdalina* L - 2 kgLimestone - 450 gWater - 3 l	Burn the limestone make a powder. Pound 2 kg of *Vernonia amygdalina* leaves and wash these in 3 litres of water to extract medicinal properties. Filter and add 450 g of limestone powder. Stir to dissolve the limestone.Prevent the animals from drinking water the evening before treatment, so they will be thirsty.To treat calves: drench 250 ml per calf the next morning. Do not allow calves to drink water until 6 hours after the treatmment.
		Urelytrum digitatum R - 1 kgLimestone - 280 gWater - 2 l	Collect about 1 kg of *Urelytrum digitatum* roots. Boil 2 litres of water with 280 g of limestone powder. When water starts boiling, add the *Urelytrum digitatum* roots and boil for 10 minutes cool and filter.To treat calves:

			drench 500 ml per calf a day, for 3-5 days.
		Carissa edulis R -0.5 kg*Curcubita maxima* L - 1.5 kg Water - 2 l	Mix one part of the root of *Carissa edulis* with 3 parts of *Cucubita maxima* leaves. Boil these in a large pot of water for 45 minutes. Filter the decoction and cool it.Drench 1 l twice a day. Repeat this treatment after 1 month.
		Leucas leaves-50g Neem leaves 50g Banana stem -100g Bitter gourd- 50gPalm jaggery-100g	Grind the cumin seeds, mustard, pepper and then mix the remaininging redients with palm jaggery and make it into a paste. Make the paste into small balls. Coat the balls with salt (100g). Put the balls into the mouth of the animal. Give it to animal once in a month.
Diarrhoea	Worms, changes in diet, poisons and dirt.Viruses, bacteria, protozoa, worms, changes in diet, poisons	*Khaya anthoteca* B -1 kg powder*Bridelia ferruginea* B - 1 kg powder*Pilostigma Anogeissus* 1kg of charcoal powder Water - 250 ml	Make a powder of 1kg each of *Khaya anthoteca B* and *Bridelia ferruginea B* . Burn the fresh stems of *Pilostigma thonningii B* and *Anogeissus leiocarpus B* and grind the charcoal into powder. Mix 1 kg of the latter powder with the first powder.To treat calves, prepare a mix of one spoon of powder per cup of water (250 ml) to treat adult cattle: two spoons of powder per 250 ml water. Administer this mixture twice a day to the animals, for 3-6 days, depending on the severity of the diarrhoea.
	Bloody diarrhoea	*Dissortis perkinsae* R - 0.5 kgWater - 1 l	Collect 0.5 kg of *Dissortis perkinsae* roots. Boil 1 litre of water and add the roots. Boil for 30 minutes, and then allow to cool and filter. Drench 250-500 ml per calf once.
	Diarrhoea caused by intestinal worms	*Psidium guajava* L - 0.5 kgGinger	Pound 50 g of ginger and 0.5 kg of tender leaves of *Psidium guajava* together and make one bolus of these

		(*ingiber officinale*) - 50 g	materials. Make enough boluses for all animals to be treated. Give 5 or 6 boluses at a time to a calf.To prevent and treat dehydration, drench calf with a large volume of water, mixed with salt, in the ratio of 250 ml (one cup) of salt to five litres of water. Drench half a litre, four times a day for 3-4 days.
	Intestinal worms especially tapeworms	*Myrsine africana* L - 0.25 kgWater - 0.5 l	Crush 0.25 kg of *Myrsine africana* leaves, mix with 0.5 l of water and drench. This is enough for an adult animal. Use half of this for calves.
		Cumin seeds -20g Poppy seeds -20g Fenugreek -20g Pepper -5 nos Turmeric- 5g Asafoetida-5g.	Roast the ingredients and make it powder and feed the animal orally.
		Onion -10 nos Garlic- 6 nos Tamarind -200g Palm jaggery- 250g	Grind the above ingredients. Make the mixture 1 and 2 into small bolus. Coat the bolus with salt (100g). Administer all bolus to the animal orally.
		Respirator diseases and problems	
Lungworm	Animals get infected by feeding on infested pasture and drinking infested water, especially during the rainy season.Animals get infected by eating	*antana trifolia* F - 2 kgWater - 1 l	Grind the fruits of *antana trifolia* into a fine powder. Mix 1 handful of this powder with 1 litre of water. Drench the animals with this liquid: 1 litre for adult cattle and 250 ml for calves.

	grass that is contaminated with lungworm larvae		
		Reproductive diseases and problems	
Inflammation of the udder (mastitis)	Teat injuries, sores, poor hygiene and sanitation, witches and wizards. Bacteria. Teat injuries, poor milking hygiene and faulty management predispose cows to mastitis	Hot wood ash -0.25 kg Water - 0.5 l	Prepare fine wood ash powder of non-poisonous wood used for cooking, by sieving. Mix the wood ash with half a litre of water and stir until a paste is formed. Tether the affected cow and milk the cow before treatment. Apply the paste on the udder of the cow and massage the affected area.
		Clematis hirsute L - 0.5 kg*Schefflera abyssinica* L - 0.5 kg Water - 2 l	Pound half a kg of the leaves of *Clematis hirsute* and *Schefflera abyssinica*. Add them to water while stirring.Milk the infected cow before treatment. Wash the udder of the cow with the prepared solution in the morning and evening for 2 days. Cow should recover during the 2 days of treatment.
		Aloe vera 200g Slaked lime -10g Turmeric powder-50g	Grind the ingredients and make it a paste. Apply it 10 times a day for 4 days over the udder. Prepare the paste freshly every morning.
Reduced milk (agalactia)	Poor feeding, disease. Poor feeding, weakness, disease, inflammation in the udder (mastitis)	*Crinum kirkii* WP 0.5 - kg*Arachis hypogea* N - 0.5 kgWater - 2 l	Pound a whole *Crinum kirkii* plant and raw nuts of *Arachis hypogea*. Soak them in 2 litres of water, while stirring.Drench every morning and evening 0.5 litres at a time, for 5-7 days. The milk yield will increase in about 2 days.
		Carica papaya F	Grind a whole green *Carica papaya,* including seeds

		-1 whole fruit *Arachis hypogea* N -0.25 kgPalm wine - 2 l	and peel. Add it to 2 litres of palm wine, together with 1 cup of raw nuts of *Arachis hypogea* and stir and filter.Drench 2 litres once a day for one week. Within half a day the milk production will increase.
Brucellosis	Infected male or female during mating.Bacteria : Animals can get brucellosis from direct contact with the infected animal or from eating contaminated food. Food can be contaminated by aborted calves, placentas and discharges after abortion.	*Kigelia africana* F -2 kg*Schefflera abyssinica* B -1 kg *Crossopteryx febrifuga* B -1 kg*Khaya anthoteca* B -1 kg *Citrus aurantifolia* B -0.5 kgSalt -18 kg	Dry and pound all components into a fine powder. Add 0.5 kg of this powder to 18 kg of salt. Feed the affected animal once a day for 1 month. It should eat as much as it wants. The animal will discharge the excessive vaginal fluids in 1-2 days.
		Kigelia africana F -2 kg powderHorse bones- 1 kg powder Salt -18 kg	Pound or grind all components into a fine powder. Add 2 kg powder of *Kigelia africana* and 1 kg powder of horse bones to 18 kg salt.Feed to affected animals once a day for 1 month. Let them eat as much as they want at any one time of feeding.
		Salvadora persica R -1 piece, 2 fingers longWater -5 l	Crush and boil a two-finger long piece of *Salvadora persica* root in 5 litres of water for 1 hour. Cool and filter the decoction. Drench the animal that has aborted: use 2 litres to drench one cow. Drench once.

Poor mothering	Heredity, painful and difficult birth, inexperience.	*Parkia biglobosa* C -100 g Sheep skin -100 g Milk from mother -1 lSalt- 2 handfuls Water -1 l	Burn the sheep skin and grind it to powder. Mix 100 g of sheep powder with 100 g of *Parkia biglobosa* C . Add salt, water and milk to the mixture.Tether the mother and bring calf in front of her. Sprinkle the solution on the head, neck and back of the calf and on the muzzle of the mother. The mother will start licking its muzzle and later its calf. It will accept the calf.
		Parkia biglobosa C -100 g*Clematopsis scabiosifolia* L -100 g Cow skin -100 gSalt -200 gFresh milk -1L	Burn *Parkia biglobosa* *CK* and the skin of a cow and grind them to powder. Also grind the leaves of *Clematopsis scabiosifolia* into powder. Mix the powders with salt in 1 litre of fresh milk.Tether the mother and bring the calf in front of her. Sprinkle the solution the head, neck and back of the calf. Open the vulva of the mother and blow air into it and close tightly until the cow begins to be uncomfortable. Blowing air into the vulva causes the animal to feel as if it is about the calf. The mother will accept the calf, will start licking it and the milk production will increase. The mother may become aggressive after accepting the calf.
Retained after birth	Diseases, such as brucellosis, a difficult birth, human assistance during the birth, dirty conditions, a lack of the mineral calcium	*Vitex doniana* B -2 kg Limestone -100 g Water -6 l	Cut 2 kg of *Vitex doniana* bark into small pieces and put it into 6 litres of boiling water with 100 g of limestone. Boil for 30 minutes. Cool and filter the decoction.Drench 6 litres at once. The retained placenta will be expelled in less than a day.

		ibiscus esculentus F -0.25 kgWater- 2 l	Pound the fruits of *ibiscus esculentus* into powder. Put 2 handfuls of this powder into 2 litres of water.Drench 2 litres of the solution. The placenta should be expelled within a day.
		Carica papaya L ten big leaves Water- 2 l	Soften the leaves in 2 litres of water and filter.Drench 1 litre in the morning and 1 litre in the evening. The next day, the placenta will be expelled.
		Salvadora persica R one arm-length (250 g) Water- 1 l	Use a knife or sharp stone to scrape the surface of an arm-long piece of *Salvadora persica* root. Crush the scrapings and soak them in a calabash (1 litre) of water for 12 hours. The water turns yellow and tastes bitter.Drench the animal. Repeat the next day if after birth does not come out.
Prolapsed uterus	A difficult birth, especially one that is assisted, heredity, in thin animals, especially during drought	SoapWaterRestraining ropeA traySafety pins or long thorns	The animal, either standing or recumbent, should be placed in a position so that the hindquarters are elevated. The protruding uterus should be cleaned carefully and washed with water. The cleaned organ should be carefully placed in a tray and pushed gently back into the birth opening. Since there is no ethnovet antibiotic known, conventional antibiotics should be administered immediately.Close the birth opening with safety pins or long thorns. The animal should be retained in a confined area or tethered for a few days, preferably standing with the hind legs higher than the front legs.
			Clean the prolapsed uterus with cold water and apply 1 kg dry sugar carefully to the outside of the prolapsed uterus before pushing it back into the birth

			opening. This helps to decrease the size of a swollen prolapsed uterus and has some antibiotic effect.
Infertility in cows	Infected uterus, aberration of libido, too little light (when animals are kept inside, in the darkness, they may not come in heat), lactation (lactating animals often do not come in heat), weakness or disease, weak legs or the vulva has two very small openings or blockage, chronic debilitating disease conditions, such as worms.		Seek help to palpate ovaries and remove cysts by squeezing gently. This will often stimulate a cow into a heat cycle.
		Arachis hypogea N -0.25 kgFresh milk -1.5 l	Grind and mix the raw nuts of *Arachis hypogea* with the fresh milk. Drench the cow once a day, for 3-5 days
Infertility in bulls	Anatomical/physiological problems of the bull, diseases, such as brucellosis	*Salix subserrata* L -2 kgSalt- 18 kg	Mix 2 kg of *Salix subserrata* powder with 18 kg salt. Feed the sterile animals once a day for 1 week.
		Emergencies and simple operations	
Wounds	Physical injuries like accidents, bites from other animals or wounds inflicted by man	*Psorospermum febrifugum* B - 1 handfulButter -5 tablespoons	Both old and fresh wounds must be washed with clean water before applying the ethnovet treatment. Grind the bark of *Psorospermum febrifugum* into powder. Mix the powder with the butter to make an

			ointment.Apply the ointment on the affected area until wound heals. This ointment also acts as an insecticide to repel flies and prevent them from depositing eggs in the wound.
		milia coccinea L -10 leaves*Aspilia africana* L -10 leaves	Soften the leaves of the plants separately until they become fluid. eep the liquids separate.Squeeze the liquid from *Aspilia africana* into the wound to stop bleeding, followed by the liquid from *milia coccinea* for actual wound healing. Treat once a day for 3 days.
		Ricinus communis S or L -0.25 kg	Crush the seeds of *Ricinus communis* and boil them to make oil. Dry leaves can also be used after being crushed into a powder.Apply the oil or the leaf power on the wound, completely covering the wound until it heals.
		Aloe barbadensis L 1 leaf	Break a piece of a leaf of *Aloe barbadensis* so that the sap begins to drip. Apply the sap on the wound. The leaf itself can also be crushed and applied.
Bone fractures	Fall of the animal, fight between animals, accident, deliberate injury caused by humans or predator	ButterBandage or clean piece of cloth Splints	Collect the materials before restraining the animal. Restrain the animal. If the skin is broken, wash the affected area with water and remove matted hair. Align bones back into their normal positions. Rub butter around the affected area.Wrap a piece of cloth around the area to keep bones in position. Place splints around the broken bone area. Tie splints gently with the bandage, without restricting the blood flow.Tether or retain the animal in a confined area. Provide high quality feed and water. Examine the

			fracture after 1 week. If the fracture has not healed, repeat the treatment and fix the bones for 2 weeks.
Broken horn	Fall of the animal, fight between animals, accident, deliberate injury caused by humans or predator	Clay soil 1 kgClean water- 2.5 lBandage or any clean piece of cloth	Collect 1 kg of clay soil from a clean place. Add the soil to 2 litres of water and heat the solution until it boils. Remove excess water, so a paste is created. Boil the remaining 0.5 litre of water too, without adding soil.Restrain the animal with the fractured horn. Cut off the broken half of the horn, if it has not fallen off. Clean the area with the 0.5 litre of clean boiled water. Apply the clay soil paste to the broken horn stump. Form and press the clay around the stump, so it sticks to the stump. Tie a bandage around the whole stump. Tether the animal for 1 week to be sure the clay does not fall off. Provide high quality feed and water. Take the bandage off, once clay has become hardened. It will take about 3-6 weeks for a full recovery.
Snake bite		*Crinum glaucum* WP -1 kgWater -3 l	Pound and soften a whole *Crinum glaucum* plant in 3 litres of water. After the plant is thoroughly softened, filter the solution.Drench 2 litres to adult cattle and 1 litre to calves for 3 days. Usesome of the solution to wash the area of the snake bite.
		Mucuna pruriens L -1 kg*Aspilia africana* L -1 kg *milia coccinea* L -1 kgWater- 5 l	Grind or pound and soak the leaves of all the plants in 5 litres of water. After thoroughly mixing, filter the solution.Drench 2 litres twice a day over 2 days. Use the residue to apply on the area of the snakebite.
		Black stone 2-3 cm in diameterMilk -50 mlWater- 0.5 l	Press the black stone on a wound caused by a snakebite, and it will stick to the wound. The stone will fall off after a few hours or a day. After it falls off,

			soak the stone in milk overnight and clean it with water. Press it to the wound again for 5 minutes. If it falls off again, then all poison has been removed from the area of the snakebite.
			Give electric shock (from cattle prod or car battery with wires) in area surrounding snakebite - many say that it neutralizes the poison also effective for bee stings.
Poisoning	Chemicals which have been used in the wrong way or in a too high concentration, eating or licking plants which have been treated with pesticides or herbicides, drinking or licking chemicals, eating poisonous plants, bites from snakes or other poisonous animals.	Charcoal -1 kg Fresh milk -4 lWater- 2 l	Grind the charcoal and mix it with 4 litres of fresh milk and 2 litres of water. Drench 6 litres of the mixture to adult cattle at one time and 3 litres to calves.
Foot and Mouth disease	Viral infection	Cumin seeds -10g Fenugreek-10g Pepper-10g Turmeric powder -10g Garlic - 4 nos Jaggery-100g Grinded coconut -1 no	Soak the cumin seeds, fenugreek and pepper for 1 hour and grind it. Then add turmeric powder and garlic and again grind and make it into paste. Add grinded coconut and mix well. Give it in 3 times/ day for 5 days orally.
		Garlic -10 no Turmeric powder	Grind all the ingredients and boil it in gingelly oil and cool it. Then, apply over the wound in legs.

		-10g Holy basil/ tulsi leaves- 10 no Indian acalypha leaves-10 no Henna leaves- 10 no Neem leaves-10 no Gingelly oil -1 l	
Ranikhet disease	Viral infection	Cumin seeds -10g Pepper-5gTurmeric powder -5g Gale of the wind/ stoneb-reaker leaf-50 g Onion- 5 no Garlic -5 no	Grind the ingredients and make into mixture. Mix the mixture with concentrate or broken rice and give it to the birds. If the birds are severely affected, make the mixture into small balls give it for 3 days orally. (For ten birds)
External parasite removal		**Mi ture** : (For one cow) *Aloe vera* 200g Leucas leaves - 50g Holy basil/tulsi -50 g Indian acalypha/ Indian nettle -50g Lantana -50g **Mi ture** (For one cow)Calamus-25g Pepper-10 no Turmeric-10g Ajwain leaves -5 no	Grind the above ingredients. Mix both the mixtures and boil in 4 litres of water until the contents become 1 litre. Then take 100ml of the boiled mixture and add 1 litre of water and spray it over the animal body in sunny days.NOTE: In 1 litre of limewater add 100g of turmeric powder and 100g of calamus powder. Mix well the contents and paint it over the walls of the shed.
Fever		Cumin seeds -10 g Pepper-10g Coriander	Soak the cumin seeds, pepper and coriander seeds in water for 1 hour and drain the water and grind it.

seeds- 10gTurmeric- 10g Small onion -5 no Betel leaves-5 leaves Drumstick leaves -50g Veldt grape-50g Holy basil/tulsi -50gGreen chirayta/ Indian Echinacea -50g Jaggery - sufficient amount.	Mix the remaining ingredients with the grinded mixture. Administer all the contents to the animal orally by coating with salt. Note: Preparation is for one cow

N Abbreviations used are: {B} = Bark, {CK} = Cake, {F} = Fruit, {L} = Leaf, {N} = Nut, {R} = Root, {SD} = Seed, {ST} = Stem, {T} = Tuber, {WP} = Whole plant. **T E A**

A H S E AB

A H International Journal of Science, Environment and Technology, Vol. 5, No 6, 2016, 4006–4012)

T Plants used for treatment of diseases, ailments and infections in India Raikwar and Maurya, 2015

Botanical Name	Common name ith useful part of plant	Ethno-veterinar Use
ryza sativa	Rice	Retention of placenta, skin diseases, strength, wounds, neck sore, post-partum complaints and cough.
Cassia auriculata	Tanners cassia (Shoot tips)	Tender shoot tips are ground with buttermilk and jaggery and given to cure dysentary to cow
annea coromandelica	Indian ash tree (Stem bark)	Stem bark is ground with ginger and garlic and the paste is given to cure fever in pigs
Cardiospermum halicacabum	Balloon plant, love in a puff (Leaves)	Leaves are ground with pepper and garlic, made into paste and given to cure fever to cow, goat
Annona squamosa	Custard apple (Leaves)	Wound healing, Foot and mouth diseases
leusine coracana	Finger millet (Seeds)	Sterility, bone fracture, dysentary and skin diseases.
erula foetida	Asafoetida (Exudate)	Relieves gastroenteritis, neck sore, paralysis, tympany, internal parasites.
Acalypha indica	Indian acalypha , Indian nettle (Leaves)	Leaf paste is mixed with common salt and applied externally to heal wounds to cow, goat, chicken
Allium sativum	Garlic (Tuber)	Wound healing
Moringa oleifera	Drum stick tree (Seeds)	Wound healing, anti-inflammatory, antipyretic
Allium cepa	Onion (Bulb)	Food poisoning, skin diseases, hoof diseases, internal parasites, diarrhoea, FMD, dysentery and loss of appetite.
Azadiracta indica	Neem, Margosa tree (Leaves)	Wound healing, lice killing, skin diseases
ithania somnifera	Winter cherry (Roots)	Immunomodulator, antistresser, weight gain
ingiber officinale	Ginger (Rhizome)	Food poisoning, tympany, sterility, FMD, skin infection, stomach-ache, arthritis, internal parasites and rheumatism.
Butea monosperma	Forest flame, Bastard tree (Bark)	Fracture healing

Curcuma longa	Turmeric (Rhizome)	Wound healing
mblica officinale	Indian gooseberry, Amla (Fruit pulp)	Antiflatulence, appetizer, digestant, immunomodulator
Cissus quadrangularis	Veldt grape (Leaves)	Leaves are ground with pepper and garlic and made into decoction. The decoction is given to cure fever to goat. Leaves are also grinded and kept before cervix to dilate it and relieve dystocia
Coriandrum sativum	Coriander leaves (Fruits)	Fruits are powdered and given after immediate pregnancy for 3-4 times to facilitate conception.
cimum sanctum	Tulsi, Holi basil (Leaves)	Wound healing, anxiolytic, immuno-modulator, adaptogen (antistressor), cures cold, constipation.
Mimosa pudica	Shy/bashful/ shrinking plant (Leaf)	Leaf is ground with pepper, onion, saffron and fed to barren cows during fever
Musa paradisiaca	Banana	Galactogogue, tympany, diarrhoea, haematuria, prolapse of uterus, heat-stroke, sterility, dysentery, loss of appetite, indigestion, mastitis, food poisoning and post partum complaints
Aloe vera	Aloe (Leaf pulp)	Wound healing, gastritis
Cocus nucifera	Coconut (Fruit)	Fruits used to treat diarrhoea, skin problems and anthelmintic.
Calotropis gigantea	Gigantic swallow wort, Madar (Root)	Root is kept in nostrils for few minutes to get relief from running nose to cow and goat

Advantages / Strengths of Ethno-veterinary Practices

- Useful for cold, skin diseases, worms, wounds, reproductive disorders, nutritional deficiencies & mild diarrhoea.
- It is freely available or at a cost in proportion to the value of the animal.
- It is easily administered, usually topically or orally.
- No residue problem

Disadvantages / Limitations of Ethno-veterinary Practices:

- Some remedies are inconvenient to prepare and use.
- Availability of plants is seasonal.
- Some practices are harmful.
- Dosages are uncertain and remedies not standard. (based on the empirical basis)
- The diagnosis may be inadequate (as it is based on symptoms) rather than underlying cause of the disease.
- Ethnomedicines are not fast acting and potent and less suitable to treat epidemic & endemic infectious diseases e.g. suitable for digestive disorders.
- Particular methods are often much localised and the scope for their further dissemination is limited.
- Cures are variable in their effectiveness according to season method of preparation, etc. and few have been validated in the same way in which synthetic drugs must be validated.
- From a technical standpoint some are totally ineffective.
- EVM has little or nothing to offer against the acute viral diseases of animals.

Tribal, rural and semi-urban people of our country are largely rely on livestock population. Due to the differences in economic status between tribal or rural people with urban areas, they apply traditional healing practices to maintain their animal health, thus, reflecting a major difference in livestock rearing which they passed down orally from generation to generation. Plants belonging to different families, which are having property of healing and preventing various disease and disorders are the one of the most commonly, used ingredients in the preparation of ethno-veterinary medicine. Therefore, ethno-veterinary practices can be best options to antibiotics and synthetic chemical drugs in livestock disease management.

R

1. Balaji, N. and Chakravarthi, R. (2010). Ethno-veterinary Practices in India: A Review. Veterinary World, 3(12): 549-551.
2. C. Varshney: www. hillagric.ac.in vpharma lectures
3. Cotton, C.M. (1996). Ethno-botany: principles and applications. John Wiley & Sons.
4. Hema Sayee, R., Gayathri, ., Femina Banu, S., owsalya, S., okila, M., Nandhini, S., Thirumalaisamy, G. and Senthilkumar, S. (2016). Ethno-veterinary medicine: A boon for animal health. International Journal of Science and Technology, 5(6): 4006 4012.
5. Jain, S. . (2000). Plants in Indian ethno veterinary medicine: status and prospectus. Indian Journal of Veterinary Medicine. 20: 1-11.
6. atewa, S.S. and B.L. Chaudhary (2000). Ethno-veterinary survey of plants of Rajsamand district. Rajasthan. J. Vasundhara, 5:95-98.
7. aur, D., Jaiswal, . and Mishra, S. (2015). Ethno-veterinary Practices in India: A Review. European Journal of Pharmaceutical and Medical Research, 2(7): 139-143.
8. Mc Corkle, C.M. (1986). An introduction to ethno-veterinary research and development. J Ethnobiol, 6(1): 129-149.
9. Patil1, U. S. and Deshmukh, O. S. (2015). Plants Used In Ethno-Veterinary Medicines by Tribal Peoples in Betul District, Madhya Pradesh, India International Journal of Science and Research. 4(10): 1536-1538.
10. Phondani, P.C., Maikhuri, R. . and ala, C.P. (2010). Ethnoveterinary uses of medicinal plants among traditional herbal healers in Alaknanda catchment of Uttarakhand, India. African Journal of Traditional, Complementary and Alternative Medicines. 7(3).
11. Raikwar, A. and Maurya, P. (2015). Ethno-veterinary Medicine: In Present Perspective. International Journal of Agricultural Sciences and Veterinary Medicines. 3(1): 44-49.
12. Schillhorn van Veen, T.W. (1996). Sense or Nonsense Traditional methods of animal disease prevention and control in African savannah. In: McCorkle CM, Mathias E and Schillhorn van Veen TW (eds.). Ethno-veterinary Research and Development, Intermediate Technology Publications, London, pp. 338.
13. Selvaraju, A., Ayyanar1, M., Rathinakumar, S.S. and Sekar, T. (2011). Plants used in ethno-veterinary medicine by malayali tribals in Salem district of Tamil Nadu, India. Medicinal Plants, 3(3): 1-7.

14. Toyang, N.J., Wanyama, J., Nuwanyakpa, M. and Django, S. (2007). Ethnoveterinary Medicine: A practical approach to the treatment of cattle diseases in sub-saharan Africa. Hanneke Mertens (Ed.). Agromisa Foundation and CTA, Wageningen, 2nd Ed. Digigrafi, Wageningen, The Netherlands.

15. ineger, H., elbessa, E., Bekele, T. and Lulekal, E. (2007). Ethnoveterinary medicinal plants at Bale Mountains National Park, Ethiopia. J. Ethnopharmacol.112: 55-70.

□□□

Chapter 17

Bovine oot Lameness and Its Impact on ertilit

R.P. Pande and Gulshan Kumar

Department of Veterinary Surgery and Radiology, College of Veterinary Science and Animal Husbandry, Uttar Pradesh Pandit Deen Dayal Upadhyaya Pashu Chikitsa Vigyan Vishwavidhyalaya Evam Go Anusandhan Sansthan, Mathura

---

Lameness in cattle and buffalo and conditions leading to limping and mild to moderate degree of pain are usually overlooked by the livestock owners and the morbid period prolongs due to insufficient management and veterinary care. The economic importance of lameness in productive daily stock is enormous and it is second most important cause of production loss, sub-performance and poor fertility the first being mastitis. Lameness due to prolonged morbidity shows major negative impact on body condition and thus, influences fertility greatly. Lame cows and buffaloes consume less feed and fodder, loose body weight and enter into prolonged periods of negative energy balance which significantly reduces fertility, particularly by increasing the interval between calving and first service and calving to conception interval.

Lame animals remain under stress and pain continuously and this indirectly affects ovarian function. Surgical conditions leading to lameness being mainly inflammatory process, like mastitis, are associated with reduced conception rate and increased number of services/inseminations per pregnancy. However, in contrast to mastitis, where tackling the inflammation and pain is easy with prompt and aggressive treatment the same is not true. This is because even simple cases hoof and foot lesions do not respond to treatment as quickly as in an udder with mastitis. Apart from causing infertility and prolonged calving interval, economic losses due to lameness also occur in the form of reduced milk yield, increased expenses of veterinary care, disposals and livestock owner s time.

Of all the causes of lameness in bovine, almost two-third are related to digits with equal share of involvement of horny tissue and and digit skin. In lame animals, involvement of hind limb digit is more than fore limb digit and outer digit more than inner digit.

The following diagram shows location and type of lesion causing lameness in bovine foot:

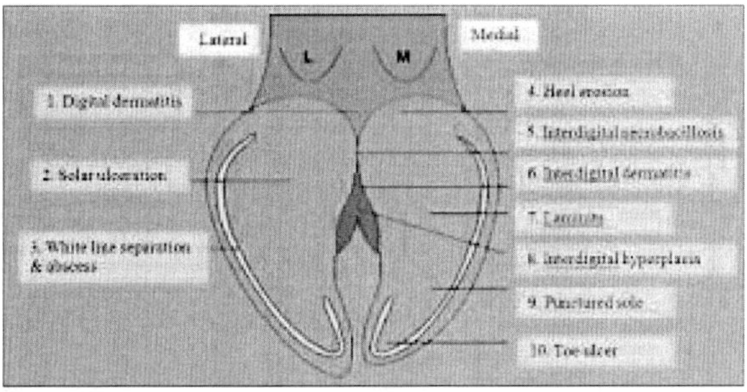

Lameness scoring LS Scoring helps in assessment of severity of lameness and in making differential diagnosis. The simplest lameness scoring is done on a scale of 0-3 as given below:

0 Normal, not lame animals

1 Slightly lame animals

2 Moderately lame animals

3 Severely lame animals, often recumbent

Brief description of Surgical Conditions

Summary of conditions of horny tissue of digits and inter-digital skin and synonyms

Inter-digital skin	Horn tissues
. **digital dermatitis** *dermatitis digitalis*	. **solear ulceration** *pododermatitis circumscripta septica*
. **inter-digital necrobacillosis** *phlegmona inter digitalis*	. **punctured sole** *pododermatitis septica traumatica*
. **inter-digital skin h perplasia** *hyperplasia inter digitalis*	. **hite line separation** *pododermatitis septica diffusa*
. **inter-digital dermatitis** *dermatitis inter digitalis*	. **laminitis** *pododermatitis aseptica diffusa*
. **verrucose dermatitis** *dermatitis verrucosa*	. **sandcrack** longitudinal or transverse *fissura ungulae longitudinalis et transversalis*
	. **heel erosion** *erosio ungulae*

1. **Digital dermatitis** Also called hairy warts or papillomatous dermatitis, it is characterized by circumscribed superficial ulceration of skin of coronary margin at heels/coronary band with granulation on sole and has a tendency to progress to verrucose dermatitis. Signs are of lameness LS 1 3. Infection of the lesion due to spirochete or bacteria may occur. The condition is treated by water jet lavage and application of oxytetracycline spray daily for minimum 3 days. Injection of tylocin, oxytetracyc line or lincomycin in appropriate dosage can aid in quick resolution of the condition. Hairy warts or severe proliferative lesions need to be resected through epidermis under local analgesia.

2. **errucose dermatitis** Also known as heel warts, it is a common form of digital dermatitis characterized by moist tissue proliferation on the dorsal and/or plantar/palmar skin, assuming a wart-like shape. Treatment is surgical removal and antiseptic dressing only if warts become large enough or ulcerated.

3. **Inter-digital dermatitis** It is the inflammation of inter-digital skin with no tendency to extend to deeper tissues occasionally associated with improper horn growth and with lameness of LS 0-1. Favoured by moist housing condition and bacterial invasion, in some cases heel bulb horn cleft may develop which may progress to solear ulceration causing severe lameness (LS 2-3). Hyperkeratosis/parakeratosis may follow and disintegration of epidermis may cause contusion of corium and secondary ulceration. Severe cases are treated by systemic and local use of oxytetracycline (injection and spray) after paring of diseased horn. For other cases foot bath or spray of copper sulphate or formalin is adequate. eeping the housing clean and dry is of utmost value.

4. **Inter-digital necrobacillosis** It is acute inflammation of subcutaneous tissues of inter-digital space and adjacent coronary band manifested by LS 1-3 with sudden onset, inter-digital swelling, spreading apart toes, scant but foul smelling pus and a split in inter-digital skin, marked by cellulitis and liquefactive necrosis. It can be managed in early stages with broad spectrum antibiotic injections and daily cleansing with disinfectant (zinc sulphate 5 10 , copper sulphate 5 or formalin 4).

5. **Inter-digital skin h perplasia** It is proliferative reaction of inter-digital skin and/or subcutaneous tissues to form a firm mass or granuloma manifested by LS 0 1 often preceded by inter-digital lesions involving single limb and associated with splayed toes a poor conformation of digits. Large lesions lead to traumatic ulceration, and contact inter-digital axial skin pressure necrosis. The condition is marked by skin hyperplasia and secondary ulceration. Treatment not necessary if lesion is small, else local caustics like silver nitrate, copper sulphate may be used followed by sulphadimidine powder under bandage for a week.

6. **Solear solar ulceration** It is circumscribed limited reaction of the pododerm (deep sensitive tissues) often characterised by an erosive defect typically at the sole-heel junction of the lateral hind claw. It forms about half of total digit lameness cases. Signs include LS 1 for first 3 months postpartum, which may be followed by LS 2-3 when granulation protrudes. Purulent infection of deep tissue, osteomyelitis and septic arthritis may follow. Under run heel horn may extend to abaxial white line and expose sensitive laminae. Treatment consist of removal of protruding tissue sparing healthy pododerm under local analgesic block and application of tetracycline powder and water proof bandage for a week with confinement in a clean place.

7. **Punctured sole** It is local or diffused sole corium (pododerm) inflammation due to excessive abrasion on rough surface, of the solear horn. Excessive horn paring and previous laminitis (coriosis) predisposes the solear horn by making it thin and abraded surface easy for foreign body penetration, which favours entry of infection upto 3rd phalanx. Signs include lameness LS 2 usually in hind limb, with solear penetration near toe or adjacent to white line and horn defect extending to solear pododerm under running and black colour pus oozing. Treatment is primarily surgical aimed at removal of foreign body, exposure of under run horn to improve drainage, local astringent dressing, broad spectrum (oxytetracycline) antibiotic injection and tetanus prophylaxis.

8. **hite line separation and abscess** It occurs mostly in peripartum period and is identified as sole wall separation at white line from laminae at mostly abaxial and less commonly axial part extending proximally with the space created, being

impacted with dirt and dung followed by development of abscess cavity at the deepest area. Signs include lameness LS 1 2, horn becomes highly sensitive to pincers pressure as deep abscesses fail to drain and in extreme cases supra coronary discharging sinuses develop. Treatment consists of paring the wall over the septic area for improving drainage, removal of all under run sole, local dressing with oxytetracycline and in some cases with severe sepsis, oxytetracycline injections. Radical surgery under nerve blocks may be considered, if involvement of coronary tissues and distal inter-phalangeal joint is present.

9. **Laminitis coriosis** This condition presents in clinical and subclinical form and is identified as diffuse acute, subacute, or chronic inflammation of pododerm involving more than one digit. Pre-disposition is by parturition, acute or subacute ruminal acidosis and possibly trauma. Signs in acute stage are a hot and painful hoof, strong digital artery pulse, generalized depression, abnormal stiff posture, reluctance to move, severe lameness of LS 2 3 and possibly recumbency and blood and serum exudation. Subacute stage is less painful (LS 1) and is characterized by stiff gait and solear and/or white line haemorrhages. In chronic stage, lameness of LS 0 1 with slipper foot malformation and horizontal lines on hoof wall, concave dorsal wall, widened white line with evidence of haemorrhages is seen. Since toe tip has no fat layer in its corium, solear ulceration and toe ulcer near the tip of third phalanx may form. Treatment in acute stage and sub-acute stage consists of NSAIDs like flunixine meglumine/ meloxicam/ketoprofen) or corticosteroids and diuretics, restriction of concentrates in ration, milk exercise on soft ground and digital nerve blocks (only in acute cases with extreme severity LS 3). In chronic cases corrective hoof trimming may be done to improve proper weight bearing on foot. Addition of sodium bicarbonate in ration, adequate exercise, good roughage quantity in ration and regular hoof care has some prophylactic effect.

10. **Sandcrack** As the name indicates, it is characterized by fissure or crack of horny hoof wall parallel to coronet pre-disposed off by overgrowth of horn and severe chronic laminitic horn rings or parallel to dorsal wall pre-disposed off by dry environment and/or trauma at coronary band. Transverse cracks are usually not associated with lameness and there is no exposure of pododerm. Single digit involvement indicates local stress but

multiple digit involvement indicates systemic cause. Longitudinal cracks are serious and may extend from coronet to the bearing surface. Longitudinal crack may also be seen as extremely painful small coronary lesion alone, at dorsal or axial wall and is easy to miss on examination. Treatment of transverse crack consists of shortening to toe to prevent dorsiflexion, cleaning and antiseptic astringent application. For longitudinal crack, removal of excess protruding pododerm, cleaning, astringent antiseptic bandaging and rest affords relief. In extreme cases, grinding a hole at proximal end and filling with resin is advised but prognosis in longitudinal or vertical crack remains guarded. Using oil on hoof in excessive dry weather may have a prophylactic role.

11. **Heel erosion** It is irregular loss of horn at bulb of heal due to contusion in the form of multiple black depressions or oblique grooves, usually in hind digits caused by chronic irritation, inter-digital dermatitis followed by bacterial infection. Signs include lameness grade LS 0 1 except in deep chronic cleft formation leading to under-run heel. Treatment consists of paring away of under-run horn, and topical use of oxytetracycline gentian violet spray and transferring the animal to dry soft floor. Systemic broad spectrum antibiotics in severe cases and formalin foot bath twice a week is also indicated.

Limping or lameness of variable degree is also seen as a condition of sudden onset in cattle and buffaloes, but in such cases it is usually preceded by fall, slip or trauma. The diagnosis in such situations is usually fracture, sprain or strain. Acute lameness due to trauma has little effect on fertility and should be dealt with accordingly.

R

1. Bovine Surgery and Lameness, 2nd Ed. by A. David Weaver, Guy St. Jean and Adrian Steiner (Blackwell Publishing)
2. Hoof anatomy, care and management in livestocks, Purdue University Cooperative Extension Service, West Lafayette, in 47907
3. Huxley, J.N. (2013) Impact of lameness and claw lesions in cows on health and production. Livestock Science,156 (1-3). pp. 64-70. ISSN 1871-1413
4. www.nadis.org.uk
5. www.msdvdetmanual.com

□□□

Chapter 18

E tension Methodologies in Identification and Control of Infectious Diseases

Amit Singh Sanjeev Kumar Singh and Rashmi

Department of Veterinary and Animal Husbandry Extension, College of Veterinary Science and Animal Husbandry, Uttar Pradesh Pandit Deen Dayal Upadhyaya Pashu Chikitsa Vigyan Vishwavidhyalaya Evam Go Anusandhan Sansthan, Mathura

Dairy farming and emerged as one of the key components of agricultural growth major factor in enhancing the socio-economic status of people of developing countries in recent years. Animal husbandry and dairy development play a prominent role by supplementing the income of rural households in rural economy particularly among the landless, small and marginal farmers. Diversification of crop farming through dairy farming can play a vital role as dairy farming provides nutrition, draft animal power, organic manure, supplementary employment and generates continuous flow of income and acts as a cushion against income shocks arising due to crop failure. With focus on developing dairy farming, it is important to impart knowledge to farmers on management practices, as majority of them lack scientific information on dairy practices. Mass media, other farmers and friends are the sources of information on dairy farming. Livestock farmers sought information largely from private rather than public sources relating to livestock production.

Participatory Rural Approaches were developed in the late 1970s and early 1980s, by researchers in international development as an alternative to conventional sample surveys. Participatory approaches are rigorous, organized and semi-structured learning experience carried out by a multi-disciplinary team and the members of the community. It s not a single event, it needs a follow-up. PRA is a way of learning as both the members of multi-disciplinary team and the members of the community try to investigate, analyse, and evaluate constraints and opportunities, and make informed and timely decisions regarding development projects. PRA are facilitated by outsiders but more than RRA, it involves rural people themselves in investigation, in the diagramming, presentation, analysis and ownership of information, in the identification of preferences and priorities, and in planning, action, monitoring and evaluation. PRA is applied most effectively in relatively homogeneous rural communities which share common knowledge, values, and belief, although it has also been used in more complex urban environments. Its short duration and low cost also make it possible to carry out a series of PRAs rather than having to rely on the results of one large survey. PRA used by a research team collect information quickly and systematically for:

- Brief analysis of a specific problem and its solution
- Assessing the need
- To identify and prioritize the work
- For effective monitoring and/or evaluation of programme
- Implementing development activities, where new information needs to be collected

There was a lot of disillusionment and discomfort with the questionnaire surveys, which constituted the pre-dominant ways of conducting rural research. They were cumbersome and tiring. The findings came quite late. There were problems with the accuracy of the data as well. These factors contributed towards the evolution of RRA.

Rapid Rural Appraisal RRA - RRA is a multi-disciplinary team approach that emerged in the early 1980s for applications in development co-operation and to makes use of simple, non-standard methods and the knowledge of local people to quickly elicit, analyze and assess information and hypotheses about rural life and rural resources that are of relevance for taking action. RRA techniques act as an alternative technique to conventional survey methods. The main aim of RRA is not to systematically capture the information, which is time-consuming and cost-intensive undertaking, but a speedy, action-oriented assessment of local knowledge, needs and potentials with an aim to examine specific problems of the area. They are also suitable for shifting the focus of conventional surveys onto essential aspects. Rapid rural appraisal is a quick approach to analyzing a situation for assessing farmer s needs by a multi-disciplinary team through a creative and structural use of investigation tools in a more accurate and cost effective manner. The quality of the results depends heavily on the team s ability to make analytical judgements on picking up key issues within a short period of time. When properly used, RRA tools can generate reliable and substantial information about problems of natural resource management.

Characteristics of RRA

1. **Rapid** It is rapid as the results are made available to the decision-makers in a short time.
2. **Eclectic** It allows picking up investigation tools that enable tailoring interview and survey techniques to meet the needs of specific information gathering.
. **Holistic** Its use makes it possible to capture a multi-disciplinary picture of a local situation.
. **Interactive** It allows adequate interaction between researchers and project clients.
5. **Inter-disciplinar** It is inter-disciplinary and includes decision makers, researchers, social scientists as well as extension workers, women and key informants to dialogue issues.
6. **Cost effective** It provides reliable and sufficient information in a relatively shorter and more flexible timeframe.
7. **More realistic** This technique is midway between formal and non-structured methods of situation analysis and hence, is a more realistic approach for a short timeframe.

Participator Rural Appraisal PRA - This concept emerged from RRA in the year 1980. It is the process of involving local people in the analysis and interpretation of rural situation, in which participants take a leadership role, in collecting, analyzing, interpreting and presenting information and impart knowledge and development insights to the specialists and extension agents. Through PRA timely, relevant, accurate and usable productive information can be available in a cost effective way. PRA helps to access the village resources quickly with the help of knowledgeable villagers themselves.

PRA is a way of enabling local (rural and urban) people to analyze their living conditions, to share the outcomes and to plan their activities. It s a handing over the stick to the insider in methods and action. The outsider s role is that of a catalyzer, a facilitator and convenor of processes within a community, which is prepared to alter their situation.

Definition It may be defined as an intensive and systematic learning experience in a community by multi-disciplinary team, which includes community members.

PRA

- Participation
- Empowerment
- Sense of Responsibility

Key principles of Participatory Rural Appraisals

1. Triangulation

This is an essential methodological concept in PRA and a form of cross-checking. Accuracy is achieved through diverse information and different kinds of sources of information, not through statistical replication. Triangulation is done in relation to:

- Composition of the team and background of team members.
- Sources of information (people, places, etc.) : The PRA should include a wide range of view points from different sources of information, such as women and men, elders and youths, various ethnic groups, diverse wealth groups and different professions.
- Methods : The PRA techniques are taken from a wide range of possible tools which are tailored to the specific requirements of the study.
- Time : ensure to visit a community in both the wet season and the dry season.

2. Multi-disciplinary team and group learning process

The members of the PRA team should have different skills and backgrounds. This could imply members from different disciplines, different sectors or a mixture of outsiders and insiders. The different viewpoint of team members will complement each other and will provide a more comprehensive picture. In this way, the team will approach the topic of the appraisal from different viewpoints, which gives new and deeper insights. All members of the PRA team are involved in all aspects of the study: design, data collection, and analysis (not just in data collection as in a conventional survey). The PRA is a learning experience in which the participants also learn from each other.

3. Flexibility and informality

Plans and research methods are semi-structured and are revised, adapted, and modified as the PRA fieldwork proceeds and when they are used in a different context.

4. Participation with community

The main aspect of the PRA is learning from, with, and by members of the community. The team should sympathise with the community members and be able to see their lives and their problems through the eyes of the community members. Most of the activities are done jointly with community members or by them on their own (e.g. planning, mapping, and analysis). PRAs are generally too short for outsiders to become insiders. Therefore, it is important to have community members (insiders) participate in the appraisal. Involving community members can greatly facilitate interpretation, understanding, and analysis of collected data.

5. Optimal ignorance and appropriate imprecision

The PRA team avoids unnecessary detail, accuracy, and over collection of data (as in sample survey) which is not really needed for the purpose of the PRA (this is decided through on-the-spot analysis). The team asks itself: What kind of information is required, for what purposes, and how accurate does it have to be

6. On-the-spot analysis

Learning takes place in the field and the analysis of the information gathered is an integral part of the fieldwork itself. The team constantly reviews and analyses its findings in order to determine in which direction to proceed. It builds up understanding and narrows the focus of the PRA, as it accumulates knowledge.

7. Off-setting biases and being self-critical

The PRA team actively seeks out the poorest, women, and disadvantaged groups in remote areas, during the worst time of the year, at any time of day, and avoids talking only to the well-off, the better-educated, the articulate, and the men. The team also has to be careful to analyse its own biases in order to prevent the PRA from turning into development tourism and collection of rumours. The team reflects on what is said and not seen, who is met and not met, and tries to identify possible sources of error and how they influence the interpretation of the gathered information. The team must also try to avoid value judgements about others.

8. Shifting attitudes and behaviour

- The use of PRA implies role reversals/shifts
- For both outsiders and local people

Methods of the PRA

illage Transect Transects are systematic walks with key informants through the area of interest, observing, asking, listening, looking, and seeking problems and solutions. The main objective of the transect walk is to understand and study the major land uses, topography, water resources, natural vegetation and different ecological zones by observing, interacting and discussing with the ey Informants (Is), while walking in the deciding direction. The findings can be mapped on a transect diagram. Most transect walks result in the outsiders discovering surprising local practices, such as indigenous conservation practices, multiple uses of plants, and a great variety of crops. The items for discussion include topics, such as soil type, water resources, crops, vegetables, fruit plants, trees and shrubs, forages, animals, land use pattern, interventions, problems and opportunities.

Agro-ecos stem map Agro-ecological or agro-ecosystem map shows the macro and micro ecological (sub-systems) features in a village. The meteorological parameters like rainfall, temperature, relative humidity and the major flora and fauna of the village and the basic land use pattern, such as crops, agro-forestry, forest cover, wasteland, animals and the natural resources like soil type, water resources (wells, river, channel, ponds, etc.), common property resources (CPRs), use of locally available resources are depicted in this map. This map helps in the preparation of perspective planning for the village development.

Social Map Social mapping is the most popular and a potent method to seeks and explore the spatial dimensions of people s realities. The focus here is on the depiction of habitation patterns and the nature of housing and social infrastructure: roads, drainage systems, schools, drinking-water facilities, etc. Social map is different from other regular maps in significant ways. For one, it is made by local people and not by experts. For another, it is not drawn to scale. It depicts what the local people believe to be relevant and important for them. Thus, it reflects their perceptions of the social dimensions of their reality with a high degree of authenticity. In spite of there being many overlaps, a social map is different from a resource map. The latter depicts the natural resources land, water sources, flora and fauna, etc. In certain cases, though, a map could be a rich combination of the two (Village map).

Resource Map Resource map was drawn after collecting information by the active participation of ey Informants (Is) of different age groups including female. Resource map describes main crops grown in the village, trees, animals, common property resources (CPRs), types of houses, school, farm implements, luxury and communication items, social resources like women groups, self-help groups (SHGs), local self-government, etc.

Seasonal Calendar This is a calendar, which indicates month wise activities related to agriculture and livelihood, threats, abundance, and shortage with regard to agriculture in a diagrammatic way. The items to be included in seasonal analysis must be of those items, which really affect the agriculture. This explores seasonal constraints and opportunities by diagramming changes, month by month throughout the year.

Seasonal Anal sis To know about the seasonal problems related to livestock seasonal analysis is carried out. In this method, the diseases affecting various animals are documented pertaining to their months of attack. Other information like availability of labour and fodder for animals are also recorded by involving the farmers. The information collected is depicted in the form of a table.

Time Line Historical analyses have been found to be a good icebreaker for field exercises and include detailed accounts of the past, of how things have changed, particularly focusing on relationships and trends. These include livestock technology histories and review, livestock breed histories, labour availability, trees and forest histories, education change, and population change. Folklore and songs are also valuable resources for exploring history.

Time Trend Time trend shows quantitative changes over the period of time and can be used for many variables of agricultural, livestock, poultry production, price, yield and areas under cultivation.

For instance, the trends in sheep and goat population in the country over a period of time could be depicted in a line diagram.

Mobilit Map The mobility map indicates the places to which the villagers go outside their village for various purposes like purchasing fodder, inputs, family needs, animal husbandry needs, getting higher education, medical needs, social relations, recreation, etc.

ealth Ranking Wealth ranking refers to placing the people on different categories according to their own criteria. The purpose is to find out the persons of the village, who belong to the rich, middle, poor and very poor group categories as perceived by the villagers themselves. Wealth ranking is based on the assumption that the community members have a good sense about fellow villagers in their own village and are able to categorize themselves. Livestock development must take into account the differences in wealth among farmers in order to determine the priorities for research and to develop the interventions and technical packages that are to be adopted by the majority of the farmers.

R

1. Jain, S.P. & Wim Polman (2003). A Handbook for Trainers on Participatory Local Development, RAP publication 2003/07, FAO Regional Office for Asia and the Pacific Bangkok, Thailand
2. Mukherjee Amitava (1995) Participatory Rural Appraisal, Methods and application in Rural planning, Vikas Publishing House Pvt. Ltd. 576, Masjid Road, Jangpura, New Delhi-110 014
3. Sally Sontheimer, arel Callens and Bernd Seiffert (1999) Conducting a PRA Training and Modifying PRA Tools to our Needs. An Example from a Participatory Household Food Security and Nutrition Project in Ethiopia, Food and Agriculture Organization of the United Nations.
4. Tiwari Rupasi, Singh. B. P and Sharma, M. C. (2008). Manual on participatory rural appraisal, ICAR-Indian Veterinary Research Institute, Izzatnagar, Bareilly.
5. Paul Narinder (2014). Participatory Rural Appraisal (PRA) report of Village- ursari, Tehsil-Bhaderwah, District-Doda (J&), Directorate of Extension, Sher-e- ashmir University of Agriculture Sciences and Technology of Jammu.

❏❏❏

Chapter 19

E tension Services Deliver to Augment Technolog Adoption

Sanjeev Kumar Singh Amit Singh and Rashmi

Department of Veterinary & Animal Extension, College of Veterinary Science and Animal Husbandry, Uttar Pradesh Pandit Deen Dayal Upadhyaya Pashu Chikitsa Vigyan Vishwavidhyalaya Evam Go Anusandhan Sansthan, Mathura

Extension service primarily involves delivering of technical know -how, instructions, and hands-on training springing from research institutions for technological adoption of innovations at the grass-root level. Extension services may be classified into three types, viz., technology transfer, advisory and facilitation.

Technolog transfer, i.e., the traditional model of the transfer of advice, knowledge and information in a linear manner.

Advisor , i.e., cadre of experts acts as a source of advice in relation to specific problems faced by the farmers.

acilitation, i.e., the aim of this model is to help farmers to define their own problems and develop their own solutions.

A number of organisations of Government of India provides extension services are: Directorate of Extension, Ministry of Agriculture, Department of Animal Husbandry, Dairying & Fisheries, Government of India, Indian Council of Agricultural Research (ICAR), National Dairy Development Board (NDDB), rishi Vigyan endra (V s), State Agricultural/Veterinary Universities, State Dairy Federations, Non-Government Organizations, State Department of Animal Husbandry (SDAH), Private Dairies, Agri-input dealers and Veterinary Pharmaceutical companies.

These organizations provide livestock oriented extension services to disseminate research innovations among the farming community. Some of the common extension services used by the extension officials to disseminate information at the grass root level are :

1. Animal Fairs

Livestock fairs enables the livestock owners of different communities and religious groups to meet at a particular place, share their ideas, sale and purchase of livestock and their goods as well as display various skills and technologies among the public. These fairs play an important role in sharing of new technology, in case if the consumer is not aware of that particular technology or its usage.

2. Kisan Goshthi / Pashupalak Goshthi

In this a livestock oriented awareness programme is held on pre-decided date and place with limited number of livestock owners. The sole purpose of this program is to create awareness regarding different livestock technologies, i.e., production oriented, management oriented, feed oriented, health oriented, etc. The livestock owners have interaction with scientific experts from various disciplines of veterinary science. There is an open-ended discussion after completion of each topic with the livestock owners and such sharing of their experiences enable them to raise their income. They are well-informed that using the right techniques at the right time farmers will enhance their monthly income by two-folds. Experts from the research institutions also get the feedback of their technologies during such interaction with the livestock owners.

3. Exhibitions

An exhibition is an organized presentation and display of items, technology in order to disseminate information through audio-visual means. All the evidence of the research innovations that influence livestock owners are displayed sequentially for better understanding among the users.

4. Technology Demonstration

Demonstration is a skilled performance of a task or technique showing precisely how it should and could be done on the job. Livestock owners are interested to see how a new idea works and also what effect it can have on increasing their production. Both purposes can be achieved by means of a livestock oriented demonstration. A demonstration will provide livestock owners an opportunity to observe, a first-hand information in relation to the differences between a recommended new practice and traditional practice. The strength of the demonstration lies in its simplicity and its ability to aware the livestock owners with concrete results. Usually two types of demonstration are used by extension agents in the field conditions, viz., method demonstration and result demonstration.

Method demonstration Method demonstrations basically show farmers how to do something. In the method demonstration, the farmer is shown step by step, for example right method of milking, dehorning, feed formulations, de-beaking in chicks, etc. The extension agent will probably be dealing with farmers who have already accepted the particular practice, but now they want to know how to do it themselves.

Result demonstration The main purpose of result demonstration is to show livestock owners how a particular new recommendation or practice is practicable under local field conditions. Comparison is the important element in result demonstration, i.e., comparison between traditional and recommended technology, such as effect of drugs on health of animals, effect of vaccination in animals, etc. Seeing is believing is an age-old expression, but it fits appropriate for result demonstration. Until a farmer has actually seen the results of a particular technology, he will not be convinced by the scientific recommendations.

5. Study Tours or Exposure Visit

Livestock owners visit dairy farms or other livestock units in other districts to see the rearing pattern of livestock in neighbouring districts, their working pattern, their marketing network, the fodders they grow, the problems they face, etc. A tour is conducted to visit a number of field demonstrations on different farms, different districts, or in different states, which attract a lot of interest and awareness among the farming community.

6. Campaign

A campaign is an intense educational activity for motivating and mobilizing a community to action, to solve a problem or to satisfy a need urgently felt by them. The duration of a campaign may be few weeks to years depending upon the nature and type of the programme. The campaign may be held for a small number of people or for the entire village/district/state or country. The campaign must be organized around a theme only once or repeatedly year after year till the goal is accomplished. The basic purpose of campaign is to provide information and education to the people so that they can improve their lives through adoption of improved and new technology.

7. Film Shows

Film shows are undoubtedly very effective crowd pullers in rural areas and is a very effective teaching aids enabling livestock owners to gain broad information about a particular aspect. They can also be used to create awareness about new technologies to very large number of people at various locations. It is very useful tool for diffusion of technology in rapid manner among the farming community.

8. Kisan Call Centre (KCC)

For speedy transmission of livestock technologies and latest technical updates among the farming community to resolve their diverse problems through an innovative means, the Department of Agriculture & Co-operation under Ministry of Agriculture, Government of India have launched the isan Call Centre Scheme on dated 21 January, 2014. The CC delivers extension services among the farming community very timely, precisely and accurately. The farmers get accurate answers for their queries, which facilitate them for better management of their livestock. The CC numbers are 18001801551 (any landline/mobile) and 1551 (from BSNL landline only).

9. Information kiosks

It is one of the ICT tool, where there is integration of livestock technology at a single place in a computer. Livestock owners get a wide range of information through farmers-friendly touch screen informative livestock kiosks. These kiosks are square shaped physical structure with touch display and a computer terminal, which provides demand-driven information with attractive pictures, animation, etc. with audio-visual backup and in brief it is very effective in transfer of information. The main role of kiosk is to enable the livestock owners to understand the application of new technologies, which will be useful to increase adoption behaviour of livestock owners.

10. Animal Health Camps

Camps are organized in remote villages where necessary extension and veterinary facilities are not available. The basic objective is to create awareness among the farming community for various livestock technologies as well as to provide better treatment facilities for their livestock. The camp is assisted with various animal husbandry experts of nutrition, management, disease control, etc. along with experts of clinical subjects. These experts disseminate livestock oriented technologies and clinical experts treat their livestock after ultrason ographic and pathological examinations.

11. Community Radio

Since long, measures were undertaken to uplift the rural people through bottom-up approach, i.e., adding the voices of grass-root level people and communities in planning, decision-making and ensuring their accountability. Recently, the government measure to empower the grassroots through community radio has added new dimensions in awareness creation thereby making society well-informed and aware for their rights and responsibilities. Community Radio Stations not only provide the platform for people residing in remote areas, who can express their views in the development agenda for their sustainable and viable development as well as to promote and protect their cultural and linguistic diversity. Community Radio is a viable tool of interaction between the various pools of knowledge interspersed between communities. Community Radio not only consolidates local traditional knowledge but also helps in empowerment of people residing at the grass-root level enabling them to show their talent, besides re-energizing local arts and culture.

Ministry of Information & Broadcasting is fully committed to nurture and support this sector so that it may reach its full potential. Since the entertaining Community Radio FM channels are unable to discuss the local problems of the community on a common platform. Hence, democratization of the airwaves through educational institutions is a sign of progressive societal change. The educational institutions must ensure the community participation in the radio and must support capacity building of communities through alive oral dialects and creating a link between the citizen & decision-makers. This two-way communication is the cornerstone of participatory democracy. Even in this age of e-communication, it is only community radio that can enter each household on a remote hill, village or island and reflect the aspirations of the people.

In this scheme, the local community will be engaged to identify livestock oriented problems through various extension methods, viz., through feedback on government welfare schemes, group-discussion sessions to identify grass-root problems and identification of remedial measures through SWOT analysis & PRA tools, communication of real inspirational stories in order to motivate them to adopt innovative technologies, folk songs to transfer innovative developments in local dialect, audio collage, docu-dramas, etc. Such identified problems may be communicated in local dialect as livestock technological programmes on community radio, in which farmers directly ask questions related to their livestock and allied problems with concerned scientists.

The programmes broadcasted through Community Radio Station (CRS) will be highly beneficial for the local community in handling day-to-day care and management of small and large animals, besides timely vaccination, timely insemination and balanced feeding which not only improves the production potential of their livestock, but also make livestock owners economically sound. However, certain livestock oriented usefulness of the programmes, which may be disseminated through community radio includes balanced feeding of livestock, management of small and large animals, knowledge about scientific dairy farming practices, prevention and control of gynaecological disorders in livestock, prevention and control of parasitic infestation in livestock, clean milk production, capacity building of livestock owners through continuous broadcasting of livestock oriented programmes, upgradation of existing breeds of milch animals, prevention and control of bacterial, viral, protozoal and other diseases of livestock, marketing of milk and milk products, SWOT analysis of various farming practices, entrepreneurial management of livestock enterprise, etc.

12. Mobile App

The mobile phone, especially the android mobile phones had made its availability in the urban, rural and even in ultra remote areas, not only for receiving the innovative technological SMS of the department of agriculture, animal husbandry, etc., but also acts as a cursor to connect the digital and physical arena. In the present digital era, the use of agile design and development principles go into developing state-of-the-art ***o e a s*** that convert our technological goals into realities. A mobile app is a computer based program design to run on mobile devices. Usually mobile phones are sold with several apps bundled as pre-installed software, but apps which are not pre-installed are usually available through various distribution platforms. The public demand forced the software developers for expansion into other categories of apps and livestock apps is the need of today for technological break-through in the area of livestock and allied activities.

The development of livestock apps is performed taking into consideration the needs and interests of the livestock owners, besides as a part of extension strategy to promote transfer of livestock oriented technologies at the grass-root level farmers/livestock owners. The apps may be prepared on various animal husbandry aspects, viz., breeding, feeding, management, disease control and marketing, which can be downloaded by the livestock owners from the app stores for effective and efficient management of livestock and allied activities. Certain areas have been identified for the preparation of livestock apps, which are enumerated as :

1. Breeding app

This app is intended to aid breeders in determining various gestation dates. It provides both, backward and forward date calculations and it is simple to use. After selecting the breed and then entering any one of the date (either date of service or date of further return to heat or date of calving) owner may get information of other breeding dates.

2. Livestock Record app

This app is a very comprehensive and user-friendly app for both, large and small animals. It will record animal weight, feeding schedule, health as well as monitors average daily gains. Besides this, it will also calculate income, expenses, losses, present assets value as well as able to generate financial statements.

3. Poison Helper app

This app will function in two ways, i.e., either by specifying the poison symptoms or by citing the poison feed-stuffs. The livestock owner may get the first hand information on identification of poison vis- -vis home-made remedial measures in adversities.

4. Heat Stress Aid app

Heat stress is the main cause of decrease milk production and reduced fertility, especially in the summer months. By citing current temperature and humidity readings, it will calculate heat stress from mild to extreme risk, besides providing tips on mitigating heat stress via management and nutrition.

5. AI Calculator app

This app helps the livestock owners and veterinarians to compare the cost and benefits of artificial insemination Vs natural service to mange reproduction in their farms.

6. Vaccination & Deworming app

This app allows the livestock owners to just indicate the date of birth of their livestock (small or large animal) thereby progressive vaccination and deworming schedule for their livestock will be displayed on their mobile screen.

7. Nutrition app

This app allows the producers to identify the best feed through calculation among various available green and roughage feed-stuffs along with their nutritional values. This app will also help the livestock owners to determine the quantity of feed to be fed among the milch and dry animals in various stages of their life.

These apps have a number of advantages among the livestock owners, which may be summarized as per below :

1. Livestock owners don't have to wait for livestock oriented information

Mobile apps provide a much faster alternative than mobile web browsing. Web browsing requires a user to launch a web browser, enter a URL and wait for the site to load, whereas it only takes a second to launch a mobile app because the majority of the information is stored in the application itself making it possible to function offline.

2. Apps are a constant reminder for their Livestock Farm Business

Mobile apps reinforce their livestock farm by increasing the livestock owners visibility in the farm with the help of app. An app gives a livestock owner more presence on a phone than a browser, because it is always visible on the phone s screen and the owners get constant alerts for daily business activities.

3. Apps increases their engagement with livestock farms

Through mobile apps the livestock owners quickly connect with the required information, they most commonly want or need.

4. Apps reduce costs

Apps reduce costs of SMS messages and paper newsletters. They simplify communications by securely, instantly and directly messaging the livestock owners. Apps reduce veterinary staff workload by disseminating the same information to a number of individual.

5. Apps boost needs and interest of the livestock owners

Apps increase interests of the livestock owners through constant instant updates of each innovations generated in our laboratories and can be able to increase its profitability in a short span of time.

6. User-friendly and free downloading

The livestock owners can freely download the app from the play store of google or other sites.

R

Birkhaeuser, D., Evenson, R. E., & Feder, G. (1991). The economic impact of agricultural extension: A review. Economic development and cultural change, 607-650.

Cole, R.R. (1999). The diffusion of innovations in agriculture: Rice technologies in West Africa, the case of the Gambia. (Dissertation/ Thesis), Pro uest, UMI Dissertations Publishing.

Dalton, G. E. (1980). The educational role of farm management extension work by state advisory services. Journal of Agricultural Economics, 31(2): 149-161.

Shah, M. M. I., Grant, W. J., & Stocklmayer, S. (2014). Adoption of Hybrid Rice in Bangladesh: Farm Level Experience. Journal of Agricultural Science, 6(7): 157.

Tripp, R., Wijeratne, M., & Piyadasa, V. H. (2005). What should we expect from farmer field schools A Sri Lanka case study. World Development, 33(10): 1705-1720.

❑❑❑

Chapter 20

udicious Use of Antibacterials in eterinar Practice

Ashish Srivastava A.K. Tripathi and Mukesh Kumar Srivastava

Department of Veterinary Medicine, College of Veterinary Science and Animal Husbandry, Uttar Pradesh Pandit Deen Dayal Upadhyaya Pashu Chikitsa Vigyan Vishwavidhyalaya Evam Go Anusandhan Sansthan, Mathura

A

In general, chemotherapy means use of chemical agents for treatment of diseases. However, the term chemotherapy is limited to use of chemicals for treatment/control of pathogens and neoplasia. As such, the chemotherapeutic agents include antibacterial, antiviral, antifungal, antiparasitic, and antineoplastic compounds.

Ideally, a chemotherapeutic agent should selectively inhibit or kill the invading pathogen or neoplastic cells without adversely affecting the host. It may do so by targetting uniquely different metabolic pathway or cell architecture of the target cell. However, in reality, this distinction is not absolute and chemotherapeutic agents also affect the host in some way or the other. Adverse effects observed in the host mostly depend upon the mechanism of action of the drug. Drugs meant to inhibit eukaryote pathogens (protozoa, fungi) have lower margin of safety as compared to drugs targeting prokaryote pathogens (bacteria) due to obvious similarity in structure and function of the pathogen and the host.

Certain clinical conditions and metabolic alterations in the host, such as dehydration, acidemia, renal insufficiency, hepatic insufficiency, etc. may also accentuate adverse effects of certain drugs.

As far as judicious use of antimicrobials particularly antibacterials is considered, the clinician must be sufficiently sure of a bacterial infection before starting the treatment. One should try to make distinction between bacterial, fungal, viral and parasitic infection.

Although it is very difficult in field practice to demonstrate presence of bacteria in every suspected case, but a proper clinical examination may help to a great extent.

When treating a bacterial infection the choice of antibiotic should be based on expected clinical efficacy, possibility of adverse effects and possibility of creating drug resistance in the bacteria. With regard to the choice of the most appropriate antibacterial, a distinction should be drawn between an empirical choice and one based on sensitivity testing.

Other important points to ponder while considering antimicrobial chemotherapy

Mechanism of Action(MOA)

MOA of important antibacterial classes is given below:

1. Disruption of cell wall e.g. Beta-lactams (penicillins and cephalosporins), glycopeptides (vancomycin), bacitracin, fosfomycin.
2. Disruption of cell membrane e.g. polymyxin B, colistin
3. Inhibition of protein synthesis by affecting ribosome function e.g. Aminoglycosides, chloramphenicol, lincosamides, macrolides and tetracyclines
4. Inhibition of DNA synthesis and replication e.g. quinolones, metronidazole, novobiocin
5. Inhibition of DNA dependent RNA polymerase e.g. rifamycins
6. Inhibition of folic acid synthesis e.g. sulphonamides, trimethoprim.

Proper understanding of MOA of antimicrobial drug is important for selecting a drug to treat a particular infection. For example, beta-lactam antibiotics cannot be used to treat mycoplasmal infection because these pathogens do not have a cell wall.

Pharmacokinetics and pharmacodynamics of the drug

Pharmacokinetic factors like dose, dosing interval, route of administration, absorption, distribution and elimination in relation to time determine the drug s serum concentration and thus, its concentration in the tissues and extracellular fluids. Pharmacodynamics describes the relationship between serum concentrations and pharmacological effects of the drug.

Most antimicrobials, when administered orally, have good bioavailability in dogs and cats with some notable exceptions, such as ciprofloxacin which has good oral bioavailability in humans but not in dogs. Oral administration of antimicrobials is not preferred in ruminants and horses, as they adversely affect the normal microflora of rumen and hindgut in these species. In fact prolonged oral administration of broad spectrum antimicrobial in hind-gut fermenter species (such as horse and rabbit) might result in life-threatening colitis and chronic diarrhea.

Solubility of the drug is another important pharmacologic factor affecting distribution of the drug in body. More polar (water soluble) drugs, such as beta-lactams and aminoglycosides are unable to cross cell membrane effectively and therefore, do not reach inside the cells in effective concentration and remain distributed in extracellular fluid only. In contrast more lipid soluble drugs, such as quinolones, tetracyclines, macrolides, sulphonamides, clindamycin, etc. cross cell membranes effectively and distribute in extracellular as well as intracellular water and inhibit intracellular pathogens also.

Elimination metabolism of drugs also influences choice of antimicrobial for treating infection of different organ systems. Some drugs undergo hepatic elimination and excreted out in bile (doxycycline, minocycline, clindamycin and macrolides), whereas some undergo renal elimination (beta lactams, quinolones, aminoglycosides, etc.). Drugs undergoing biliary elimination are not suitable to treat urinary tract infections and may prove detrimental in case of hepatic insufficiency/failure. Drugs undergoing renal elimination are, therefore, suitable to treat urinary tract infections but their dose should be reduced while treating any infection in animals suffering from renal failure.

Drugs that are poorly absorbed from gastro-intestinal tract (gut acting antimicrobials) should be preferred to treat infections limited to GI tract with no signs of systemic invasion e.g. oral neomycin, oral colistin, sulphaguanidine, sulphaquinoxaline, etc.

B S

Ability to clinically identify important bacterial diseases and common bacteria causing those diseases in different animal species is important to design empirical chemotherapeutic regimen. However, laboratory identification of the pathogen involved should always be carried out, where facility is available and treatment should be designed/ modified accordingly. As far as choice of the drug is concerned for treating a particular type of infection, the clinician should be aware of local pattern of antibacterial sensitivity/resistance of the bacterium. It has been observed that same bacterium is sensitive to different antimicrobials at different locations. If drug sensitivity of the bacterium is known, then it is better to select a narrow spectrum and effective antimicrobial. Drug sensitivity pattern of microbes can change with time. Therefore, it is important to periodically test for it to remain updated.

B B

Antibacterials can be broadly classified into bacteriostatic (those only inhibiting the proliferation of bacteria) and bactericidal (kills the bacteria). Bacteriostatic drugs include tetracyclines, chloramphenicol, macrolides, lincosamides and unpotentiated sulphonamides. Rest of the drugs have bactericidal action.

As bacteriostatic drugs rely on host s immune system to clear the infection, use of bacteriostatic drugs is not suitable in immuno-suppressed animals (e.g. along with glucocorticoids, in parvoviral enteritis, post *Trypanosoma evansi* infection, etc.) and in peracute bacterial infections.

Antibiotics can be divided into three main groups based on the parameters, which best predict their clinical efficacy:

1. Those with concentration-dependent activity: aminoglycosides, quinolones and metronidazole
2. Those with time-dependent activity: beta-lactams and tetracyclines
3. Those with both concentration- and time-dependent activity: clindamycin and macrolides

For drugs having concentration-dependent activity, dose of the drug is more important than frequency of administration. These drugs are more effective, if their tissue concentration is much more than the minimum inhibitory concentration (MIC) for the target bacteria. Practically, this means the drug should be given at higher end of the recommended dose range. For time dependent drugs, the time for which their tissue concentration remains above the MIC for the target bacteria is important. To achieve this, the frequency of drug administration is more important and depends upon the elimination rate of the drug. Due to this, most of the beta-lactam drugs need to be given 3 to 4 times a day, which sometimes is challenging in field practice.

A very important point to consider while deciding the dose of drugs in animals is availability of reliable reference. It has been observed that pharmaceutical companies regularly push different compounds and suggest arbitrary dose for that in different animal species. However, relevant pharmacokinetic data are not available for such compound to arrive at a universally accepted dose. The solution is to refer to reliable references like veterinary codex and formularies.

Two or more antimicrobial drugs may be given simultaneously to:

- Treat mixed bacterial infections in which the pathogens are not sensitive to a single drug.
- Achieve synergistic antimicrobial activity against resistant bacteria e.g. *Pseudomonas aeruginosa*
- Reduce adverse effects of a single antibiotic, which if given alone, might require higher dose and thus more possibility of toxic side effects.

When two antimicrobials are combined, the combination might act either in additive or in synergistic way. Usually, two bacteriostatic drugs act in additive way, whereas bactericidal drugs act in synergistic way. However, a bacteriostatic drug should not be combined with a bactericidal one, as it reduces the proliferation and thus, susceptibility of pathogen to the cidal drug. Another important point to consider while selecting a combination is spectrum of activity of the components of the combination. Consider a case of mixed sepsis due to disruption of intestinal mucosal barrier (e.g. in acute parvoviral enteritis). In this case, the invading bacterial population might consist aerobes, anaerobes, gram positive, gram negative i.e. all sort of bacteria and clinical condition might not provide luxury of time to wait for results of blood culture and drug sensitivity. Hence, one has to select a combination of antimicrobials to contain all possible pathogens, such as a 3rd generation cephalosporin an aminoglycoside metronidazole.

There is one more aspect of combination chemotherapy that needs further deliberation is that of commercial fixed dose combinations (FDC), such as streptomycin penicillin and ampicillin dicloxacillin. The problem with FDCs is that adequate dose of neither of the component is available. Worldwide, FDCs are now being withdrawn from the market. It is a better strategy to combine two drugs at their respective recommended dose.

T G

Recently, it has been observed that use of 3rd generation cephalosporins (particularly Ceftriaxone) has spiked in veterinary practice, even for seemingly innocuous infections. On one hand, this has aided in development of resistance in previously susceptible bacteria and on the other hand, this has certain serious clinical implications while treating acute endotoxemia (say haemorrhagic septicemia in ruminants). We all know that cephalosporins are beta-lactam antibiotics killing bacteria by destroying its cell wall. In case of Gram negative bacteria (as *Pasteurella*) lipopolysaccharide (LPS), which is essentially the endotoxin responsible for initiation of systemic inflammatory response syndrome (SIRS) is an integral part of cell wall. As Gram negative bacterial cell is destroyed by the drug, there is massive release of LPS into the circulation, further aggravating the sepsis. Therefore, use of other bactericidal drugs with site of action other than cell wall (such as aminoglycosides and quinolones or a combination thereof) should be preferred.

A

Adequate tissue perfusion is necessary before diffusion of antibiotics into infected tissue can occur. Effective concentrations of antibiotics cannot, therefore, be guaranteed in the extremities of patients with hypovolemic shock. It can also be difficult to achieve effective concentrations of antibiotics in abscesses and granulation tissue. Certain tissue types do not permit ready diffusion of antibiotics from the blood to the tissue due to the presence of anatomical barriers e.g. blood-brain barrier (BBB). Antimicrobials that readily cross the BBB include 3rd generation cephalosporin, chloramphenicol and sulphonamides.

Antimicrobials usually accumulate differentially in body tissues even without any anatomical barrier. For example, ceftiofur tend to accumulate in lungs and uterus in bovines and therefore, is better suited to treat pneumonia and metritis but not mastitis. Local factors like presence of pus or necrotic tissue can reduce an antibiotic s efficacy by binding and inactivating it. Production of biofilm on surgical implants can protect bacteria against antibiotics and phagocytosis.

Continuous and long term usage of antibacterials (particularly oral use of broad spectrum drugs e.g. Amoxi-Clav) results in significant disruption of GI microbiota. In this situation, overgrowth of pathogenic clostridia: *Cl. Difficile* and *Cl. Perfringens* is fairly common often leading to fatal enterocolitis. The disease is particularly severe in hind gut fermenters like horses and rabbits.

R

The regulatory authorities in Europe have licensed fluoroquinolones and cephalosporins for treatment of common infections of the urinary tract, skin and superficial wounds in companion animals. However, it is well known from both human and veterinary medicine that the use of both fluoroquinolones and 3rd-generation cephalosporins increases the development of extended spectrum beta-lactamase (ESBL)-producing E. coli and methicillin-resistant staphylococci, both of which are highly clinically relevant. There is a real risk that these and other multi-resistant bacteria will spread, if we do not limit the use of fluoroquinolones and cephalosporins now and in the future. Antibiotics can be divided into five categories, based on their critical relevance to human medicine along with the risk for development and spread of resistance of high clinical relevance from companion animals to humans.

The first category comprises of those antibiotics with a relatively narrow spectrum and limited risk for the development and spread of dangerous resistant bacteria in companion animals (e.g. penicillin, macrolides and streptomycin). The second category contains antibiotics with a somewhat broader spectrum and a limited risk for spreading resistance of high relevance from companion animals to humans (amino-penicillins, lincosamides, tetracyclines, sulphonamides and nitrofurantoin).

First-generation cephalosporins and amoxicillin clavulanate are placed in the third category due to their broader spectrum than the amino-penicillins and because their use can encourage selection of multir-esistant bacteria. Rifampicin is increasingly used as an alternative medication for treatment of human MRSA infections in some countries. Gentamicin is also included in this group due to its importance in treating human infections, such as endocarditis.

The risk for spreading antibiotic resistance which can lead to treatment failure is even higher in the fourth category, which consists of third-generation cephalosporins, fluoroquinolones, amikacin and metronidazole. These antibiotics should be used with caution both to preserve their clinical effect in veterinary medicine and to prevent the selection of resistant bacteria with high clinical relevance and zoonotic potential. Metronidazole is critical in managing *Clostridium diffcile* infections in human hospitals.

The fifth category comprises the most critical drugs, namely the carbapenems, vancomycin and linezolid. Use of these should be restricted to rare instances of serious multiresistant infections, which cannot be managed in any other way.

A

Drugs prohibited by the United States Food and Drug Administration (US-FDA) in food animals (as of May 2015) are chloramphenicol, clenbuterol, diethylstilbestrol, dimetridazole, ipronidazole, other nitroimadazoles, furazolidone, nitrofurazone, sulphonamide drugs in lactating dairy cattle (except for those specifically approved), fluoroquinolones, aglycopeptides (e.g., vancomycin), phenylbutazone in female dairy cattle ≥ 20 mo old, cephalosporins (except cephapirin) in cattle, swine, chickens, or turkeys for disease prevention. It is well known that a lot of above mentioned drugs are freely used in food animals in India, which may be due to its cost effectiveness, ease of administration, efficacy against the suspected infection or just due to easy market availability.

Cost of treatment has major bearing on treatment outcome particularly in the farm animal practice, where it directly affects owner compliance. Consider a case of staphylococcal mastitis most of us would agree that amoxicillin sulbactum will be more effective than amoxicillin alone. However, former will cost approximately three times the latter one and whole regimen of three to five days will become unaffordable and in all probability, the owner will abandon the recommended treatment. Here, it is clear that we will get a poor treatment outcome in spite of selecting a better drug.

A

Adverse effects reported for common antimicrobials is given below:

A	A T
Aminoglycosides	Nephrotoxicity, Neuromuscular blockade, Ototoxicity, fetotoxicity
Beta-lactam	Immune mediated diseases & allergy, rarely acute renal failure
Fluoroquinolones	Chondropathy in growing animals, Retinopathy in cats
Chloramphenicol	Bone marrow suppression & aplastic anaemia
Macrolides	GI microflora disturbance (mainly by erythromycin), GI hypermotility
Lincosamides	GI microflora disturbance, Oesophagitis in cats (by oral clindamycin)
Sulphonamides /-Trimethoprim	Folate deficiency & anaemia, skin eruptions, thrombocytopenia and dry keratoconjunctivitis in dogs, crystalluria and functional hypothyroidism in dogs
Tetracyclines	Cholestasis and Oesophagitis (oral Doxycycline) in dogs and cats
Nitroimidazoles	Neutropaenia & CNS toxicity (metronidazole)

□□□

Chapter 21

Strategies to Control Ecto and Endo-Parasitic Infections in Dair Animals

itendra Ti ari Pradeep Kumar and Da a Shanker

Department of Veterinary Parasitology, College of Veterinary Science and Animal Husbandry, Uttar Pradesh Pandit Deen Dayal Upadhyaya Pashu Chikitsa Vigyan Vishwavidhyalaya Evam Go Anusandhan Sansthan, Mathura

---

Parasites are a natural component of the ecology, where dairy animals like cattle and buffaloes have evolved. Parasites need these animals for their survival and do not kill their host in most of the cases, however, during the infective phase of their lifecycle, they cause huge loss to the animal owner in terms of production losses. The traditional approach to parasite control in Indian perspective has been to wait until a clinical problem develops in the herd. By the time symptoms or clinical disease develops in a few animals, substantial production loss has already been occurred in the herd due to sub-clinical parasitism. In many cases sub-clinical disease can occur in a herd in the absence of clinically affected animals. Therefore, timely detection and control of sub-clinical parasitism is very much required to avoid losses.

Parasites of cattle and buffalo are broadly classified into ecto and endoparasites based on their position on or inside the host body, respectively. These parasites are usually controlled by chemical intervention using anthelmintic and acaricidal drugs. However, relying on drugs is expensive, increases the quantity of chemicals in the environment and intensifies selection pressure for the development of resistance in parasitic population. The emergence of drug resistance in parasites of cattle has been increasingly common and needs to be control before it is too late.

For strategic control of parasites and controlling development of resistance against the available drugs, alternative control measures including herd management, pasture management, herbal control, host resistance, biological control and use of natural dewormers are suggested by different workers. However, each class of parasites differ in their lifecycle, type of organ affected and their virulence. Therefore, before implementing an alternative control measure in a particular area, it is essential to have thorough knowledge about types of parasite present locally. In the following text, we will discuss about different classes of endo and ecto parasites and respective control strategies against each of them.

E

As the name indicates these parasites reside inside the body of the animals and thereby causing various types of harm. These parasites usually compete with the host for the ingested food or directly suck the host blood. A few other parasites can also cause mechanical destruction of the host s tissues like liver or lung. Most often, these parasites do not cause any typical clinical symptom or mortality in their host and remains there unnoticed for years making huge loss to the owners. On the basis of number of cells in the body, the endoparasites are classified into metazoan and protozoan. The metazoan parasites are further classified into phylum platyhelminthes and nemathelminthes on the basis of body morphology.

Nemathelminthes or Round orms These are cylindrically elongated parasites that seem rounded in the cross sections of the affected tissues of host giving the more common name roundworms . This is the largest group of endoparasites affecting a vast range of tissues of their hosts. Discussing each parasite, here is beyond the scope of this chapter, therefore, only the most prevalent and economically important parasites of cattle and buffaloes are enlisted here:

- Abomasum worms: *aemonchus, Trichostrongylus, Mecistocirrus*
- Duodenum worms: *Ascaris, Trichostrongylus, Nematodirus, Cooperia, Strongyloides*
- Large intestine worms: *esophagostomum, Trichuris*
- Small intestine worms or Ancylostomidae (hookworm): *Ancylostoma, Bunostomum*
- Lungworm: *Dictyocaulus*

Plat helminthes or lat orms As the name indicates, flatworms are dorsoventrally flattened parasites that resides the gastro-intestinal tract of their host. For better ease of understanding this phylum is further classified into class Trematoda and Cestoda.

Trematodes: Amphistomes, *asciola, Schistosoma*

Cestodes (tapeworm): *Taenia, chinococcus, Moniezia* (duodenum)

Proto oans : These are unicellular parasites that affect a wide range of host s tissues and thus, be classified into enteric protozoans, haemoprotozoans and tissue protozoans. The enteric protozoans are most frequently found affecting the cattle and buffalo population, especially the young animals. Enteric protozoan: *imeria*

H

Parasite	Infected Organ	S mptoms
aemonchus	Abomasum	Anaemia, oedema under jaw and abdomen, weakness, reduced weight gain
Trichostrongylus	Abomasum, duodenum	Same as *aemonchus* and also diarrhoea and weight loss
Cooperia	Duodenum	Same as *aemonchus*
Bunostomum	Duodenum	Oedema, anaemia, weight loss, diarrhoea
Strongyloides	Small intestine	Anorexia, enteritis, diarrhoea
Chabertia	Large intestine	Anemia, diarrhoea with blood
esophagostomum	Large intestine	Dark green diarrhoea edema
Dictyocaulus	Lungs	Sticky nasal discharge, difficulty breathing, cough
Moniezia	Small intestine	Weight loss
asciola	Bile duct, liver	Oedema, weight loss, diarrhoea
Amphistomes	Rumen, reticulum, duodenum	Enteritis, haemorrhage in faeces, foetid diarrhoea, anorexia
imeria	Intestinal tract	Diarrhea, dehydration, weight loss, anorexia and occasionally death

Control of Internal Parasites

The basic principle of a parasite control programme is to keep the challenge to livestock by the pathogenic parasites at a minimum rate. The development of such programmes requires a thorough knowledge of the types of parasites present, herd structure and grazing management, parasite seasonal availability and survival and the weather conditions in particular areas.

Control of Trematodes

Any method that reduces the number of host snails or prevents stock from grazing in fluke habitats will aid in control. Theoretically snails could be poisoned, but killing all snails is virtually impossible and the environmental consequence of using a molluscicide is unacceptable, as they are similarly toxic to other organisms in the same habitat. Strategies that can be used to reduce the habitat of the fluke snail include fencing off areas that contain the snail and providing alternate water supplies to the animals. Control of snail population by alternative methods like biological control can also be useful without any side, effect. Introduction of large numbers of ducks into rice fields after harvest can be an effective method to reduce the snail population. The ducks eat the snails and the fluke species specific to the ducks compete with the fluke species of ruminants in the infection of snails. It is reported that snails infected with duck flukes will not become infected with flukes of livestock.

The introduction of edible snail species like *elix aspersa* and *elix lucorum* unsuitable as intermediate hosts into the habitat of the host snails may prevent the flukes from completing their lifecycle. There are reports that some plants like *Thevetia peruviana, Alstonia scholaris, uphorbia pulcherima and uphorbia hirta,* have potent molluscicidal activity against freshwater snails. Planting of plants having molluscicidal properties along streams and irrigation channels can reduce number of snails in a population. Good drainage and the building of dams at appropriate sites in marshy and low lying areas may reduce the snail problem. Also, keeping livestock away from pastures contaminated with metacercariae and establishing proper watering facilities to prevent animals from drinking from lakes, ponds and streams might be helpful in controlling snail population in a herd.

Control of fluke within cattle requires the use of chemical drenches. The timing and frequency of drenching will vary between locations and seasons. In most situations, two drenches in May June and September will provide adequate control. The number of fluke-infected cattle can be reduced by treating cattle 6 8 weeks after introduction to at-risk areas to ensure the fluke lifecycle is not completed. Fluke drenches vary in the stage of the fluke lifecycle that they control. The three most widely used drenches contain triclabendazole, nitroxynil or clorsulon, however, only triclabendazole kills all stages of the liver fluke.

Control of Cestodes

For different cestode parasites, dairy animals act differently either as the definitive host or as the intermediate hosts. Cestodes like *Moniezia, Thysaniezia and Avitellina* species infects the dairy animals in the adult stages are considered virtually non-pathogenic. Therefore, specific treatment for these parasites is not recommended. In case of severe infections, it is advisable to modify the treatment and control strategies selected for nematodes to include the use of a broad spectrum anthelminthic that controls both tapeworms and roundworms. Praziquantel drugs can effectively control tapeworms and it is a drug of choice for cestode parasites. Control may also be directed at the intermediate host, the oribatid mites. It has been shown that the habitat of the mites can be destroyed by ploughing and where this is feasible, newly sown pastures can be kept free of tapeworms for several years.

Many of the dog cestode parasites infect the ruminants as intermediate hosts. Conditions like Cysticercosis, Coenurosis, Hydatidosis are frequently seen in dairy animals due to these parasites. To prevent infection of dairy animals, all final hosts, namely man (*Taenia saginata*) and dogs (*T. ovis, T. hydatigena*) should be treated according to need. In addition, humans should be educated in the use of high standards of personal hygiene to prevent the spread of eggs. Drugs which have shown efficacy against larval cestodes include praziquantel, mebendazole and albendazole. Control of cysticercosis and the adult tapeworms is, therefore, based on the prophylaxis of the infections.

Control of gastro-intestinal nematodes

The gastro-intestinal nematode infection usually coincides with grazing and seasonal changes. To control helminth infections, it is to ensure that rise in pasture infectivity, which naturally occurs as the grazing season, is reduced in an area. Move cattle from highly infected to minimally infected pastures before there is a major effect on performance. Alleviate the impact of parasitic helminths in cattle grazing infected pastures. For this mixed or alternate grazing with cattle and sheep can reduce the infectivity of pasture with host-specific nematodes. Early season administration of anthelmintics ensures that few gut worm eggs or lungworm larvae are deposited on pasture up to mid-February, by which time the majority of overwintered infective larvae will have died.

Assessment of risk factors and production losses caused by helminths in cattle and buffaloes

Risk factor	High	Medium	Lo
Age (grazing seasons)	1 year (First grazing season)	1-2 years (Second grazing season)	2 years (adult)
Weight gain (2 years old) two months after turnout	0.7 kg/day	0.7-0.8 kg/day	0.8 kg/day
Faecal worm egg count in weaned calves two months after turnout	200	50-200	50
Field type	Permanent pasture	Silage/hay aftermath	Newly sown, ungrazed
Snail habitats	Widespread	Patchy	Isolated/none
Faecal fluke egg count in adult	20	1-20	0
Fasciolosis diagnosed	Previous year	5 years previously	Never
Lungworm diagnosed	Previous year	5 years previously	Never

Coccidiosis is a disease caused by a microscopic protozoal organism of *imeria* spp. that lives in the small and large intestine of young cattle. Coccidiosis is most common in calves three weeks to six months of age. The most damaging coccidia organisms in cattle are *imeria zuernii* and *imeria bovis*. Severe infection produces profuse, dark, watery diarrhoea, resulting in dirty tails and hindquarters. Infected animals dehydrate and some become recumbent and may die. Recovered animals often have a long period of low food consumption and poor weight gain.

Multiplication and development of *imeria* in the intestinal wall damages the lining of the gut. The first sign of the disease is profuse, watery diarrhoea that contains blood, clots and shreds of intestinal lining. Affected animals become depressed, dehydrated and weak and show signs of sudden onset of severe, foul-smelling diarrhoea which may be blood-stained.

imeria cause few problems in unstressed grazing cattle. In most cases, coccidiosis can be prevented by reducing faecal contamination of the environment, minimising stress and risk factors. To avoid the transmission, unaffected calves should be moved to a fresh environment and consideration given to the provision of coccidiostats in the ration or supplement. All calves with diarrhoea should be isolated in an area, where contamination can be managed and treated. The principle reason for death from coccidiosis is dehydration. The first priority, when treating sick calves is to restore fluids lost in diarrhoea, and oral electrolyte solutions should be administered.

Tips for Integrated Parasite Control on Dairy Farms

Under typical farming conditions, cattle are frequently infected with several parasite species simultaneously, which can affect clinical manifestations, their impact and control options. In addition, the seasonality and epidemiology of different parasites frequently overlap, so it may be appropriate to address their control simultaneously.

Before planning for parasite control on a dairy farm, one should know about the type of parasitic infection present on the farm and when and how they impact the dairy enterprise. For controlling the parasites discriminate use of drugs in its proper dosing and route is usually sufficient. However, relying on chemicals is expensive, intensifies selection pressure for the development of parasite resistance and increases the quantity of chemicals in the environment.

Drug Resistance Resistance to antiparasiticides has become an increasing problem worldwide that suggests the change in current approaches to treatment and control. Important tools in combating the spread of anthelmintic resistance are methods of detecting it, while it is in its prime. At present, monitoring anthelmintic resistance relies almost entirely on the Faecal Egg Count Reductions Test (FECRT). This technique will be of great benefit to those responsible for managing anthelmintic resistance in the field. Resistance development at dairy farms can be managed following management practices given under:

1. **Promoting refugia level** : This term is used to describe the proportion of a parasite population that is not exposed to a particular drug, thereby escaping selection for resistance. Basically, this would entail not drenching a portion of the flock, perhaps 20 of the flock that appeared the fit. This allows the unselected worms to continue to produce offspring and dilute the effects of offspring of resistant worms from treated 80 of the flock.

2. **Changing anthelmintic groups** Switching to anthelmintics from a group with a different mode of action, when resistance has been discovered is another tactic. Using formulations that contain two anthelmintics, each with a different mode of action has also proved successful in extending the life of the combined chemicals. The genetic principle behind this strategy is that resistant genes are rare in the population, so it is extremely rare that a single parasite has genes for both the drugs.

Integrated Endoparasite Management

It is a method of controlling parasites in a population of animals by using a combination of chemical and non-chemical methods. Non-chemical methods include providing safe pastures for young, vulnerable stock, good herd management practices, best breeding strategies, appropriate biological control measures and ensuring adequate nutrition so that stock can develop immunity to these parasites. Integration of more than one measure, like scientific utilization of alternative control techniques and appropriate chemical control measures is essential to achieve the sustainable control on the parasites.

A. Herd Management

1. **eaning of Calves** The age at which young animals are weaned is an important factor in regard to parasite resistance. It has been observed that milk-fed calves are distinctly less infected by *aemonchus, Cooperia* and *esophagostomum* than the weaned calves. Ideally, females should calve during periods, when risk of contamination is low, so that young animals are exposed as late as possible to potentially contaminated pastures.

2. **Nutritional Management** Types of diet and availability of vitamins, minerals and other nutrients are directly related with susceptibility of animals to the parasites. Vitamin A, D and B complexes and minerals like zinc, iron, cobalt, sodium, potassium, phosphorus, etc. are essential in developing the immunity against parasites. The zinc deficient animals have impaired cell mediated cytotoxicity and T helper cell function. Cobalt deficiency promotes parasitism, as it is essential for vitamin B12 synthesis. Iron supplements are also very important, where animals are affected by blood sucking worms, like *aemonchus* and *Bunostomum*. The animals should always have access to mineral block and vitamin

supplements to compensate for the mineral deficiencies in pastures. Animals on low protein diets are more susceptible to infection because they produce less immunoglobulin IgA.

3. **Animal Housing** The animals having good living conditions resist or tolerate better against internal parasites as compared to animals kept under poor housing conditions. Animal shed having high humidity and low light favours the accelerated growth of parasites population. Water should be clean and free from faecal matter and watering areas should be situated in well-drained places with gravel or even cemented floors. Facilities of proper drainage in the animal shed reduce the chances of survival of the parasites. The newly introduced animals should be quarantined for 4 6 weeks and if required, administer the anti-parasitic drugs. Always keep the manure by making heap so that eggs, larvae, cyst, or other stages of parasites are killed due to heat generated during composting. The bedding material should be allowed to decompose along with manure for better control of parasites, as it acts as important source of various parasitic infections like *imeria.*

B. Pasture Management

Safe pastures are those pastures that have a low level of larval pasture contamination. Preparation of safe pastures requires good planning so that young stock can be rotated onto a new pasture every few months. These pastures can be prepared in a number of ways:

1. **Cross-species gra ing** The most commonly available method of providing worm-safe pasture is cross-species grazing with sheep and cattle. Each grazing period should be longer than two months and preferably six. Grazing cattle pastures with sheep from December to June has been shown to significantly reduce contamination with *aemonchus* and *Cooperia* roundworm larvae.
2. **Pasture rotation** It consists of dividing the pastures into parts of land of varying sizes called paddocks and frequently moving the animals from one paddock to another to optimize grass use. The objective is to not put the animals back into the same field until the risk of infection has diminished. Theoretically, this means that parasitism will decrease, if the number of parcels of land is increased or the rotation time is increased.

3. **Gra ing time** The drier the grass, the more parasites will stay at the base of the plants. It is estimated that in wet grass, larvae can be found over 30 cm away from the pats, whereas they venture only a few centimetres away, when the grass is dry. The risk of infection is greatly lowered by waiting until the dew has lifted or until the grass has dried after rain before putting animals out to graze.

C. Herbal Control

Several plants have anthelminthic properties, and were in fact a part of the traditional husbandry before synthetic dewormers were commonly adopted. These plants contain active principles, which are highly potent against parasites and therefore, can be used successfully to control a wide variety of parasites. Some of the plants with known anthelmintic properties are Wormwood (*Artemisia vulgaris, Artemisia cina*) Wild ginger (*Asarum canadense*) Goosefoot (*Chenopodium ambrosioides*) Common juniper (*Juniperus communis*) Crucifers (mustard family), Cucurbits (seeds of squash, pumpkins), Fern (*Dryopteris filix mas*), Tobacco and its derivatives nicotine, nicotine sulphate.

D. Natural Dewormers

1. **Diatomaceous earth** Diatomaceous earth is made from the remains of fossilized marine algae called diatoms. The product is mined and reduced to powder form. This powder acts as tiny pieces of glass that tear the shells of insects and other arthropods. Addition of diatomaceous earth in the ration of animals help in supplementing minerals and is also relatively inexpensive.

2. **Copper sulphate** has a strong deworming action against certain parasites, particularly *aemonchus contortus* and *Trichostrongylus axei*, which affect the abomasum. Copper sulphate is administered in a 1 solution in water, in the amount of 30 ml/ 22.5 kg of live weight for calves to a maximum of 100 ml. Likewise, Copper oxide particles (administered as a bolus) have been shown to reduce worm infections in ruminant.

E. Biological control

Biological control has many obvious advantages. For example, it is applicable to the range of nematode parasite species for all classes of livestock. It will provide the opportunity for livestock producers to capitalize on the increasing demands by consumers for chemical-free livestock products. Also, it is difficult to envisage the development of resistance mechanisms by nematodes to biological control. Nematophagous fungi like *Arthrobotrys oligospora* and *Duddingtonia flagrans* is now emerging as the most promising non-chemotherapeutic control option of nematode parasites of livestock. Practical methods of fungal deployment are now being developed, such as feed supplements, feed blocks and controlled release devices.

F. Host Resistance

Resistance to nematode parasites can be improved by selection, but only recently have efforts been made to include resistance as a trait in commercial livestock breeding programs. Host resistance is heritable and so, it is possible to make genetic progress in a breeding program. One of the most-widely used measures of resistance is faecal worm egg count, as it directly suggests the total number of adult parasites in an animal.

There is as much difference within breeds as between breeds. As a rule approximately 20 per cent of the herd sheds 80 per cent of the eggs onto pasture. Thus, selection of animals, especially the sire on the basis of FEC and further selection of their progenies for generations can be a fruitful tool for selection for parasite resistance. For example, in the University of New England flock, one sire had extremely low FEC in repeated faecal examinations and its progenies were also found resistant to the nematode infection. That ram named as Golden Ram was then used to develop worm resistant flock of sheep.

Ecto parasites Losses in livestock production due to ectoparasite infestations are huge. The hot humid climatic conditions of India favour the enormous growth of arthropod population around the country. Dairy animals in our country are frequently affected by a range of arthropod ecto parasites and nuisance pests, which can cause significant productivity losses and severely compromised animal welfare.

E

Ecto parasites of large ruminants are morphologically classified into two class *viz.* Insecta and Arachnida. Both these class are of economic importance as their infestation causes irritation, blood loss, nascence and anorexia to the hosts. Moreover, these ecto parasites particularly the ticks also act as vectors for other pathogens of the animals. The major ecto parasites of cattle and buffaloes are given under with their possible control strategies.

lies A wide range of adult flies may feed on the blood, sweat, skin secretions, tears, saliva, urine or faeces of cattle to which they are attracted. They may do this either by puncturing the skin directly or by scavenging at the skin surface, wounds or body orifices. Biting and nuisance flies can also induce avoidance behaviours in hosts which disrupt normal grazing and resting patterns. Flies may also be of importance because of the infestation by their larvae, a condition known as myiasis, but this is relatively rare in cattle and is usually only seen where there is a pre-disposing wound or skin lesion.

Lice Lice are permanent ecto parasites of their host, have populations that increase over winter and can survive for only relatively short periods in the environment. Four species of lice viz. *Bovicola bovis, inognathus vituli, aematopinus eurysternus* and *Solenopotes capillatus* usually affects the cattle population. Lice are opportunistic and heavy infestations usually occur in cattle already stressed from other factors. The louse infestation causes considerable irritation to the host animal. The skin reaction can cause hair to loosen and the cattle react to the irritation by rubbing or scratching, which may produce wounds or bruises that lead to secondary skin infections. Besides causing direct harms, louse like *inognathus vituli* is capable of transmitting bovine anaplasmosis and dermatomycosis. However, under conditions of adequate nutrition, lice have little or no effect on weight gain.

Control of lice infestation Treatment for lice is only suggested when more than two lice per square centimetre are present. It is not important to identify the lice species present, as lice control chemicals are usually effective against all species. A range of pour-on or spot-on synthetic pyrethroids (e.g. deltamethrin or permethrin) is available for louse control, with pour-on and injectable ivermectin also commonly used. Injectables may have only limited activity against chewing lice and are more effective against sucking lice.

Most insecticides registered for use on cattle are not active against louse eggs. This means that after treatment, eggs can still hatch and these newly hatched nymphs must be killed by the residual effects of the treatment. If, however, the residual efficacy of the product applied is short, less than two weeks, the newly hatched nymphs can continue the infestation. Where this is the case, a second treatment will be required.

Mites Parasitic mites inhabit either on the surface or inside the layers of the skin and feed on host tissue or associated secretions. Their presence often provokes an inflammatory response which results in intense itchiness and this, in turn, can lead to further tissue damage and inflammation. The clinical manifestations of mange are, therefore readily observed through the presence of inflamed skin, hairloss, inflammatory discharges, scratching and self-inflicted trauma. *Chorioptis, Psoroptes, Sarcoptis* and *Demodex* are the general mainly responsible for mange in cattle. Mite populations are highest in the winter and may regress over summer. Transmission from host to host is primarily by physical contact, but may also occur through contact with a contaminated environment (bedding, housing, trailers, etc).

Control of mange Treatment can be done by spray dipping topical application of nonsystemic acaricides and oral, topical, or injectable formulations of systemic drugs. Spray dipping is time consuming but useful for small herds. Injectable ivermectin in repeated doses for three times are also very effective in treatment of different mange except *Chorioptes*. Hot lime sulphur dips or sprays may be used with treatment repeated at 12-days intervals as needed, usually for a maximum of three treatments. Certain spray formulations of permethrin are labelled for use against mange mites in cattle, but it is generally not considered the compound of choice. Other available treatments for the control of mange, including flumethrin pour-on (2 mg/kg, repeated 10 days later), 0.3 coumaphos, 0.1 phoxim, 0.075 diazinon, and 0.025 0.05 amitraz.

Tick It is estimated that ticks cost the indian dairy industry in excess of 150 million annually. Heavy tick infestations result in anaemia, licking and rubbing at bite sites (tick worry), tick sores, ulceration, lack of energy, rapid weight loss and death. Ticks can also transmit tick fevers caused by *Babesia, Theileria* and rickettsial organisms like *Anaplasma*. Each engorged female adult tick feeding on a cow can reduce milk yield by 9ml and weight gain by 0.6g per day.

Control of tick infestation Tick control is difficult because the ticks spend most of their life-cycle away from the host, sheltered in the cracks and crevices of the dairy and at the base of thick damp vegetation. A reduction in the tick population can be achieved through pasture improvement, drainage and scrub clearance, although this is a long term exercise requiring sustained effort and when alternative hosts, such as wild ruminants are present population management is even more problematic.

Treatment and control Integrated control of ticks combines the use of tick resistant cattle, chemical treatments, tick vaccines and tick-safe pasture. In endemic areas, the mere presence of ticks should not be the trigger to treat with chemicals. Cattle can tolerate low burdens of ticks without losing production. Treatment is recommended, when there are more than 30 ticks on one side of an animal.

A range of injectable and pour on acaricides like synthetic pyrethroids and MLs may give protection. For effective control of tick population, these products need to be re-applied at regular intervals during the tick season to achieve sustained protection. Also, spraying in dairy is also recommended for the removal of life-cycle stages present there.

A vaccine against cattle tick (TickGARD) is available against *Rhipicephalus Boophilus microplus*. It kills ticks slowly, as they engorge on blood. The vaccine must be given every 10 12 weeks throughout the year. This requirement makes its use more practical in frequently handled cattle. Because of the strong natural tick immunity of *Bos indicus* breeds, the vaccine is likely to be more beneficial in *Bos taurus* breeds and their crosses.

I E

The clinical response and irritation caused by these arthropods vary widely between individual animals. Heavy infestations are usually associated with young or older animals in poor health. The selection of appropriate measures for the control of these parasites requires correct identification of the parasite, understanding of the epidemiology and life cycle of the parasites, assessment of the cost/ benefit of the intended outcome and an assessment of the current resistance status of the parasite to the insecticides and acaricides.

Animals are likely to be infected with a range of both, endoparasites and ectoparasites simultaneously and it is important to consider strategies that integrate treatment for individual farms, to minimise treatment costs and optimise impact. Low intensities of infection with some ectoparasites, for example lice, may have little clinical significance and eradication from a herd is likely to be difficult and may be unnecessary. Monitoring burdens in animals and spot treatment of heavily infested individuals may be sufficient to prevent infestations building up over winter and reduce unnecessary treatments of individuals with low burdens.

The use of insecticides is the basic procedure for controlling most ectoparasites, but alternative methods are also being developed to enhance the efficacy and reduce the adverse effects of insecticides. These methods are classified as ecological control (modification of the environment of the parasite), biological control (predation, parasitism, action of pathogens, etc.), genetic control (release of sterile males, hybridisation, genetic manipulations) and mechanical control (insect traps, use of repellents). The application of such methods depends on the biological and ecological characteristics of the ecto parasite, and they may act directly or indirectly, affecting mortality and/or reproduction.

□□□

Chapter 22

Creating A areness about Disease Preventive Measures Disease Data Collection Disease Reporting and Maintaining Biosecurit Provisions

Barkha Sharma Singh Parul and Udit ain

[1] Department of Veterinary Epidemiology and Preventive Medicine, [2] Department of Veterinary Public Health, College of Veterinary Science and Animal Husbandry, Uttar Pradesh Pandit Deen Dayal Upadhyaya Pashu Chikitsa Vigyan Vishwavidhyalaya Evam Go Anusandhan Sansthan, Mathura

---

India has a large animal population comprising, as per Livestock Census (2003), 485 million of livestock and a one-time count of 489 million poultry. Livestock plays an important role in India s economy, contributing (alongwith fisheries) 5.21 to the country s GDP and 31.6 to the agriculture GDP in 2007-08. The livestock sector has immense potential. It has emerged as the key driver of agricultural growth in the country.

The biggest impediment to growth of this sector, however, is the large-scale prevalence of diseases, such as Foot and Mouth Disease (FMD), Haemorrhagic Septicaemia (HS), Black uarter (B) in cattle, Enterotoxaemia, Peste des Petits Ruminants (PPR) & Sheep-Goat Pox in sheep and goats and Swine Fever in pigs, which drastically affect the productivity of animals. The presence of animal diseases also deters domestic and foreign investment in the livestock sector. These diseases not only wreck havoc on the existing stock but also constrain market access to our livestock sector, in spite of the fact that we have ample scope to participate in the global trade. The economic impact of the diseases in livestock results from both, morbidity and mortality and the consequent production losses. This includes the direct losses due to mortality, reduced production in terms of milk, meat, wool, hide and skins, as well as indirect loss due to abortions, subsequent infertility, sterility, and deterioration of semen quality.

A significant number of these livestock diseases can easily be spread to humans e.g. as food-borne infections, and to wildlife.

Infectious diseases are also a major cause of poor animal welfare. Within livestock production, it is too late to undertake actions only after clinical signs of disease have developed. Instead, a continuous focus on disease prevention is needed, which also minimizes the need for use of antimicrobials and any subsequent risks of problems with antimicrobial resistance. The importance of prevention is emphasized in the new EU Community Animal Health Strategy, which has been named Prevention is better than cure .

B R P

Correct Diagnosis and Appropriate Scientific Skill

All actions should be based on correct diagnosis. Basic clinical training and skill as well as access to qualified diagnostic laboratory services are, therefore, essential. In addition, the outline of a suitable strategy for disease-preventing health control and its implementation is specialist work that requires deep insights into veterinary pathology and microbiology and an understanding of the epidemiology and pathogenesis of the disease and of the situation associated socio-economic situation.

Recording of Disease Occurrence

Control and prevention of animal diseases also require insights into disease occurrence. A system for the monitoring and surveillance of disease occurrence should, therefore, be established. In health control at herd level, disease-recording systems can be based on observational results, such as the recording of lesions at slaughter or production data, such as weight gain, pregnancy and farrowing rate. Such data, despite often being of a non-aetiological type, are valuable tools as a basis for further evaluation of possible involvement of specific infectious diseases.

Strategies for Prevention and Control of Diseases

Total Exclusion from Exposure – Eradication

The most extreme and safest way to prevent an infectious disease is by eradication of the pathogenic microbe in a country or on regional level. The requirement for an eradication procedure is that the epidemiology of the infection concerned is known. An eradication procedure has to be based upon good monitoring and surveillance systems and associated reliable diagnostic techniques and capacity that allow the identification of infected animals or holdings. Access to management and technical infrastructure is necessary to stop the spread of the infection and eliminating its source is essential. Of particular importance is consideration of the requirements for preventing re-introduction of the infection, once eradication status has been achieved.

Partial Exclusion from Exposure – Prevention

This method should always be applied in animal production, at least for endemic infections. The concept is to minimise the microbial exposure to a level below the infective dose, or decrease it to such an extent that immunity is induced in exposed animals but no clinical disease develops. This limits further spread of the infectious agent from the primarily exposed animals to in contact animals so that secondary clinical outbreaks are prevented.

Methods empirically and/ or scientifically found to promote this concept are:

1. Optimising Hygiene

The application of basic concepts of hygiene, which can be defined as measures taken to prevent sources of pathogens building up and methods applied for preventing their exposure to possible target animals. In animal production, this should primarily focus on preventing exposure to the manure.

2. Isolating Sick Animals

The isolation of sick animals is a basic measure for limiting the exposure of excreted pathogens to neighbouring animals.

3. Avoiding Introducing Sick Animals into a Herd

For the same reason as sick animals should be isolated, they should not be traded or introduced into other herds. Transport itself is known to be a factor that can trigger the exacerbation of a subclinical infection to fulminant status and associated excretion of the pathogen.

4. Quarantine

uarantine is the isolation of animals that are either infected or suspected of being so, or of non-infected animals that are at risk. Animals should be introduced into a herd only if they come from disease free herds of the same or higher health status.

5. Test and slaughter

The productivity of animals usually is decreased, when they are chronically diseased. If a disease is infectious, affected animals can be a source of infection to others. In such circumstances, it may be economically and technically expedient to slaughter the affected animals.

Pre-emptive slaughter : Cutting of infected animals during epidemics is often accompanied by the slaughter of animals that may have been exposed to infection and therefore, be at risk of developing disease.

The blanket culling of animals on premises immediately surrounding an infected farm (contiguous culling) is a particular category of pre-emptive cutting that also aims to get ahead of the disease before clinical signs occur.

Slaughter of animals in epidemics is usually accompanied by other procedures designed to reduce the risk of transmission (e.g., disinfection, and destruction of carcasses by burning or burial) this is termed **stamping out** .

6. Vaccination

Strategic vaccination : These three strategies are applied in countries that do not routinely vaccinate. Vaccination may be deployed strategically to prevent incursion of disease from endemic areas. **Emergenc vaccination** is done to check the spread of disease, when epidemics occur using high potency vaccines. First, animals in an area surrounding an infected region are vaccinated to provide a circumjacent barrier against spread of infection this is **ring vaccination**. Secondly, a barrier, not completely circumscribing an infected region, may be created (**barrier vaccination**). Thirdly, vaccination can be practised both, within and around a region, where an outbreak occurs this strategy (which includes ring vaccination) is **suppressive or dampening-do n vaccination**. **Mass vaccination**

includes vaccinating every animal for a particular disease. This is done to control a disease in endemic areas.

Points to be noted during vaccination

- Animals should be in good health at the time of vaccination.
- The cold chain of the vaccines, wherever prescribed, should be maintained till the time of administration to the animal.
- The manufacturers instruction on the route and dosage should be strictly followed.
- A minimum vaccination coverage of 80 of population is required for proper control of the disease.
- It is beneficial to deworm the animals 2-3 weeks before vaccination is carried out for better immune response.
- Vaccination should be carried out at least a month prior to the likely occurrence of the disease.
- Vaccination of animals in advanced pregnancy may be avoided even though in most cases nothing untoward may happen.

7. Therapeutic and prophylactic chemotherapy

Antibiotics, anthelmintics, other drugs and hyperimmune serum are used (therapeutically) to treat diseases, and are administered (prophylactically) at times of high risk to prevent disease and thus, to increase productivity.

8. Movement of hosts

Animals can be removed from high risk areas, where infections are endemic. This control strategy is implemented in tropical countries, where hosts are seasonally migrated from areas in which biological vectors are active.

9. Restriction of movement of hosts

The movement of animals is often restricted during epidemics and eradication campaigns to reduce the risk of disease transmission.

10. Control of biological vectors

Infectious diseases transmitted by biological vectors can be controlled by removing the biological and mechanical vectors.

Biosecurity

Biosecurity is the application of management practices that reduce the opportunities for infectious agents to gain access to, or spread within, a food animal production unit. Biosecurity can also be extended to the national level, with the aim of excluding pathogens and pests from a country. During epidemics, biosecurity is also relevant to preventing infection being taken from animals on infected farms to healthy animals on clean farms. Biosecurity encompasses cleanliness, disinfection, reduction of exposure (e.g., maintenance of perimeter fencing, testing of animals before inclusion into a herd, isolation of new additions and diseased animals, and waste management), management of personnel (limiting visitors, adequate training of staff), and ensuring that animals can be traced.

Replacing Live Breeding Animals by Semen and Embryos

The genetic status of a herd has traditionally been improved through importation of live breeding animals. In most countries, this method has historically led to the introduction of a number of economically devastating diseases. Even if the risk for introduction of epizootic diseases has decreased as a result of international co-operation, this is not the case for the endemic diseases. However, this risk is considerably decreased, when the importation of live animals is replaced by semen and embryos.

Adequate Disease Monitoring and Surveillance

Control and eradication programmes require effective surveillance of diseases. **Disease surveillance** is an epidemiological practice by which the spread of disease is monitored in order to establish patterns of progression. The main role of disease surveillance is to predict, observe, and minimize the harm caused by outbreak, epidemic, and pandemic situations, as well as increase knowledge about which factors contribute to such circumstances. A key part of modern disease surveillance is the practice of **disease case reporting**.

Surveillance can be defined as Ongoing systematic and continuous collection, analysis and interpretation of health data allowing epidemiologists to follow in time and space the health status and some risk factors associated with diseases for a given population, for use in the planning, implementation, and evaluation of disease control measures . Monitoring is the routine collection of information on disease, productivity and other characteristics possibly related to them in a population.

Surveillance, in contrast, is a more intensive form of data recording than monitoring, and has three distinct elements:

1. Gathering, recording and analysis of data
2. Dissemination of information to interested parties,
3. Action can be taken to control disease.

In modern times, reporting incidences of disease outbreaks has been transformed from manual record keeping, to instant worldwide internet communication.

Organizations like the World Health Organization (WHO) and the Centers for Disease Control and Prevention (CDC) now can report cases and deaths from significant diseases within days - sometimes within hours - of the occurrence. Further, there is considerable public pressure to make this information public.

Disease Data Collection

Data collection is the core of disease monitoring and surveillance systems (MO&SS) and whenever data are used, the data quality is of great concern. As with any other data collection, if the data on disease are collected accurately and representatively and the MO&SS is designed to monitor the disease, the monitoring or surveillance may be referred to as active (primary data are collected). Passive monitoring or surveillance is then referred to when data collected for other purposes (existing or secondary data) are used. Passive data are prone to selection bias. Census data may be passively available for use of information system, however, the accuracy of these data needs to be assessed, before they are used.

Methods of data collection

1. Observation-clinical examination, postmortem, diagnostic imaging
2. uestioannaire
3. Use of documentary sources-clinical records, laboratory results.

Data obtained by first two methods is the primary data, whereas the data obtained by the third method is secondary data. A number of surveys, registries, cohort studies, administrative data, and vital statistics are used by different stakeholders to gather different kinds of information about diseases. A registry is one of the most powerful tools employed to record chronic diseases. There is great potential for the use of electronic health records (EHRs) as sources of surveillance information.

The data related to disease and associated factors are utilized for epidemiological investigation. nowledge regarding the suitable sources for a particular disease is very essential before collection of data. In well-developed countries, the data obtained are reliable and actual but this is not the case in developing and under-developed countries, where diagnostic infrastructure is lacking.

Data collected for health-related purposes typically come from three sources individual persons, the environment, and health-care providers and facilities. Moreover, data collected for non-health related purposes (e.g., taxes, sales, or administrative data) might also be used for surveillance of health-related problems. Because a researcher might wish to calculate rates of disease, information about the size of the population under surveillance and its geographic distribution are also helpful.

Sources of data

1. Government Veterinary Hospitals
2. Govenrnment Organized farms
3. Central Government Institutes
4. Private Livestock farms
5. Slaughter houses
6. Veterinary Colleges
7. Poultry farms
8. Pharmaceutical Companies
9. Private Pet Clinics
10. nacker ards
11. Government Bulletins

Nature of data : The data collected should be accurate, the right type, and unbiased.

Co-operation : The lack of co-operation can pose a problem to surveillance and other epidemiological investigations. The reasons for collecting information may not be clear to potential suppliers of data and so, they may be discouraged. Thus, it is very important that the objectives of data gathering should be explained to all who are involved in it. Motivation may be difficult to maintain in long-term data collection. Co-operation is also unlikely, if data collection is laborious or time-consuming, for example completing a complex or cumbersome questionnaire. Thus, the method of data collection should be as simple as possible within the constraints of the requirements of the data collection program.

Cost of data collection : The collection of data always incurs a cost, and this is particularly relevant to active surveillance. Costs include laboratory examination charges and postal charges, when the data are collected by postal questionnaire. The value of data, therefore, has to be judged in the context of the costs of collecting them.

Traceabilit : Refers to the ability to trace the history, application, or location of an item by recorded identification. Tracing systems have become a priority for national and international veterinary services. The starting point for a tracing system is animal identification, which has increased in sophistication with the development of electronic microchip implants both in livestock and companion animals, ruminal boluses, electronic ear tags, and genetic markers. Individual-animal identification, linked to details of diagnostic tests, movements and livestock holdings, then forms the basis of a system for documenting an animal s history and current location.

Disease Reporting in India

At present, an animal disease is primarily recorded by the veterinary doctor working in a Government hospital / dispensary on the basis of clinical diagnosis. This information is passed on to the Taluka / Block level and then to the District and the State veterinary authorities. Disease information is also generated from the disease diagnostic laboratories at the District, State or Regional level on the basis of laboratory diagnosis. Finally, information from State level is transmitted to the Central Government, i.e., the Department of Animal Husbandry, Dairying & Fisheries (DADF) in New Delhi. The DADF notifies the World Animal Health Organization (OIE) and other international organizations, as appropriate.

The present system of animal disease reporting is not satisfactory for the following reasons:

The disease reporting is neither timely nor complete. As a result of reliance on postal means of communication, the reports and returns take considerable time and some are also lost in transit. Hence, the compiled information does not represent true picture of the disease situation at any given point of time. The veterinary services available in the country are grossly inadequate. As a result, a large portion of the livestock owners do not have access to the Government veterinary services. These people rely on either the traditional systems of veterinary medicine or the private veterinary services. These incidences of animal diseases remain out of the reporting system. Their number is believed to be significant. In order to bring about desired change to the existing situation, a computerized system of animal disease reporting is being introduced, linking each Taluka/Block, District and State Headquarters to a Central Disease Reporting and Monitoring Unit at the DADF in New Delhi. This computerized system, proposed to be called National Animal Disease Reporting System (in short NADRS), enables fuller and timely reporting of the animal disease situation in the country, enabling its effective management.

N

A notification is the reporting of certain diseases or other health-related conditions by a specific group, as specified by law, regulation, or agreement. Notifications are typically made to the state or local health agency. Notifications are often used for surveillance, and they aid in the timely control of specific health problems or hazardous conditions. When reporting is required by law, the diseases or conditions to be reported are known as **notifiable** diseases or conditions.

Individual notifiable disease case reports are considered confidential and are not available for public inspection. In most states, a case report from a physician or hospital is sent to the local health department, which has primary responsibility for taking appropriate action. The local health department, then forwards a copy of the case report to the state health department. In states that have no local health departments or in which the state heath department has primary responsibility for collecting and investigating case reports, initial case reports go directly to the state health department. In some states, all laboratory reports are sent to the state health department, which informs the local health department responsible for following up with the physician.

The livestock sector has immense potential. It has emerged as the key driver of agricultural growth in the country. The presence of animal diseases has immense impact on domestic and foreign investment in the livestock sector along with economic losses due to morbidity and mortality and the consequent production losses. These diseases not only wreck havoc on the existing stock, but also constrain market access to our livestock sector, in spite of the fact that we have ample scope to participate in the global trade. To control and prevent the livestock diseases, it is very important to have continuous monitoring and surveillance of animal diseases. And the foremost requirement for any such work is availability of authentic and reliable data and proper reporting. The interpretation and collation of collected data is necessary to draw any type of conclusions regarding the morbidity, prevalence, incidence and mortality from the disease. As a result of the information that would emerge from this, it would be possible to develop disease forecasting models, leading to development of disease prevention strategies, ultimately leading to reducing the global burden of the diseases.

R

1. shirsagar DP, Savalia CV, alyani IH, umar R and Nayak DN (2013) Disease alerts and forecasting of zoonotic diseases: an overview, *Veterinary orld* 6(11): 889-896.

2. LeBlanc,S.J. Lissemore, . D., elton, D. F., Duffield, T. F. and Leslie, . E. (2006) Major Advances in Disease Prevention in Dairy Cattle. J. Dairy Sci. 89: 1267 1279.

3. DADF (2012). National Animal Disease Reporting System. User Manual, District and State level Users. Animal Health Informatics Division. National Informatics Center, Deptt. of Information Technology,Ministry of Communications and Information Technologies, Govt of India.

4. Christensen, J. (2001) Epidemiological concepts regarding Disease Monitoring and Surveillance. Acta Vet. Scand. 94: 11-16.

5. WHO (2006).Communicable Disease Surveillance and Response Systems: Guide to monitoring and evaluating.
6. Lefran ois T., Trotman, M., Gongora, V., Hackshaw, .H., alloo, M. and Pradel, J. (2012). Innovative strategies for strengthening regional animal health networks. Conf OIE
7. Dufour B. & Hendrikx P. (2009). Epidemiological Surveillance in Animal Diseases, World Animal Health, 2009, 386 p.
8. Willeberg, P. (2012). Animal Surveillance Applications: The Interaction of Science and Management. Prev Vet. Med. 105: 287-296.
9. Zepeda, C. Salman, M and Ruppaner, R. (2001). International Trade, Animal Health and Veterinary Epidemiology: Challenges and opportunities. Prev Vet. Med. 48: 261-271.
10. Thrusfield, M.and Christley, R. (2018). Veterinary Epidemiology. th Edition, Blackwell Publication, London.

□□□

Chapter 23

Preventive Care Measures for Dair Animals accination De- orming and Biosecurit

Barkha Sharma Singh Parul and Udit ain

[1] Department of Veterinary Epidemiology and Preventive Medicine, [2] Department of Veterinary Public Health, College of Veterinary Science and Animal Husbandry, Uttar Pradesh Pandit Deen Dayal Upadhyaya Pashu Chikitsa Vigyan Vishwavidhyalaya Evam Go Anusandhan Sansthan, Mathura

Milk production has become a way of life in India owing to involvement of about seventy per cent of small and marginal farmers and landless labourers in animal husbandry and dairying. It is a known fact that Indian economy is agriculture based and animal husbandry has the potential to increase the income of a marginal farmer to the level at which he can easily sustain himself and his family. In majority of rural households, women of the house holds are involved in taking care of livestock, empowering them by providing gainful employment in the area. With an annual production of 138 million metric tonnes during 2013-14, India has been on the top in the world in milk production since 1997. The main sway of the dairy cattle management should be to harness maximum production in the form of milk yield according to the genetic potential of the animal. It is important for the dairy farmer to adopt scientific practices that would lead to increased productivity at optimum costs to make dairying a profitable and sustainable venture and for this to happen, the farmer should be aware of the correct practices pertaining to animal health, breeding and feeding.

The novel goal of The National Dairy Plan-I (NDP-I), launched by the Government of India to double the milk production in the country by 2020, would require focused efforts in all the areas of livestock management to increase productivity at minimum cost. Indigenous Indian cows are sturdy with respect to disease and climate tolerance but they lack high milk yield as compared to exotic breeds. Focus should, thus, be to improve the genetic potential of indigenous breeds by increasing the coverage of artificial insemination (AI) using disease free semen from high genetic merit bulls. There is also an urgent need to optimize the utilization of feed resources in order to reduce the cost of milk production through balancing the ration of animals.

The paradigm shift from treatment of clinical illness to disease prevention in last 25 yrs is perhaps the single biggest advancement in dairy health. Only a healthy animal can be expected to give its maximum output. Diseased animal is a burden to the farmer. Thus, health management is the most important task in dairy management. It includes promotion of health, improvement of productivity, and prevention of disease in animals within the economic framework of the owner and industry, while recognizing animal welfare, food safety, public health, and environmental sustainability. Timely intervention is, therefore, pivotal in reducing the economic losses due to diseases but prevention is significant in harnessing the full production potential of the animal. Accordingly, disease prevention is no longer the sole domain of veterinarians. The combined efforts and best practices of nutrition, housing, and whole farm management systems are required to deliver effective health management and disease prevention. Veterinarians are, therefore, evolving from task oriented providers of therapy to advice-oriented consultants.

L H H

The relationship between the health of dairy cattle and that of humans doesn t need to be emphasized. A number of zoonotic diseases can be transmitted through these foods. Thus, the major goal of dairy industry is production of wholesome and safe milk and dairy foods. Milk is a potential source of zoonotic bacteria like *Salmonella, isteria,* and *Campylobacter.* The possible associations of Johne s disease in cattle with Crohn s disease in humans and bovine spongiform encephalopathy with variant Creuztfeld-Jacob disease, as well as the possible contribution of antibiotic use in cattle to the development of antimicrobial resistance in human pathogens are important concerns. Additionally, more indirect links between cattle and people through consideration of environmental or ecosystem health (e.g., fecal shedding of *scherichia coli* O157:H7) are likely to expand the concept of disease prevention in the future. Increasing indiscriminate and non-judicious use of antimicrobials has raised another concern in the form of increasing resistance to all the available antibiotics used for treatment of diseases. This antimicrobial resistance (AMR) can be horizontally transferred between microbes, animals and humans, as the genes responsible are generally located on plasmids.

Disease Prevention

Of late, focus has shifted from treating individual animals to disease treatment and prevention of diseases in groups, herds and populations. With the looming threat of bioterrorism and continuously emerging and remerging zoonotic diseases, roles played by environment and ecology have become a significant component of disease prevention efforts. There is renewed interest in eradication of neglected zoonoses like brucellosis, tuberculosis, etc., especially in developing countries like India and South East Asia and Africa, which are considered as hotspots for the emergence of new diseases.

Disease prevention in a dairy herd requires more than keeping cows up-to-date on vaccinations, controlling parasites and maintaining a clean facility. Apart from these important duties, emphasis on basic biosecurity measures and training of employees is a must. The health of cattle on a dairy is an essential part of good husbandry and a well-being program. An animal s well-being should include freedom from pain, injury, and disease. A dairy maintains the health of the cattle by providing appropriate nutrition, housing, disease prevention, and detection along with well-designed treatment programs.

Udder Health

Clean wholesome milk requires a healthy udder free from mastitis and other ailments. Thus, a continuous monitoring to check the condition of udder is required. Till now, Somatic cell counts (SCC) has been used as an indirect indicator of intra-mammary infection to monitor bulk milk quality. But emerging molecular and genetic techniques promise huge advances in the field of quick diagnosis of any infection in the next 25 yrs. Recognition of the importance of immune function for mammary and uterine health continues to grow. Prevention of retained placenta, metritis, endometritis, and mastitis through enhanced immune function are still elusive, but increasingly refined recognition of where to focus investigative efforts is likely to yield more specific and effective preventive strategies in the foreseeable future.

Calf Health

Improved calf health depends upon timely and adequate colostrums feeding, and swift removal of calves from the dam to calf hutches to avoid passing on of infections of adult animals to susceptible young ones. Best possible management practices (e.g., tube-feeding 4 L of colostrums at birth) and strategies to monitor management (e.g., systematic measurement of serum total protein prophylactic medication to prevent parasitic diseases) are needed to have healthy calves at farm. Health should be maintained through preventive care programs augmented by rapid diagnosis and treatment, when necessary. As per the standards, for any given dairy herd at any given point of time, the calf mortality rate should be less than 5 . All calves should receive colostrum or colostrum replacer and given healthy diet to promote health and reduce the risk of disease. They should be protected from seasonal weather extremes. Enough space should be provided for them to stand, lie down, and turn around without difficulty. Continuous access to adlib fresh water at least twice a day or as necessary to maintain proper hydration and adequate calf rations to provide the required nutrients for maintenance and growth (and to stimulate rumen development). Calves should be handled, moved, and transported in a manner that reduces the risk of the potential for injury, discomfort, or disease.

Good Science Based Animal Husbandry Practices

Most diseases can be prevented by the same measures that enhance production. Taking good care of animal health does not only mean treating an animal, when it is sick. It also means helping the animal to avoid becoming ill because it takes a long time for the animal s body to heal. Consequently, production losses may continue for long time even after the animal has seemingly recovered. Some general preventive measures are maintaining hygiene (Cleaning and disinfecting), free access to clean and fresh water, regular feeding with good quality nutritious feed, shelter for protection against bad weather (rain, wind and cold, or intensive sunshine), regular light exercise and a peaceful environment. Basic sanitation practices include keeping the surroundings of animal facilities clean, cleaning waste removal implements frequently, and emptying waste containers. Facilities should be free of standing water, excess manure, unnecessary farm items, and clutter. Some parasitic infections, such as coccidiosis and cryptosporidiosis, can cause serious health problems. It is recommended that a regular parasite control program to be developed. A clean environment is the best tool for combating parasite infections.

The goals of sanitation for animal facilities are to:

- Minimize animal disease through clean facilities.
- Minimize generation of odours and dust
- Minimize pests and parasites
- Minimize spread of pathogens

Animal Monitoring

Observation is the key to identifying health issues early in order to provide effective treatment. Animals should be observed daily to assess their haircoat, behaviour changes (includes vocalization), abnormal respiration, feed and water consumption, nasal or ocular discharges, manure consistency, locomotion and milk abnormalities, etc.

Inducting a new animal into the herd

Quarantine (Isolating the animal)

Any newly purchased animal should be kept in isolation without contact with the other animals atleast for 3 weeks. One should attend to the newly purchased animal only after attending the herd that too after a proper wash and cloth change. Routine deworming and vaccination should be done during the period of quarantine. For lactating animals, milking of the newly purchased animal should be done separately and, only done after the milking of all the other animals in the herd. The quarantine premises should be cleaned and disinfected before inducting another animal(s).

Testing during quarantine

All animals should be tested for Brucellosis, Tuberculosis, Johnes disease and subclinical mastitis before inducting into the herd, while in quarantine. If found positive for subclinical mastitis, they should be treated and re-tested till negative results are obtained. In case these animals do not become negative for SCM on subsequent tests, they are most probably chronically infected. If any of the animals comes positive to any of the above tests, it should not be inducted into the herd. They should be maintained separately and disposed off at the earliest. There is no cure for these diseases and these are easily transmitted to healthy animals on contact. An animal testing negative does not necessarily mean, it is free from disease.

Vaccination

Vaccination is an essential component of disease prevention plans and is most effective, when planned according to the particular needs of a farm. Strategic vaccination program includes determining what diseases to vaccinate against, when to vaccinate to get most protection levels and identifying who will benefit most from vaccination. Vaccination is necessary to protect animals from diseases, like FMD, enterotoxemia, anthrax, etc. Some vaccines can give life-long immunity against a particular disease but most vaccinations have to be repeated after a certain amount of time to ensure protection. Our country is endemic to many diseases that cause severe economic losses due to drastic reduction in the production capacity. Some of the diseases are even highly fatal. Timely vaccination on mass scale covering a large proportion of the susceptible population (at least 80) can easily control the targetted disease.

Following diseases can be prevented by timely and proper vaccination:

a) Foot and Mouth Disease (FMD)
b) Haemorrhagic Septicaemia (HS)
c) Black uarter (B)
d) Brucellosis
e) Infectious Bovine Rhinotracheitis (IBR)
f) Rabies
g) Anthrax
h) Theileriosis

Foot and Mouth Disease (FMD)

It is a highly contagious viral disease, which spreads through contact, contaminated water, feed and air, caused by aphtho virus of picornaviridae family. Disease is rarely fatal for adults but there is sharp drop in milk production, and fertility in females and draft power of males, which are severely impaired for life after recovery from disease. The disease is usually fatal in calves due to myocarditis. It also affects sheep, goat which are usually sub-clinically affected and may serve as maintenance hosts. Pigs are amplification hosts, multiplying the virus around 3000 fold. Animal suffers with fever, vesicle formation followed by raw ulcers, serous nasal discharge and excessive salivation. Vesicles may be seen on tongue, dental pad, lips, gums, etc. Vesicle in inter-digital cleft may lead to lameness. Lesions on teat may lead to mastitis. Loss in condition may persist even after recovery. All animals aged 4 months and above should be vaccinated once in 6 months. Infected animals should be immediately separated, since all excretions and secretions from infected animals contain the virus. All feed and fodder in contact with the infected animal should be destroyed. All equipment, used should be cleaned and disinfected with 4 sodium carbonate solution or as suggested by a veterinarian. Healthy animals should not be handled by persons in contact with infected animals. The infected premises should be disinfected with 4 sodium carbonate solution or with the disinfectant. Vaccinating sheep, goat and pigs would control the disease to a better extend. Since the disease is a viral disease, treatment is only symptomatic, the disease will run its course. Emollients may be applied on lesions to soothe pain.

Haemorrhagic Septicemia (HS) or Shipping Fever

This is an acute bacterial disease of cattle and buffaloes, which usually occurs during monsoon. Buffaloes are generally more susceptible than cattle. Mortality rate may be as high as 80 . Germs of this disease survive longer in humid and waterlogged conditions. The disease is characterized by high temperature, sudden decrease in milk yield, salivation and serous nasal discharge with a typical grunting sound emanating from the animal due to severe oedema of the throat region. There is difficulty in breathing. Death usually occurs in 1-2 days of showing symptoms, in case treatment is not provided. Animals with clinical signs, particularly buffalo, rarely recover. In endemic areas, most deaths are seen in older calves and young adults. Preventive measures include segregating the sick animal from healthy ones and avoiding contamination of feed, fodder and water. Crowding should be avoided, especially during wet seasons. Treatment is usually ineffective unless treated very early, that is during the stage, when fever sets in. Few animals survive, once clinical signs develop. Case fatality approaches 100 , if treatment is not followed at the initial stage of infection. Adjuvanted killed vaccines given to all animals which are 6 months and above of age annually, before the onset of monsoon in endemic areas will help to prevent the disease in the herd.

Black Quarter(BQ)

This is an acute disease of cattle characterized by emphysematous swelling usually in heavy muscles. Buffaloes usually suffer from a milder form. Contaminated pasture appears to be major source of infection. Healthy animals in the age group 6 months to 2 years are generally affected. There is sudden high fever (107 F-108 F) and the animal stops eating and ruminating. Characteristic hot and painful swelling develops on loin and buttocks causing lameness. Swelling sometimes affects shoulders, chest and neck also. When pressed, a crackling sound is heard because of the gas accumulation in the swellings. Death occurs within 24-48 hrs. of appearance of symptoms. At this juncture, swellings become cold and painless. Vaccination of all animals which are 6 months and above of age annually before the onset of monsoon in endemic areas should be done. Burning the upper layer of soil with straw to eliminate spores may be of help in endemic areas. Sprinkle lime over carcass at the time of burial. Treatment may be effective in initial stages of infection. However, in most cases treatment is not effective.

Brucellosis

An important zoonotic bacterial disease of cattle and buffalo causing loss in milk production, loss of calf, birth of weak or diseased calf, repeat breeding and even mastitis. Humans may also get the disease from consumption of raw milk of infected animal or contact with uterine discharges. The disease is very much prevalent in India, both in humans and animals. Abortions occurs typically after 5th month of pregnancy. In an infected animal, chances of abortion reduce with number of calvings. No abortions may be observed after 4th calving, but dam and calf remain infected. Placental retention may lead to infection and even death of the animal. Females calves (not male calves) between 4-8 months of age should be vaccinated with S 19 modified live vaccine. Only one vaccination is required in its lifetime to protect it from brucellosis. Any abortion from 5th month onwards should be suspected for brucellosis. Ideally, such animals should be culled. If culling is not possible, isolation of the animal immediately for a minimum of 20 days after calving/abortion is recommended. The aborted foetus, placenta, contaminated bedding, feed, etc., should be buried (at least 4 feet deep) after a liberal sprinkling of lime. These materials contain very high bacterial loads and if disposed improperly, cause the spread of disease by contaminating food sources (pasture, feed, water, etc.). Disinfect the shed after isolating the aborted animal. There is no effective treatment, once the animal is infected since the bacteria remains in the body of the animal. Disease in humans is curable provided proper treatment regimen is followed.

Infectious Bovine rhinotracheitis (IBR)

It is an important viral disease affecting domestic and wild cattle and buffaloes occurring in three forms : respiratory, genital and encephalitic, the first two being more common. There is a high prevalence of this disease in India, but vaccine is not available. It causes abortions, ROP, moderate reduction in milk production and even death in calves. Infection can be transmitted through semen. Coughing, profuse bilateral serous discharge from nostrils and pyrexia, rhinitis, conjunctivitis (one or both eyes) with profuse ocular discharge are major symptoms seen. In genital form, vulva gets swollen with papules which later become ulcers. Abortion is common at 6-8 months of pregnancy. Uncomplicated cases of respiratory and genital forms usually resolves in 5-10 days. Infected animals may carry the virus throughout its lifetime. The brain may be affected in calves below 6 months causing high mortality.

Theileriosis

It is a haemoprotozoan disease transmitted by ticks affecting mostly young exotic and crossbred cattle. Indian breeds of cattle (Zebu) are comparatively resistant. Buffaloes suffer with a mild form of disease. Typical symptoms are fever, swollen peripheral lymph nodes, pallor of mucous membranes, anaemia, nasal discharge, jaundice, salivation, rapid and shallow breathing. Cattle lose condition rapidly. Some animals show nervous signs characterized by stepping gait, head pressing, recumbency, unconsciousness and death. To prevent the disease, regular tick control is the most effective way. Treatment works only if done in initial stages. Delays may result in death. Vaccination of all exotic and crossbred animals aged 3 months and above, once in its lifetime is recommended.

Points to be noted during vaccination

Animals should be in good health at the time of vaccination. The cold chain of the vaccines, wherever prescribed, should be maintained till the time of administration to the animal. The manufacturers instruction on the route and dosage should be strictly followed. A minimum vaccination coverage of 80 of population is required for proper control of the disease to develop herd immunity. It is beneficial to de-worm the animals 2-3 weeks before vaccination for better immune response. Vaccination should be carried out at least a month prior to the likely occurrence of the disease. Vaccination of animals in advanced pregnancy may be avoided even though in most cases nothing untoward may happen.

Reasons for Vaccination Failure

1. Lack of maintenance of cold chain from the time of manufacture till vaccination.
2. Poor immune response in weak and improperly fed animals.
3. Lack of herd immunity due to only a few animals being vaccinated.
4. Poor quality of vaccine - uality will deteriorate, if repeatedly thawed and cooled.
5. Low efficiency or ineffective vaccine May occur in case of strain variation (e.g. FMD).
6. Presence of maternal antibodies.

There are certain other diseases which cause severe economic losses, but there are no vaccines available. A few of these diseases are self-limiting and proper care and treatment during infection may aid in recovery. Besides these, there are some diseases which are incurable and the only option is to isolate and remove infected animals from the herd to prevent infection spreading to other animals. The clinical symptoms are seen only later in the disease and animals can spread the infection before exhibiting any symptoms. These diseases include Johne s Disease (JD), Bovine Tuberculosis (bTB), Aflatoxicosis, Ephemeral Fever (3 day sickness) and Foot rot.

Biosecurity

Biosecurity measures prevent infectious diseases from entering a herd. By implementing general management and vaccination practices, animal herds can be prevented from endemic as well as exotic diseases. Good farm biosecurity practices are generally important in order to prevent the spread of disease within the modern farm animal holdings.

Some biosecurity measures to prevent disease spread by visitors at animal holdings:

- Use thoroughly cleaned and disinfected boots or disposable shoe covering before entering the premises.
- Clothing available at the holding, or protective clothing should be washed at 60 C as minimum before next visit.
- Hands are thoroughly washed after the visit.
- Equipment used in contact with animals, manure or other similar matter must be cleaned and disinfected before use on another animal holding.
- Conclude a health advisory agreement with a veterinary practitioner.
- Develop a biosecurity plan that outlines how the herd is protected against infectious diseases.
- Purchased breeding stock must be quarantined.
- Housing for piglets and slaughter pigs to be divided into sections.
- Veal calves must be inserted in stable sections, where the all-in-all-out principle is applied or alternatively in quarantine sections.
- Large sow herds and dairy herds may have upto three suppliers of animals per rolling 12 months.

Quarantine

Every farm should have a month-long quarantine policy for new arrivals or the animals leaving the farm for showing, breeding or emergency veterinary visits, before rejoining the herd even if the newcomers are up-to-date on all vaccinations. The feeding, cleaning and milking of quarantined cattle should be done at last to minimize exposure to the closed herd or calves.

Isolation

Immediate isolation of any cow or calf showing any signs of disease should be done. That means it should not have contact with any healthy livestock, including animals in quarantine. An animal showing signs of serious illness requires immediate veterinary care. Necropsy should be performd on any cow who dies of unknown causes.

Cleaning and disinfection of animal trucks

Vehicles used for transport of cattle, pigs, sheep, goats and poultry must be cleaned and disinfected after each transport. The driver must keep a log of the sanitary activities at all times. These procedures can be checked at slaughter houses, assembly centres, at animal holdings or at police checks.

Even on the best managed farms, unexpected health and production problems do arise from time-to-time. The best way to manage them is to detect them early. For that, surveillance programs should be incorporated in health and production management programs to monitor the problems before considerable financial damage has occurred. Better surveillance and monitoring of diseases along with a good herd management plan is essential to have the maximum benefits from a dairy herd. India has the world s largest livestock population with 58 per cent of buffaloes and 15 per cent of cattle. Owing to this huge bovine stock, though India has managed to attain *numero uno* position in milk production, the full potential of Indian milch herd remains unattained. Over the last three decades (1982 to 2012), average productivity of Indian cattle and buffaloes has grown from 1.9 to 3.9 kg per day, and from 3.7 to 6.2 kg per day, respectively. The average daily milk yield for crossbred cattle is better at 7.1 kg per day, but still significantly lesser than the best of global standards. Developed nations like U , US and Israel have per capita production at 25.6, 32.8 and 38.6 kg per day, respectively. The major causes of low productivity in India are both, intrinsic (low genetic potential) and extrinsic (poor nutrition/feed management, inferior farm management practices, ineffective veterinary and extension services and inefficient implementation of breed improvement programmes). Government initiatives, such as the National Project on Cattle & Buffalo Breeding (NPCBB) have contributed significantly to strengthening artificial insemination (AI) services. After all, these gargantuan efforts, AI services cover only 25 per cent of dairy animals. Further, over the years, emphasis has been on crossbreeding, with limited attention to improvement of indigenous breeds. Imbalanced nutrition due to lack of farmers knowledge about appropriate use of existing feed resources is also a major factor. Unavailability of high quality veterinary services, trained manpower and lack of mobility are an important constraint in acquiring the desired impact. An authentic, concurrently updated database for prevalence and emergence of diseases is essential for identification, onward prevention and control. A fairly large infrastructure of vaccine and diagnostic production units, semen stations and AI breeding farms, largely owned by the government, can be more efficiently utilised by way of appropriate participation of the private sector. There is a need for devising and implementing low cost technologies (for feeding, healthcare diagnostics, cow comfort and milking) that are suited to Indian dairy farming, thereby improving yields. Effective delivery of extension services is critical to achieve higher milk productivity. Extension activities also need to address farmer education on preventive measures, improved animal feeding and farm management practices. Currently, less than 1 per cent of the total plan budget for the animal husbandry sector is allocated for extension activities. Progressive farmers also need to be trained to act as extension agents for disseminating technical knowledge. A significantly spruced up breeding programme, efficient feed management interventions, broad-basing the scale and scope of veterinary services, adoption of superior farm management practices and an efficient extension network are the five pillars, on which the dairy sector shall be efficiently poised to achieve the full potential of the Indian dairy herd.

R

1. shirsagar DP, Savalia CV, alyani IH, umar R and Nayak DN (2013) Disease alerts and forecasting of zoonotic diseases: an overview , *Veterinary orld* 6(11): 889-896.

2. LeBlanc,S.J. Lissemore, . D., elton, D. F., Duffield, T. F. and Leslie, . E. (2006) Major Advances in Disease Prevention in Dairy Cattle. J. Dairy Sci. 89: 1267 1279.

3. Shome, R, Nagalingam, M and Rahman, H. (2012). National Control Programme on Brucellosis: Aims and Strategies: PD ADMAS. Technical Bulletin.

4. DADF (2012). National Animal Disease Reporting System. User Manual District and State Level Users. Animal Health Informatics Division. National Informatics Center, Dept of Information Technology,Ministry of Communications and Information Technologies, Govt. of India.
5. Singh, A. (2014). Common Cattle Diseases: Symptoms, Treatment and Prevention, Dairy ear Book. 77-85.
6. Christensen, J. (2001) Epidemiological concepts regarding Disease Monitoring and Surveillance. Acta Vet. Scand. 94: 11-16.
7. Heymann, D and Dar, O.(2014)Prevention is better than cure for emerging infectious diseases. BMJ 348:g1499
8. Park, J.H. (2013). Requirement for improved vaccines against Foot and Mouth Disease Epidemics. Clinical and Experimental Vaccine Res. 2: 8-18.
9. Rehman, H. (2011). Vision 2030: PD ADMAS.
10. WHO (2006).Communicable Disease Surveillance and Response Systems: Guide to Monitoring and Evaluating.

❑❑❑

Chapter 24

Livestock Entrepreneurship as a Means of Self-Emplo ment and Empo erment

Sanjeev Kumar Singh Amit Singh and ija Kumar

[1] Department of Veterinary & Animal Husbandry Extension, College of Veterinary Science and Animal Husbandry, Uttar Pradesh Pandit Deen Dayal Upadhyaya Pashu Chikitsa Vigyan Vishwavidhyalaya Evam Go Anusandhan Sansthan, Mathura, [2] Department of Veterinary Extension, ICAR-CIRG, Makhdoom, Farah

Livestock Entrepreneurship is a new applied branch, which enables the veterinarians to start their own enterprise. This branch primarily deals with the concept of livestock entrepreneurship, basic theories of entrepreneurship, avenues for veterinarians in private/ public sectors, essential qualities needed for livestock entrepreneurship along with the modalities for starting a business, different kinds of Indian institutes offering training programmes for entrepreneurship activities. This branch also offers information to a veterinarian in respect to preparation of a livestock project, preparation of financial statements of livestock farm and how to find out the worthiness of the programme will be elaborated in this programme. How a veterinarian can fulfill the expectation of their clients to run their business successfully is also informed.

The knowledge of livestock entrepreneurship among veterinarians not only instill confidence in their minds to start a new venture, but also highlight certain basic qualities which are essential for livestock entrepreneurship, i.e., in respect to preparation of a livestock project, to evaluate the techno-economic feasibility of various livestock projects, how to approach banks for loan and avail them, how to prepare financial statements (Balance sheet, Profit and Loss statement Cash-flow statement, etc.) of the livestock farm. Besides this, the vast knowledge of entrepreneurship enables a veterinarian to not only operate his farm successfully, but also enables him to enables him to stop its production at shut down point level.

There is tremendous improvement in the skill level of veterinarians, since this branch provides training regarding essential qualities required for being a successful entrepreneur. He easily identifies business opportunities underlying in the livestock sector, able to prepare livestock based projects for various livestock enterprises. Being a master and having thorough knowledge, he is able to assess the techno-economic feasibility of livestock projects as well as identify the financial worthiness of livestock farms. He is also able to make an improvement in purchasing various sustainable items for the livestock farm, besides successful marketing of its products by satisfying the customer needs.

In dairy farm economics, output is considered to be created by the amalgamation of various factors of production such as land, labour, capital and organization. In the production, process, each factor is rewarded, i.e., land is paid in terms of rent, labour is rewarded with wage while capital is paid in terms of interest. Therefore, an entrepreneur combines all these factors of production judiciously besides assuming risk and uncertainty linked with the production process and for this activity, he is paid in terms of profit. Thus, we can very well say that entrepreneurship develops a veterinarian to become an entrepreneur, i.e., an individual who has possession of an enterprise or venture and accepts significant accountability for the inherent risks and the outcome. He may also be termed as an economic agent who amalgamates various factors of production, such as land, labour and the capital, thus produces a product to earn a handsome profit.

Thus, this branch enables a veterinarian to become innovative and identify the market opportunity and exploit them rapidly by efficiently organizing the available resources to accomplish an outcome in the form of profit for its enterprise.

Entrepreneurial Qualities needed for Veterinarians

Before establishing an enterprise, a veterinarian must possess certain basic qualities to become a successful entrepreneur. Some of the essential qualities are discussed as hereunder :

Success and Achievement : The entrepreneurs are self-determined to achieve high goals in business, which strengthen them to overcome the obstacles, suppress anxieties, repair misfortune and decide expedient in order to run a successful animal husbandry enterprise.

Opportunit E plorer : A common criterion among successful entrepreneurs is their focus on opportunity rather than on resources, structure or strategy. This quality equip them with more profitability, as he immediately launches a new innovative product in the market as per consumers needs, interests and desires.

Integrit : Integrity and reliability are like glue and fiber that bind successful personal and business relationships and make them endure. Their innovative products are highly reliable and consumers have faith and full integrity in their products and purchase them with full assurance.

Optimistic and Confident : As entrepreneurs, they often face obstacles as well as down periods. During these difficult days, their self-confidence and optimism/behaviour helps them to get out of the crisis in a short span of time.

Risk Taker : Since an entrepreneur always faces uncertainties, hence, he always accepts risk. They always select a moderate risk situation, rather than gambling or avoiding risk. They very well know how to manage risks, without making its impact on their health.

Energetic : There is always a heavy workload and rising demands of the enterprise gave them a stressful life, but entrepreneurs willfully face them by maintaining their energy levels. Many entrepreneurs fine-tune their energy levels by monitoring their diet and follows fitness regime and relax their body at a particular time.

Opportunit E plorer : Entrepreneur always identifies opportunities. He seizes the opportunity with both hands and converts them into realistic achievable goals. It may be in the form of new product, newer methods of production or marketing strategies.

Perseverance : Entrepreneur makes efforts and works hard till the goal is successfully accomplished. They are undeterred by uncertainties, extreme risks and difficulties coming in the way of achievement of final goal.

acing Uncertaint : After launching an innovative product before the consumers, the entrepreneurs always face uncertainty. But their achievement orientation lends them to successfully tackle any unfamiliar situation. They go ahead with solutions for the problems even when the guidelines are not available.

Seek eedback : Entrepreneurs are quick learners and requires prompt and immediate feedback of their innovations in order to improve them continuously so as to cater according to the ever changing consumers needs, desires, taste and preferences.

Independence : Entrepreneur likes to be their own master and wants to be responsible for their own decision and never wants interference of others. An entrepreneur is a job giver and not a job seeker and don t want to follow others or being dictated by others.

le ibilit : As per the prevailing situations an entrepreneur takes time-to-time decisions in various activities of its enterprise. They never hesitate in revising their decision, which shows that they are open minded and not a rigid person.

Planner : Entrepreneur frames realistic business plans and set goals and follow them rigorously to achieve the objectives within a stipulated period of time. They plan meticulously and execute it.

Self-Confidence : Entrepreneur are self-confident and they direct their abilities towards the accomplishment of goals with the help of his strengths. Self-confident individual are usually self-assured of their personal judgements, their abilities, their power, etc. and have a positive belief to accomplish their business tasks.

Motivator : A distinguishing character which separates entrepreneur from the other individuals is his ability to motivate his workers. Entrepreneur influences and initiates their workers and enables them to think and act in his way. They can improve the productivity of their employees only by motivation.

Stress Taker : A entrepreneur always faces a lot of physical and emotional stress in day-to-day functioning of his enterprise. He has the ability to keep himself cool even under severe tense situations.

Self-starter : Being a master of his innovation, the entrepreneur has the ability to take his own initiative, work independently and develop his own ideas.

Commitment : It is the willingness of an entrepreneur to make personal sacrifices to work for long hours for the sake of its enterprise. He is totally dedicated and committed for his enterprise for maximization of his entrepreneurial benefits.

ision : Entrepreneurs know the path and direction they have to travel. They have clear vision of what their farms can be and go after it.

Team ork : Entrepreneurs always believe in teamwork and motivate it among the workers for better productivity and thereby profitability.

Self-Employment Avenues in Livestock Entrepreneurship

A veterinarian graduate after completing his degree approaches various channels in search of a job, i.e., in the form of a veterinary officer or pursues masters degree to get JRF or performs job in a private sector, etc. Besides this, there are other areas, where a veterinarian utilizes his degree to earn a handsome income. Some of the self-employment avenues are discussed as per below:

Livestock Farms

The veterinarians can start their own livestock farms with the help of their vast technical knowledge, i.e., they apply various scientific management techniques on their own farms. WTO (World Trade Organisation), GMP (Good Manufacturing Practices) and SPS (Sanitory and Phytosanitory) measures are of great importance for export of livestock commodities for maintaining the quality and food safety measures. If veterinarians start their own scientifically managed livestock enterprise, they can exploit this opportunity, since he is aware of proven scientific management techniques. He is the person who can better improve productivity of their animals, which would lead to overall quantitative and qualitative improvement of livestock sector.

Feed Manufacturer

The veterinary graduates being fully aware of balanced ration of livestock, they can start their own feed mill units for various livestock and poultry species. Demand for commercial feed availability for various unconventional poultry species, such as uail, Emu, Ostrich, etc. is less, but for other species it is a nice business.

Fodder Supplier

The main constraint which hampers the growth of livestock production is the inadequacy of nutritious fodder. As there is more than 60 fodder deficit in India, a veterinarian can purchase the fertile land and produce quality fodder and supply them to the nearby livestock farmers and earn a handsome profit. They can also start seed/fodder banks in the potential areas.

Farm Equipments Manufacturer / Dealer

A number of farm equipments are required for the operation of livestock farms enterprise. For example, in case of dairy farms chaff cutter, milking machine, feeding manager, etc. are required. Poultry farmers need debeaker, vaccinator, automatic feeder, waterer, etc. The demand for farm equipments is increasing day-by-day with the wide-spread adoptation of intensive livestock and poultry farming system in rural and urban areas. A veterinarian can either start their own enterprise for manufacturing of farm machinery equipments or they may also act as dealer for supply of such equipments directly among the livestock owners.

Dog breeder

Dog breeding is an ever green field with potential opportunities in urban and semi-urban areas. Dogs with good pedigree record fetches good price and the veterinarians can readily exploit this opportunity. Dog breeding can be done in association with veterinary consultancy services in urban areas and offers excellent earning opportunity for the veterinarians.

Hatchery

A veterinarian can also start its own hatchery, but requires higher investment in the initial phase, but offers good return after the business is well-settled.

Pet Animal Clinic / Large Animal Clinic / Mobile Clinic

It is the widely practised by the veterinarians, which offer them good earnings in both, rural as well as in urban areas.

Livestock Products Processor

Value addition to the livestock products, such as milk, egg, meat, and fish have huge profit potential. Value of the products get increased manifolds during processing and thereby provide excellent returns.

Veterinarians can start their own milk parlour, where they can sell processed milk and milk products like flavoured milk, khoa, ice cream, etc. They can also establish a meat centre where fried chicken, mutton khima, etc. could be sold. Marketing of this value added products could be done with their own brand name and they can start chain of parlours/hotels after successful launch of its brand.

Farm consultant

Livestock farm consultant is a lucrative avenue. Veterinarians with skill and knowledge can earn well in specialized dairy farms, stud farms, breeder farms, hatchery, sheep/goat farms. After some years of experience in managing such farms, they can start their own farms independently or with partnership.

Contract Farming

Contract farming is a emerging system, where the livestock farmers are given all the inputs, such as chicks/animals, feed, medicines, technical inputs, etc. Farmers have to rear the chicks/animals and the integrator will take care of the marketing activities. Veterinarians can join with livestock owners and venture into contract farming.

Leather Industry

Leather industry is so far unexplored by the veterinarians, since it offers great profit potential. The skin and hide from animals are usually purchased by the inter-mediaries in the villages at a throw away prices and are sold to the processors after taking a huge margin. The processors add value to the raw skin and make products and export/sell them at a very high price. The veterinarians can perform the role of inter-mediaries in leather industry.

Agents for By-products utilization

The livestock feed manufacturers and pharmaceuticals require several ingredients, such as bone meal, fish meal, blood meal, etc. which they are getting from the agents on contract basis. A veterinarians can also make intervention in this area. They can make a tie-up and could meet the requirements of feed manufacturers at a reasonable price and can also earn money.

Veterinary Pharmaceutical Industry

It is also a lucrative opportunity, but requires huge investment. A veterinarian may get exposure in the pharmaceutical industry and gains learning experience after some years, he can initially start a small drug enterprise with fewer drugs/medicines, which can later on be expanded according to the needs of the local farmers.

E O

A veterinarian can get skilled information in respect to development of an enterprise through various entrepreneurial development programmes initiated by the government of India. These programmes help the entrepreneurs in strengthening and fulfilling his motive by acquiring skills and capacities to promote and manage his enterprise efficiently and effectively. It also makes him capable to analyze environment, select and formulate a project, procedure of setting-up of small scale enterprises, acquisition of basic management skills, etc. Some of the entrepreneurial development programmes initiated by the government are discussed as hereunder:

National Institute for Enterpreneurship and Small Business Development (NIESBUD)

The National Institute for Entrepreneurship and Small Business Development (NIESBUD) was established in 1983 by the Ministry of Industry (now Ministry of Small Scale Industries), Government of India, as an apex body for co-ordinating and overseeing the activities of various institutions/agencies engaged in entrepreneurship development, particularly in the area of small industry and small business. This institute was registered as a society under Government of India Societies Act (I of 1860).

Enterpreneurship Development Institute of India

The Entrepreneurship Development Institute of India (EDI) was set up in 1983 as an autonomous body and not-for-profit institution. This institute is sponsored by apex financial institutions, namely the IDBI Bank Ltd, IFCI Ltd. ICICI Ltd and State Bank of India (SBI). It is also registered under the Societies Registration Act, 1860 and the Public Trust Act, 1950.

Indian Institute of Enterpreneurship (IIE)

With an aim to undertake training, research and consultancy activities in the small industry sector focusing on entrepreneurship development, the Indian Institute of Entrepreneurship (IIE) was established in the year 1993 at Guwahati by the erstwhile Ministry of Industry (now Ministry of Small Scale Industry), Government of India as an autonomous national institute.

Ministry of Small Scale Industries

Ministry of Small Scale Industries is the nodal Ministry for formulation of policy, promotion, development and protection of small scale industries in India. The Ministry of Small Scale Industries (SSI) designs and implements the policies through its field organizations for the promotion and growth of small scale industries.

Small Industries Development Organisation (SIDO)

SIDO was established in 1954 on the basis of the recommendations of the Ford Foundation of USA. Its role is mainly as an agency for advocacy, hand holding and facilitation for the small industries sector. It has over 60 offices and 21 autonomous bodies under its management. These autonomous bodies include Tool Rooms, Training Institutions and Project-cum-Process Development Centres. SIDO provides a wide spectrum of services to the small industries sector. These include facilities for testing, training for entrepreneurship development, preparation of project and product profiles, technical and managerial consultancy, assistance for exports, pollution and energy audits, etc. SIDO provides economic information services and advises government in policy formulation for the promotion and development of SSIs.

The National Small Industries Corporation Limited (NSIC)

The National Small Industries Corporation Ltd., is an ISO 9001:2000 company, which was established in 1955 by the Government of India with a view to promote, aid and foster the growth of Small Industries in the country. NSIC continues to remain at the forefront of industrial development throughout the country, with its various programs and projects, to assist the small scale sector in the country. The Corporation provides integrated technology, marketing and financial support to Small Scale Sector.

National Institute for Small Industry Extension Training (NISIET)

The NISIET, was set-up in 1960 by the Government of India and has taken gigantic strides to become the premier institution for the promotion, development and modernization of the SME (Small and Medium Scale Enterprise) sector. It is an autonomous arm of the Ministry of Small Scale Industries (SSI).

Small Industries Development Bank of India (SIDBI)

Small Industries Development Bank of India (SIDBI) was established in April 1990 under an Act of Indian Parliament as the principal financial institution for promotion, financing, development of industry in the small scale sector and co-ordinating the functions of other institutions engaged in similar activities. Since its inception, SIDBI has been assisting the entire spectrum of SSI Sector including the tiny, village and cottage industries through suitable schemes tailored to meet the requirement of setting up of new projects, expansion, diversification, modernization and rehabilitation of existing units.

T I I

The hadi and Village Industries Commission (VIC) is a statutory body created by an Act of Parliament (No.61 of 1956 and as amended by Act No. 12 of 1987) and was established in April 1957. The basic objectives of the VIC include the social objective of providing employment, the economic objective of producing saleable articles and the wider objective of creating self-reliance amongst the poor and building up of a strong rural community spirit. The VIC is charged with the planning, promotion, organization and implementation of programs for the development of khadi and other village industries in the rural areas in co-ordination with other agencies engaged in rural development, wherever necessary.

❑❑❑

Chapter 25

Undersatnding the light one and Point of Balance in Animals for their Safe Handling

ajuvendra Singh Rajneesh Sirohi and D.N. Singh

Department of Livestock Production Management, College of Veterinary Science and Animal Husbandry, Uttar Pradesh Pandit Deen Dayal Upadhyaya Pashu Chikitsa Vigyan Vishwavidhyalaya Evam Go Anusandhan Sansthan, Mathura

For safe and stressfree handling of animals, make sure the animals can see you. Do not make sharp, loud noises. Do not rush the animals. Use cattle prods and other equipment as little as possible. And yes, try to think like a cow, sheep, goat or horse. Step out of the human world and become a prey animal. If you think like a prey animal, pretty soon you start getting the prey animal to think more like a human. Therefore, it is important for farmers working with livestock to anticipate and understand livestock behaviour to minimize stress to the animal and to create a safe working environment. A common misconception is that low stress must mean no pressure. That is absolutely false. All animals respond to appropriate application and release of pressure. There are times, when significant pressure must be applied to get the animals to move how and when you need. Pressure, used appropriately, does not cause long-term, harmful stress. Animal reactions to humans and other animals are guided by instincts. Animal handlers must be aware of natural animal instincts to handle livestock in a safe, stress-free environment. Thus, a good handler must understand two key principles: (1) flight zone and (2) point of balance.

T

In simple terms, the flight zone is an animal s personal space. It is the minimum distance the animal will try to maintain between itself and any perceived threat. It is an area found with all animals, but most commonly associated with cattle and horses. Thus, a flight zone is a bubble like area around an animal that, if invaded by a handler, will cause the animal to move away (Fig. 1).

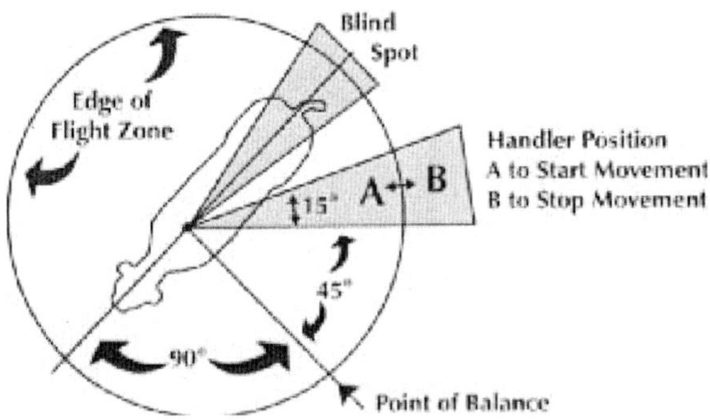

Flight zone of an animal

Thus, flight zone gives reason to the important concept of flight distance in safe handling of livestock. It can be described as a circle of safety around an animal, which reduces stress on the animal and reduce the likelihood of injuries to handlers as well as to the animals. When a person penetrates the flight distance/ zone, the animal will move. Thus, it is the minimum distance from an animal that a handler must maintain for the animal to feel comfortable. A good stockman knows when to penetrate this zone and when to retreat so that the animals move quietly in the desired direction. The flight distance may vary between animals the flight distance of a range cow may be as large as 90 metres (300 ft), while a feedlot animal has a flight zone of between 1.5 and 7.5 metres (5 and 25 ft.). Thus, a dairy cow that is accustomed to human interaction on a daily basis has a smaller flight zone than an animal out on the range. The flight distance is also affected by handling techniques bad experiences with a handler will result in an increased flight zone. An understanding of the flight zone will allow handlers to move animals calmly and safely.

The flight distance is smaller along the side of the animal, whereas, it is larger when the animal is faced head on. The flight zone of the animal remains surrounded with a pressure zone. The pressure zone is an area around the flight zone which when is intruded, creates a psychological pressure on the animal and it becomes alert without creating any attempt to fly away until and unless the intruder trespasses the outer boundry of flight zone (Fig. 2).

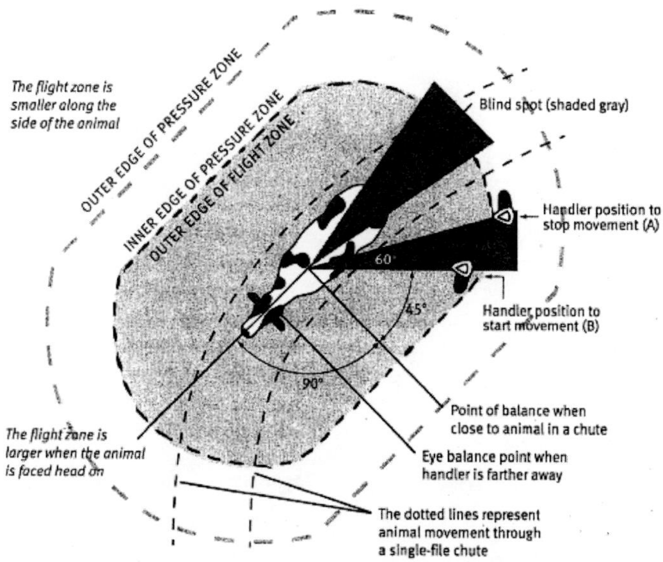

Flight and pressure zone of an animal

Point of Balance

Point of balance is a factor related to flight zone, and working with a cow s point of balance will also help you move a cow more safely (Fig. 2). The point of balance is located at the cow s shoulder, at which pressure in front of that point will cause the animal to stop or back up, and vice versa. To move a cow forward, you should be positioned behind its shoulder. If you need to move the animal backward, position yourself in front of the shoulder. Whether moving a cow forward or backward, work at the edge of the cow s flight zone and at angle of 45 to 60 so that you stay within the animal s field of vision, which is known as **Handler s Movement one** (Fig. 3). If the handler is positioned at a point located at 90 from the longitudinal axis of the animal, will not move in either direction.

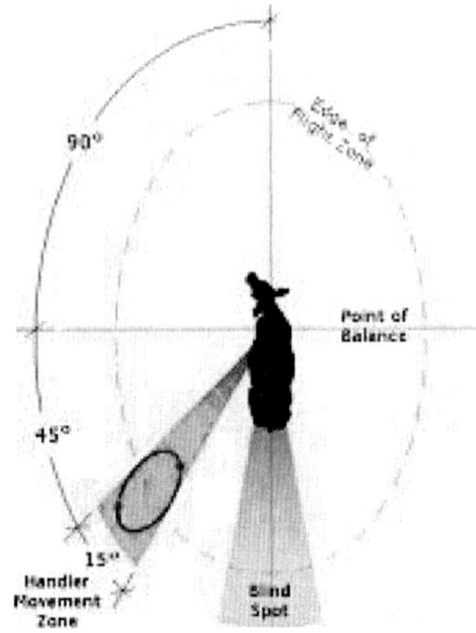

Point of balance and handler movement zone

To move a single man forward, the handler must be behind the point of balance and stay out of the blind spot directly behind the animal. When handler is close to the animal, the point of balance is at the shoulder. When the handler is farther away, the point of balance may move forward to just behind the eyes. When the handler is at the outer edge of the pressure zone, the animal becomes aware of the handler s presence and turns around and looks. When the outermost edge of the flight zone is penetrated, the animal moves away.

Blind Spot

Large animals have a blind spot on the front along with a binocular vision area. They have monocular vision area on their both the sides. The angle of binocular and monocular area varies as per the different species of animals. Large animals also have a blind spot located directly behind them. Animals cannot see the objects in this area and will usually kick, if they become aware of any activity in this area (Fig. 4).

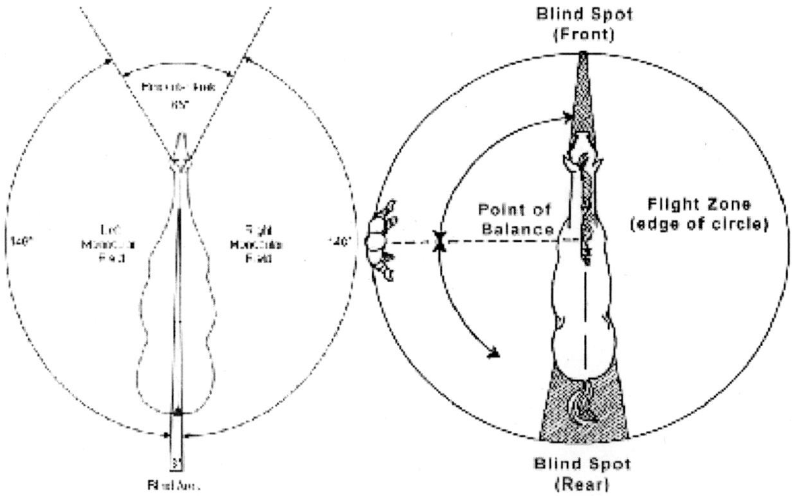

Visual fields and blind spots of an animal

Using the concept of flight zone and point of balance in animal handling

The handler s body position should always be relative to the animal s personal space and point of balance. An animal will respond to an invasion of its personal space. The approaching pressure will affect the animal s reaction to the handler. When an animal becomes stressed, it takes 20 to 30 minutes to calm down.

By using the point of balance, animals can be easily moved in desired directions without stress. When a handler is outside the flight zone but inside pressure zone, the animal will turn and face the handler to understand his or her intentions. All species of livestock will move forward, if the handler stands behind the point of balance. They will back up, if the handler stands in front of the point of balance. Many handlers make the mistake of standing in front of the point of balance, while attempting to make an animal move forward in a chute. Groups of livestock will often move forward without prodding, when the handler walks past the point of balance in the opposite direction of each animal in the chute. If the animals are moving by themselves, leave them alone. When a stockman is at the edge of the flight zone and properly balanced, only slight movements are needed to control the animals in a low-stress manner. To make animals speed up, walk against their direction of travel to make them slow down, walk with them. As you pass the point of balance, notice how each animal responds to your movement and position.

A good stockman will stay quiet, when working livestock. If animals are not doing what you want, it is not because they can t hear or see you. It is because you are in the wrong place doing the wrong thing. Do not yell and scream, and do not make wild movements. Move calmly, purposefully and in straight lines. Livestock will be able to predict your movements and respond accordingly. If you move like a predator (hesitating, followed by sudden movements and in curves around them), the livestock will treat you like a predator.

The most important aspect of handling any livestock is to be able to recognize and interpret an animal s reactions. The animal s body language will indicate its probable actions. Livestock remain immobile, when first threatened. Their first reaction is to stand and assess the situation. If frightened, their natural instinct is to escape. Livestock try to maintain other animals within their vision. They have a field of view of 300-330 degrees and have the ability to see threats from almost all directions.

Social order in the herd is usually established at an early age and maintained by threats and butting. When herds are mixed, social order has to be re-established, so aggression occurs until a new order is established. This may hinder movement of stock. Within a herd, there is an order of dominance. This can be seen in action at the water or feed through, where certain animals are always first to drink or eat. Other animals tend to stand back until the dominant animals have finished. Dominance may also be seen, when livestock are on the move. The same animals will usually lead the herd. They will also be the first to enter gateways. Crowding will also increase aggression as the animals try to maintain personal space. Social behaviour varies with age, breed and sex Bos indicus and Bos indicus cross cattle are more sensitive/temperamental than British or European breeds.

Arousal is the state of activity of animals and ranges from deep sleep to fight/flight. Handling techniques raise the level of arousal. However, if you control the level of arousal, you control the animal. Problems occur, when this arousal is too high. Highly aroused (stirred up) animals are more likely to make sudden violent movements, and they behave in a self-protective way either by running away or fighting back. Highly aroused animals are also more responsive to further stimulation (a mature bull, ram or buck which is highly aroused needs little provocation to attack). It is desirable to keep animals as calm as possible, so they can move quietly. When necessary, however, handlers may temporarily raise arousal for particular purposes, such as forcing lead animals through a gateway.

The usefulness of instinctive (natural) behaviour is that it is predictable and requires no training of the animals. The instinct to escape is helpful, when handling livestock that are raised under extensive conditions and have little contact with people. With infrequently handled animals that are flighty and have less chance of learning the flow system of paddocks and yards, instinctive behaviour is used so that animals escape to where you want them to be. To do this, the stockperson must learn the rules of position and movement. A person moving alongside animals at just the right moment can turn a herd exactly when needed, but someone positioned wrongly can cause havoc (Fig. 5).

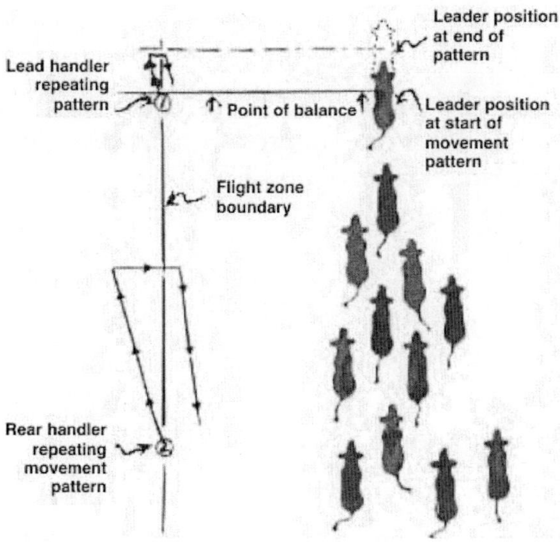

Working pattern of handler to keep animals calm and move them easily

Livestock move most effectively, if they can see the handler at all times. Attempting to drive animals by standing directly behind them is often not efficient because they turn and look at the handler. An animal is best driven (forward), when the handler is situated at a 45-60 degree angle from a line perpendicular to an animal s shoulder. This same principle applies to driving herds of animals. The flight distance varies with the tameness of the animal. The distance may be larger for feral animals and smaller for animals handled oftenly. Very tame animals are difficult to move because they no longer have a flight zone. If a handler shouts and excites them, this can enlarge the animals flight zone. A good stockman is patient. eep doing the right things until the animals respond correctly. After you have mastered the art of stockmanship, you can usually move animals quickly, when you need to. But realize that if you make livestock do something before they are ready to do it, then it is no longer low-stress handling. Train livestock how to behave every time you are with them. Go to the pen or pasture and use these techniques to just move them around, teaching them to respond. If possible, move livestock on their way to feed or to another pasture. Always make your livestock walk past a gate. Do not let them run wildly, or they will hurt themselves and you, tear up your gates and be stressed, when they finally stop. When moving livestock from a pasture, ignore the few animals that may quit the herd. If you drive the main herd in a low-stress manner and do not chase the few on the edge, they will usually come back to the herd of their own will.

Ranchers who do not follow these guidelines and rush their animals, harass them with noise or prod them unnecessarily risk raising their stress, increasing sickness and lowering production. The basic elements of animal handling are the handler, the stock and the facilities. These elements are all inter-dependent. An understanding of these dependencies is essential for continued improvement in livestock handling. Research and practical observations have identified factors pertinent to each element. These are as follows:

1. Handler

Desirable attributes for handlers are a positive attitude to stock, an understanding of animal behaviour, the ability to recognize and interpret animal actions, and allowing sufficient time for operations. Visual thinking skills are essential to horse training and livestock handling.

2. Livestock

Livestock differ in their ease of handling due to factors including previous experiences, breed characteristics, sex and physiological state. Animals think by visual association.

3. Facilities

Poorly designed or maintained facilities can lead to confusion and stress on livestock. There is a higher incidence of stress and injury to both, stock and handlers in a poorly constructed facility. The basic element of design is to allow for good stock flow. The larger the facility and the more diverse the livestock history, the more important it is to correctly design the facility.

Since humans are predators, it is imperative that we understand how livestock think, react and communicate as a herd. Armed with this knowledge, we can guide animals to a chosen location and reduce stress of handling in confined areas without invoking fear from the livestock.

R

Grandin, Temple, and Catherine Johnson. Animals in Translation. Orlando: Harcourt Inc., 2006.

Grandin, Temple. Behavioural Principles of Livestock Handling. Professional Animal Scientist, December 1989, pages 1-11, American Registry of Professional Animal Scientists.

Grandin, Temple. Thinking the Way Animals Do, Western Horseman, November 1997, pp. 140-145.

Grandin, Temple. Livestock Handling and Transport, 1993 CAB International, Walling-ford Oxon, United ingdom.

Smith, Burt. Moving Em. A Guide to Low Stress Animal Handling. Hawaii: The Graziers Hui, 1998.

❑❑❑

Chapter 26

Basic Bod Scoring in Selection and Purchase of Animals

Sat endra Pal Singh Madhu Ti   ari and Deepak Sharma

Department of Animal Genetics and Breeding, College of Veterinary Science and Animal Husbandry, Uttar Pradesh Pandit Deen Dayal Upadhyaya Pashu Chikitsa Vigyan Vishwavidhyalaya Evam Go Anusandhan Sansthan, Mathura

Body scoring is a means of accurately determining body condition of dairy cows, independent of body weight and frame size. It is very important in assessing the health status of an animal. It is an important criterion for purchasing of new animal in the farm.

P

Choice of Breed

The type of breed farmers want to rear depends on the ways and means available with the livestock owner and the fitness of the breed to the local environment. The already existing breed on your farm is usually the best choice. The breed that is most popular in the community is usually the one that has proven most profitable for the area. The choice or the breed is liked best, should be taken seriously after one has studied and learned about the breeds.

Source of animals

Animal should only be purchased from farms known to conduct regular TB, JD and brucellosis and positive animals removed periodically. It is always good to purchase animals from the owners farm complex rather than from cattle markets as probability of the animal being infected to diseases is more at these places.

Observe following general signs before purchase

E es Crusty or bloodshot eyes with runny (discharges) should be avoided and animal with bright and clear eyes should be selected.

Nose Cool, moist muzzle, with frequent licking breathing should be regular and not laboured beware of discharge, coughing, wheezing or irregular breathing.

Coat Clean and un-matted shiny coat, absence of ticks/lice, other parasites.

eight Prescribed mean weight for the breed don t purchase week or debilitated animals.

Attitude Contended and curious and always alert animal to be purchased should not stand apart from the herd bad temperament animal should be avoided.

Mobilit Limps while walking are unacceptable unbalanced gaits or hunched posture, when sitting are also undesirable rising process from seated state should be with ease.

Udder Healthy size does not always matters animals having prominent milk veins, udder seated forward and not too meaty. While walking, it should not sway much on sides.

Bod score This is an important indicator of the health of the animal. A body score between 3-4 indicates that animal is in good health.

Histor Detailed history of the animal is required while purchasing an elite animal on number of calving, previous year total lactation yield. Animal history should be checked for any certain disease incidences, like hypocalcaemia, mastitis, ROP, dystocia, prolapse of uterus, etc.

Age Though not directly related to health, the farmer should also ensure the age of the animal by referring to its dentition.

Selection of animal before purchase

Judging of an animal in cattle show is an art. It is better to raise own herd by breeding his own animals. Important guidelines for selection of dairy cows are as follows :

- Always purchase an animal based upon its breed characters and milk producing ability from cattle fairs.
- To know the complete history of animal one must purchase an animal with availability of pedigree sheet.
- The maximum yield by dairy cows is noticed during the first five lactations. Farmer should always select the animals of first or second lactation and having a month old calf at foot.
- To check the production by a particular animal, it is advised to do three complete milking.
- A docile cow should be purchased so as to felicitate the easy milking by any one.
- It is better to purchase the animals during the months of October and November.
- Peak yield can be reached around 90 days after calving, then it starts decreasing.

Breed characteristics of high yielding dairy cows

- Attractive, feminine and animal with vigorous qualities should be selected.
- Animal body should have balanced and even blending of all parts, it should carry an impressive style and carriage.
- Proportionate wedge shaped appearance of the body is preferred.
- It should have bright eyes with lean neck.
- A good udder is evenly attached to the abdomen.
- Animals having fine network of blood vessels on skin of udder should be selected.
- All four quarters of the udder should be well-demarcated with well placed teats.

Selecting animals for Commercial Dairy Farm - Suggestions

- Under Indian scenario one can find a commercial dairy farm consisting of minimum twenty animals (ten cows, ten buffaloes) and this strength can easily go upto hundred animals divided in ratio of 50:50 or 40:60. Always carry a SWOT (strength, weakness, opportunity and threats) analysis before planning for an expansion of your existing dairy farm.

- Most of the middle income household prefers low fat milk. It is always good to go for a commercial farm and have mixed type milk (Indian/Crossbred cows and buffaloes kept in separate rows under one shed).
- Conduct a thorough study of the immediate market, where you are planning to market your milk. Mixed milk of cow and buffalo after standardization can be sold as per needs of market. Local customers and hotels give more preference to pure buffalo milk. Hospitals, and patients, and families with infants prefer cow s milk.
- Good quality cows are available in the market or their native tract and its cost according to its production, lactation number and breed type.
- They are more docile and can be handled easily. Good milk yielding Indian breeds (Sahiwal, Tharparkar and Gir) and crossbreds (Holstein and Jersey crosses) have well-adapted to Indian climate.
- The fat percentage of cow s milk varies from 3.0-5.0 and is lower than Buffaloes (6.0).
- In India, there are good buffalo breeds like Murrah and Nili ravi, which are suitable for commercial dairy farm.
- Some farmers don t sell milk directly to customers, but they go for Ghee (butter oil) and butter preparation for fetching good price from customers, buffalo milk is preferred for these preparations. Buffalo milk is also a choice for making tea, a welcoming drink prepared in every Indian household.
- Buffaloes have ability to thrive on more fibrous crop residues hence, there is a chance for lessening the feed cost involved.
- Buffaloes maximally mature late have inter-calving period of 16 to 18 months. It is known that male buffalo calves earn little value.
- Showers/foggers with fan are must for buffaloes, as they lack natural cooling, that s why buffaloes love to wallow in mud and water tanks.

Steps in selecting a dairy animal

Following steps should be followed in selecting a dairy animal:

- Breed character
- Body confirmation
- Body weight
- Ancestors performance
- Reproduction capacity
- Health condition
- Age
- No. of lactations
- Past performance of the animal
- Free of chronic disease
- Cleanliness of teeth
- Legs and toes free of injuries
- Good eye sight
- Whether animal is dry or lactating
- Date of delivery
- Month of pregnancy
- If non-pregnant, how many times it came into heat
- Animal should follow owners, instructions
- The udder should be in good shape and easy to milk

The animal should not have the following:

- Poor growth
- Late maturity
- Not coming into heat
- Repeat breeder
- Long gap between two lactations
- Incurable chronic diseases
- Retained placenta
- Low milk production
- Unable to give milk without calf

Body Condition Scoring (BCS)

The body condition scoring is an intuitive appraisal of the energy deposit in adipose tissues of a dairy animal. It is an acceptable, non-invasive, quick and inexpensive method to estimate degree of fatness. A less score might be an indication of ailments or malnutrition, while a high score may indicate high chances of breeding and metabolic complications.

Body Score 1

- These animals are extremely thin, no fat in brisket or tail dock.
- All skeletal structure is visible.
- Hairs are very coarse and dull.
- These animals may be diseased and survival during stress is doubtful.

Body Score 2

- These animals are thin. Vertebrae, hips and pin bone are prominent.
- In these animals, some tissue covers around tail dock, hip bones and the flanks.
- Muscle tissue evident, but not abundant,
- These animals look healthy, but in well condition.

Body Score 3

- These animals having only slightly visible ribcage. Hook and pin bone visible, but not prominent.
- Fat deposit behind shoulder and brisket area.
- This body condition is ideal for calving.

Body Score 4

- Skeletal structure difficult to identify.
- Obvious fat deposits behind shoulder and tail head.
- Flat appearance to the top line.
- Folds of fat starting to develop over ribs and thighs.

Body Score 5

- Animal is obese, flat appearance dominates.
- Brisket should be heavy and bone structure not noteable.
- A fold of fat should encompass the tail head and hip bones completely a flat back layered completely with fat
- Mobility impaired by large fat deposits.

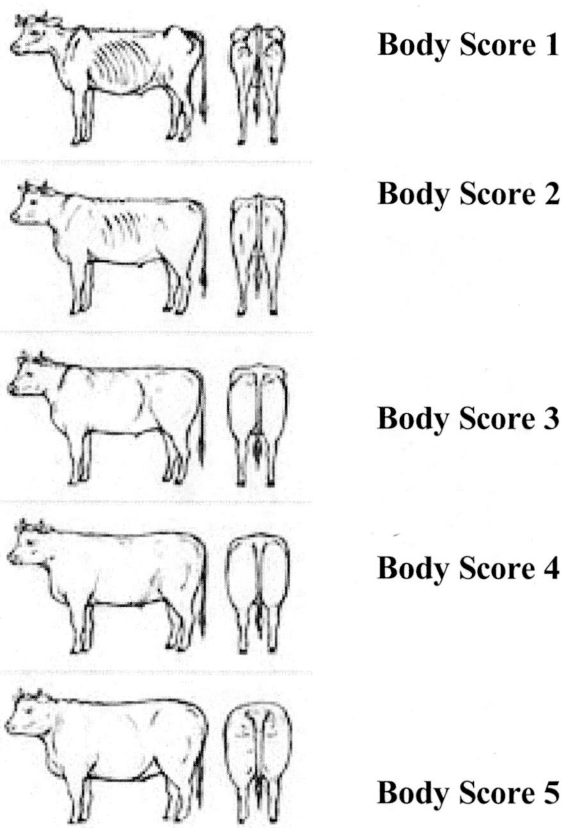

Body score condition (rear and side view)

Scoring	Vertebrae at middle of the back	Rear view of the hook bone (cross-section)	Side view of the line between hook and pin bones	Cavity between tail head and	Interpretation
Score 1 - Severe under-conditioning					Not in good health. Will not milk well or reproduce.
Score 2 - Frame obvious					Health may be OK. But milk production low and poor reproduction.
Score 3 - Frame and covering well					High producing, but fat may not be enough for peak production.
Score 4 - Frame not very visible					May have more metabolic problems at calving.
Score 5 - Severe over-conditioning					Extremely fat and will have metabolic and breeding problems.

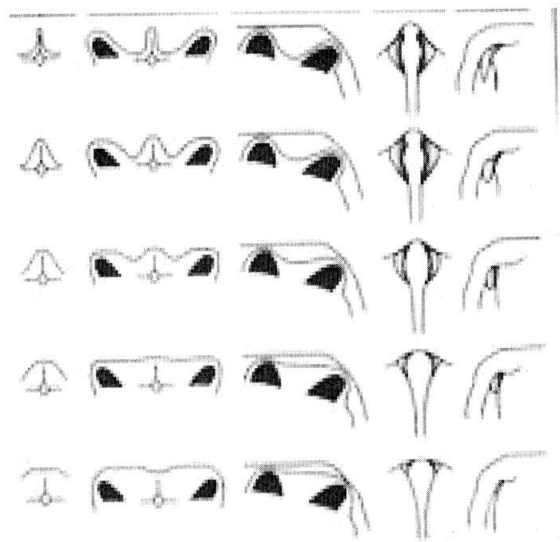

Dairy cattle judging

In cattle judging, animals are ranked as per their closeness to ideal dairy conformation. An ideal dairy animal should be able to live a long trouble free productive life. Dairy score for cattle judging in fairs, shows, or exhibitions is based not only on apparent look of the animals, but on score points (score card) given for qualifying traits with respect to:

1. Frame (15)
2. Dairy character (20)
3. Body capacity (10)
4. Feet and legs (15)
5. Mammary development (40)

While judging a dairy cow, we should overlook the breed type but keep in mind the categories. The similar principles cover to dairy cow of the same breed and category.

1. Frame of the animal: points allotted= 10

The frame of an animal is awarded a highest of 15 points. Frame includes bony cage of the cows except feet and legs. For selection important body traits are rump, stature, front end, back and breed characteristics, respectively.

The rump which is the base for the udder includes the hip, thurls, and pins. A wide, long and nearly level rump is said be ideal, as it forms space for udder development.

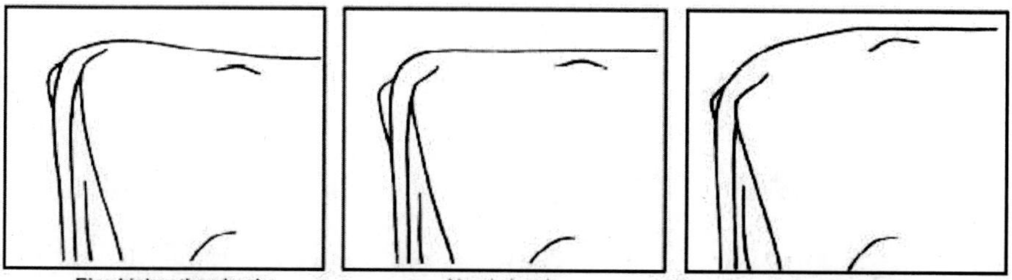

Pins higher than hooks | Nearly level | Severe slope

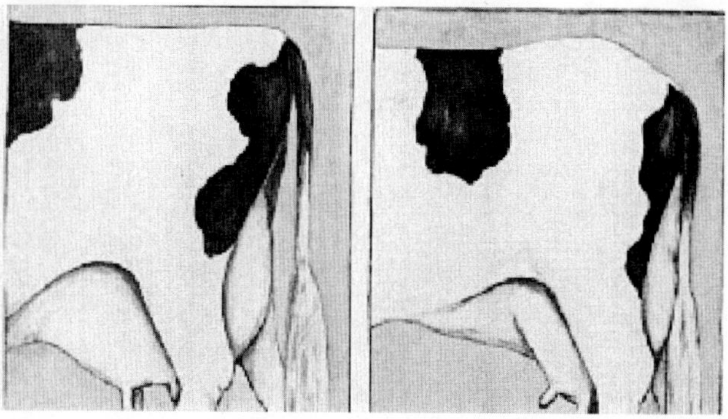

A contrast in rump and pelvic development. Note the long, smooth, level development of the rump, with pin bones placed high and on a level with hips.

Thurls should be wide apart and pins should be high and wide. Capacity is evaluated by the height and length of leg bones. Superior animals with their udders high up are usually taller and are given preference.

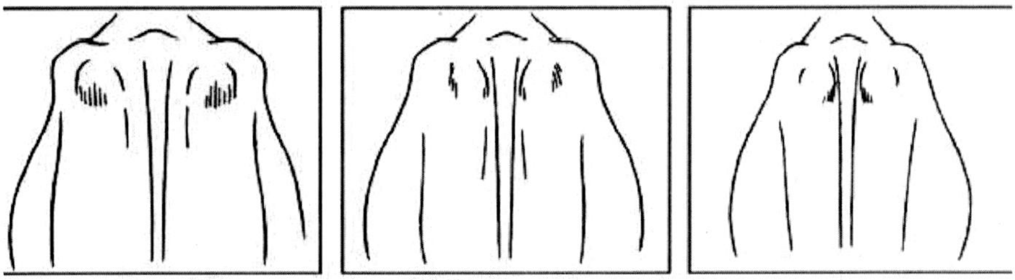

Pin bone development (Rear view). Pin should be high and wide apart.

The front end is evaluated by depth of chest and smooth mixing of shoulders to the body wall providing the dairy animal the appearance of balanced, style and smoothness. Finally, the cow should exhibit an overall breed characteristic.

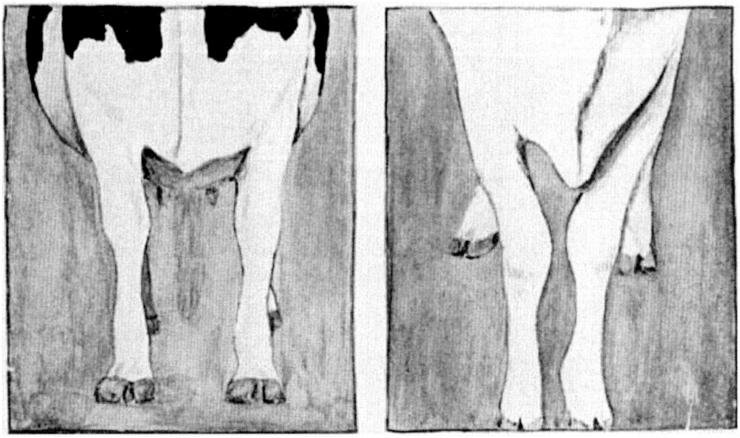

A contrast in chest development with respect to depth and width (front view)

2. Dairy character: Points allotted = 20

This category has a total of 20 points. Here, the traits to look for are of a cow that can produce a lot of milk and evidence of milking potential. Ribs, thighs, withers, neck and chine, respectively are observed to gain insight about the characters like angularity, openness and cleanness. A long neck with open rib cage, sharp withers, rump and a lean top line are ideal body traits for a dairy cow. Neck should be long, lean, blending smoothly into shoulder. Flank should be deep and refined. The hip bones and pin bones should be sharply defined. Thighs should be incurving to flat and wide apart from rear view without excess fat. The skin should be thin, loose and pliable.

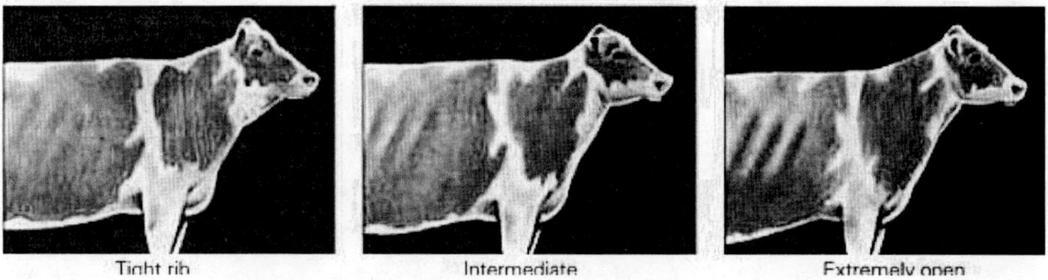

Illustration of different type of rib in dairy animal.

Loss of weight after calving is imperative and after this body of cow tends to appear angular in presentation. This means that parts of the skeleton, such as the withers, shoulders, backbone, hips, and pin bones, project more from the body and appear to be much sharper. The best dairy cows are, as a rule, the most angular. Angularity is one of the best indicators of dairy character. The body should be straight and structured rather than rounded. One should use the following triangles as a guide to help you to select an angular dairy cow:

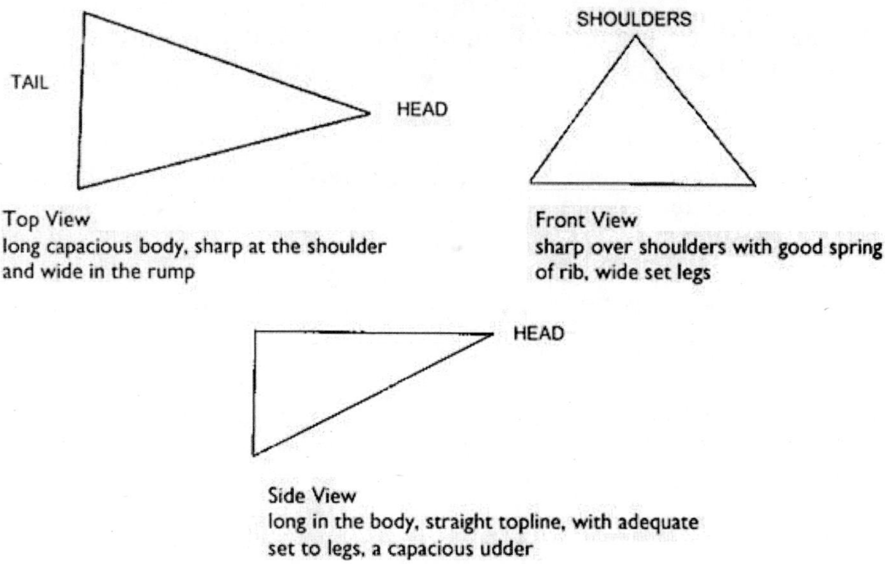

Illustration of triangle as a guide to judge the angularity of dairy cow

3. Body capacity: Points allotted = 10

Appraisal of body capacity is usually done out of 10 points. The heavier the size, the more capacious is the ability of animal to take in more feed and produce more milk. Capacity of body is decided by the length, width and depth of the animal. Animal having higher body capacity would be stronger, vigorous, wide chested. The ribs should have position as angled slightly backwards towards the udder, well-spread and deep. Width of the barrel tends to increase towards rear it, should be long and deep. Heart girth should be large, deep and well strong.

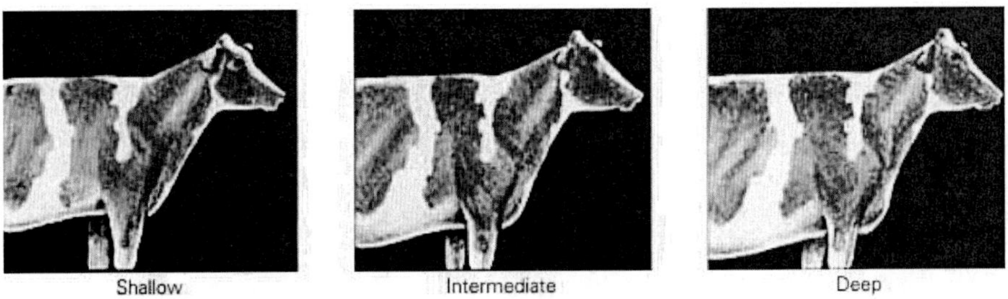

Illustration of different Barrel (body capacity) in dairy animal.

4. Legs and feet's: Points allotted = 10

Legs and feet are judged out of 15 points. Mobility and strength are important terms as to evaluate the feet and legs. A long and fluid stride with the rear feet nearly replacing the front feet is desirable. Feet should be short, compact and well-rounded with deep heel. Squarely placed fore legs with medium length are ideal. From a rear view, the hind legs should be straight wide apart with feet squarely placed and angle should be nearly perpendicular from hock to pastern. If seen from the side, the rear legs should have a moderate angle to the hock. The hock should be flat with no swelling. Cow with a short and strong pastern with a moderate upright angle should be selected.

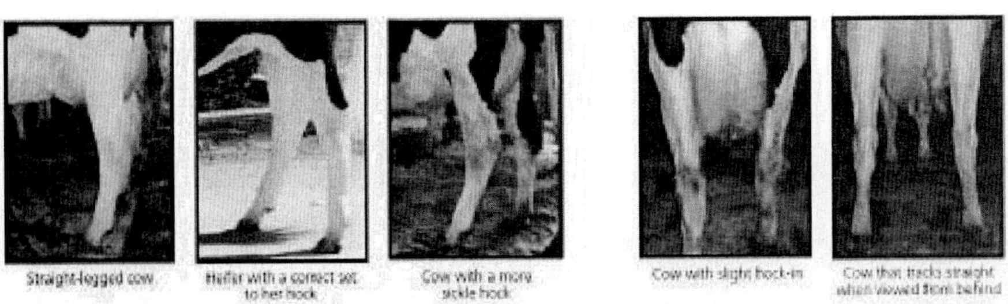

Different hind leg condition in dairy animal (rear and side view)

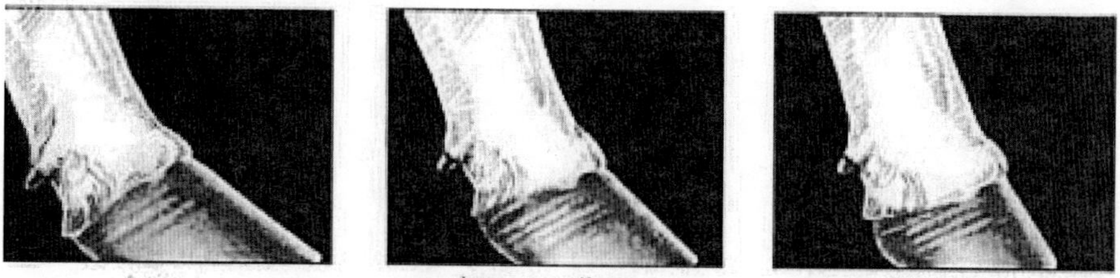

Low Intermediate Steep

Different type of foot angle (side view)

5. Mammary system: Points allotted = 40

Being the most important part of a dairy cow the udder is awarded out of 40 points. Traits that contribute to high milk yield and long productive lifespan are emphasized. The mammary system should have following characteristics:

Udder : A well-balanced udder with symmetry and acceptable size and capacity are desirable in a dairy cow. It should be firmly attached. The skin should be soft, pliable, and loose. Udder should be symmetrical and moderately long, wide and deep. Consideration is given to an animal s age and stage of lactation, when evaluating udder capacity. It should be soft and spongy, when milked out, indicating high proportion of secreting tissue. As the cow grows older, her udder becomes deeper and larger. oung cows less than five years old having their udder hanging below the hocks should be discarded.

Udder depth : An udder with an adequate capacity and clearance with a moderate depth relative to the hock is important. A well, levelled udder with no quartering at floor is desirable in dairy cows.

Udder gets its support from median and lateral suspensory ligaments. The median suspensory ligament is situated between the halves of the udder. The lateral ligaments are present on the sides of the udder. Due to weakness of these ligaments, the udder hangs below the hocks. An undesirable udder conformation is absence of cleft between the quarters it happens due to weak median suspensory ligaments and causes the udder floor to be flat and teat becomes pointed out teats, which are difficult to milk.

Udder te ture : Udder should be always soft, pliable and elastic. After milking, the udder should be well-collapsed.

ore Udder : The fore udder should be moderately long, firm, strongly attached and blend smoothly into the body wall. A longer

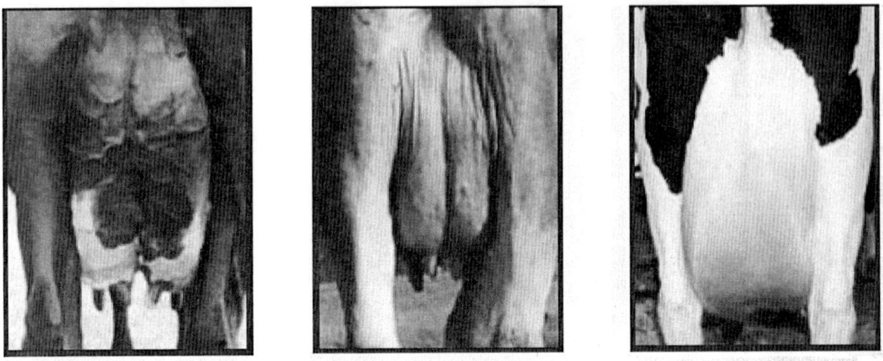

Mature udder with strong cleft | Shallow udder lacking depth and capacity in the rear quarters | Udder lacking strength of the median suspensory ligament

Illustration of different Udder cleft condition in dairy animal

fore udder attachment provides for more capacious udder. It should be evenly wide from front to rear and be balanced with the rear udder. The udder should have little movement, when the cow is walking.

Rear Udder : The rear udder attachment should be wide and high, firmly attached. It should be balanced in proportion to the fore udder attachment. The rear udder should have a slightly rounded appearance and be uniform in width from the top of the attachment to the floor of the udder with even balance of the quarters.

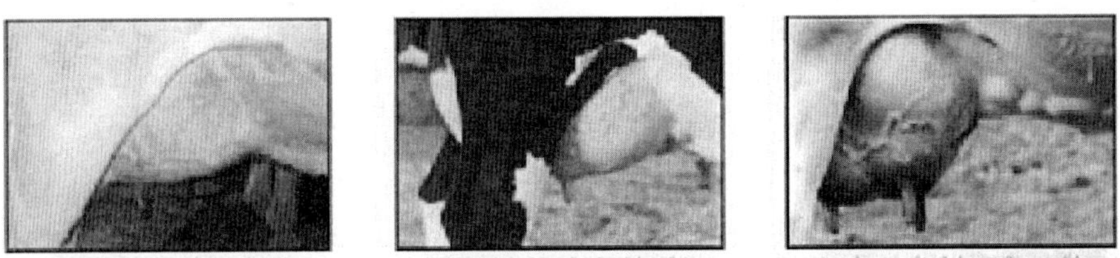

Tightly attached fore udder | Adequately attached udder that could blend more smoothly into the body wall | Poorly attached, loose fore udder

Illustration of different fore udder attachment condition in dairy animal

Teats : The teats should be four in number, uniform in size and symmetrically placed on the four quarters of the udder. The teat size and length should be suitable for easy milking (1 to 2 inches long). When cow is standing, all teats at same height from floor. All four teats should be squarely placed situated at the corners of the udder, Teat should be pointed slightly inward before the udder is filled, and they should hang straight down, when the udder is full.

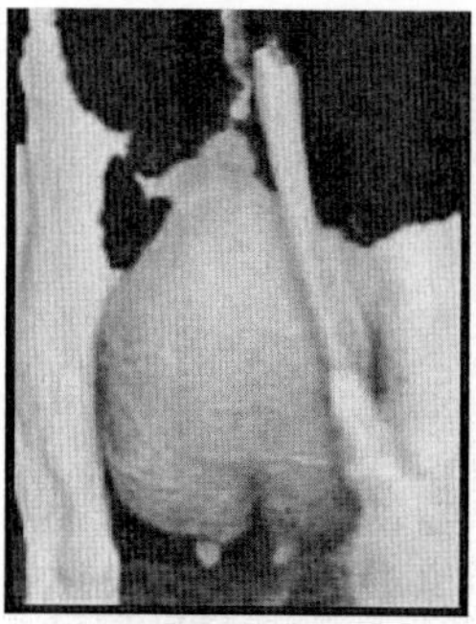

High, wide rear udder with strong udder cleft

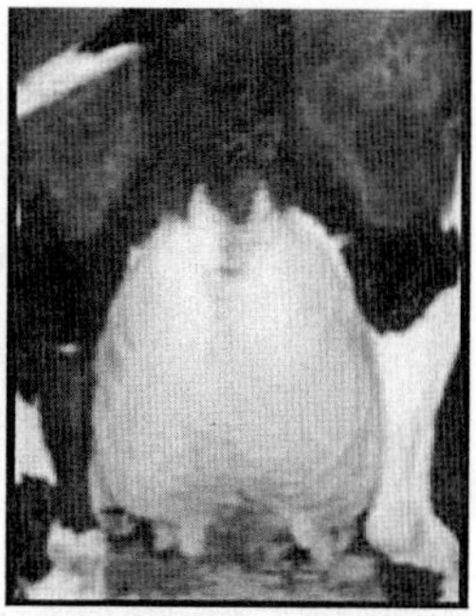

Lower rear udder that gets narrow at the top

A contrast in rear udder attachment condition of dairy animal

Teat with undesirable characteristics: very small in size or short, or extra-large teats having less space in between, interfering in milking more than four teats or extra openings interfering with milking, leaky teats, when udder is full lumps or warts on the teats.

Mammar vein Milk vein: Mammary vein should be long large and tortuous. Large veins with many branches extending forward from the udder milk wells (openings in body wall through which veins enter body) large to prevent constriction of blood flow:

On the basis of the score points, grades are awarded to the animal according to merit as follows:

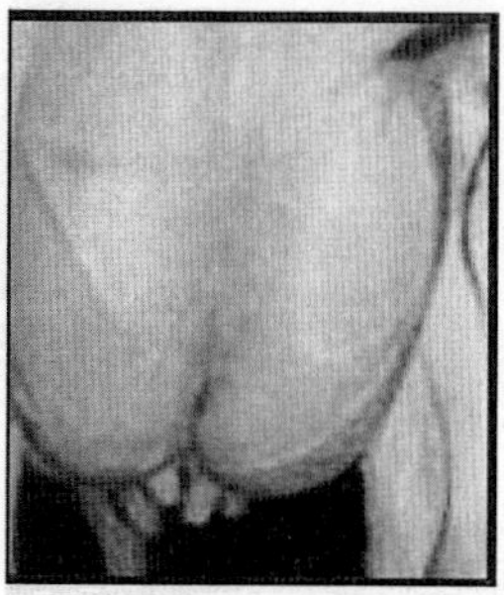

Teats set too close together

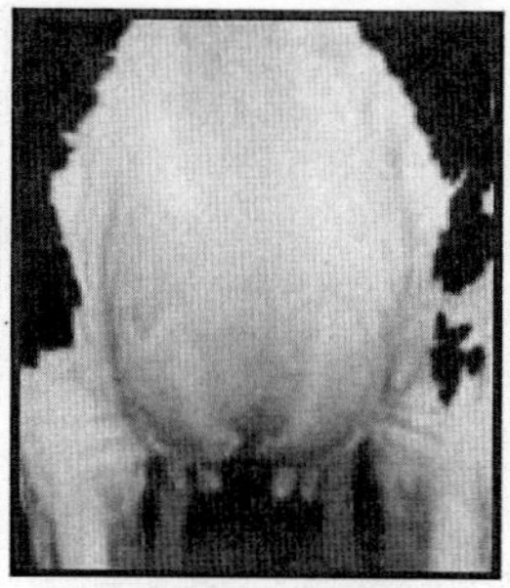

Centrally placed

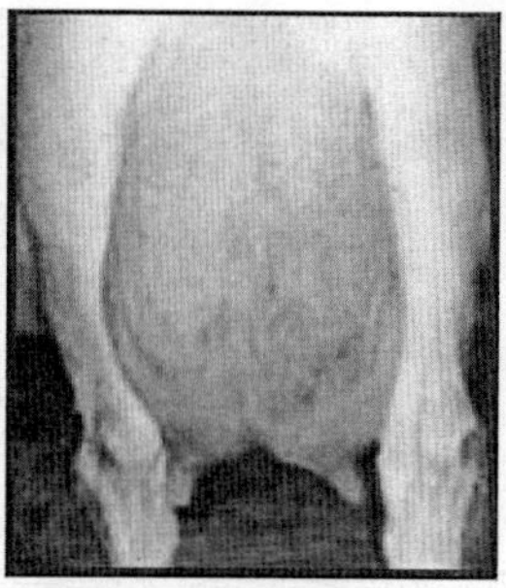

Rear teats set too wide

Illustration of different teat condition in dairy animal

Score	Grades	Score	Grades
90 and above	Excellent	70-80	Acceptable
85-90	Very good	60-70	Fair
80-85	Good	Below	Poor

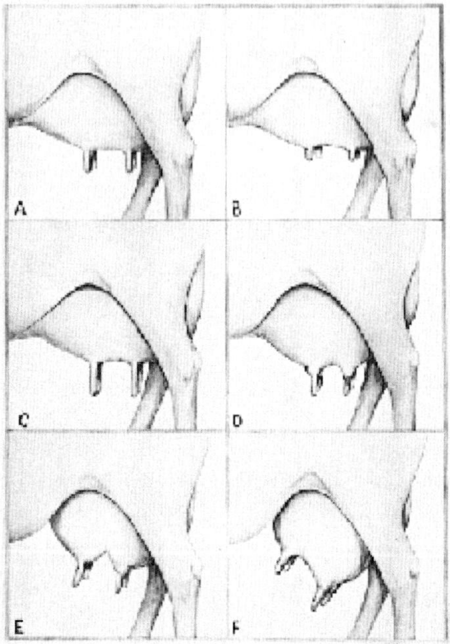

Illustration of different Udder and teat condition in dairy animal. (Ideal udder. (Udder ideal in shape and size, but teats too short. (Teats too long. (Teats have enlargements at the base which interfere with milking. (Udder "cut-up" or strictured between front and rear quarters, and front also weakly attached to body. (Udder tilts forward, with capacity of front quarters much less than that of rear. Note extra teat, which is likely to interfere with milking.

R

General Observation of animals, Section 1.: In Handbook of Good Dairy Husbandry Practices by National Dairy Development Board (NDDB), Gujarat, India.

Nevens W. B., uhlman A. F. (1934). Selecting dairy cattle, circular 422, University of Illinois, College of Agriculture, Urbana, Illinois.

South Dakota dairy judging guide (2010). South Dakota State University, College of Agriculture and Biological Sciences, South Dakota Cooperative Extension Service.

Stamschror J. (2000). Judging dairy cattle, University of Minnesota.

https://www.gov.mb.ca/agriculture/rural-communities/4h/pubs/judge-dairy-factsheet.pdf Judging dairy cattle (2015). 4H Manitoba, Canada.

❑❑❑

Chapter 27

Risk Management Tool of Dair armers Livestock Insurance

Amit Singh Sanjeev Kumar Singh and Rashmi

Department of Veterinary and Animal Husbandry Extension, College of Veterinary Science and Animal Husbandry, Uttar Pradesh Pandit Deen Dayal Upadhyaya Pashu Chikitsa Vigyan Vishwavidhyalaya Evam Go Anusandhan Sansthan, Mathura

I

Animal Husbandry and Dairying, along with agriculture, continue to be an integral part of human life, since the start civilization process. Animal Husbandry and Dairying activities have contributed to the food basket and by providing draught animal power and thus, helping in maintaining ecological balance. This sector have played prominent socio-economic role in India comprising of an important productive asset and source of income for about two-third of India s farm households (Birthal, 2008). The supplemental income derived from rearing of livestock is a great source of support to the farmers facing uncertainties of crop production, apart from providing sustenance to poor and landless farmers. According to estimates of the Central Statistics Office (CSO), the value of output livestock sector at current prices is about 28.5 of the value of output from agricultural and allied sector. The total Bovine population (Cattle, Buffalo, Mithun and ak) is 299.9 million numbers in 2012, which shows a decline of 1.57 over previous census. The total Buffalo contributes around 21.23 of the total livestock population and total cattle contributes around 37.28 of the livestock population and the total livestock population decreased by about 3.33 over the previous census.

T Livestock Population of India

S. No.	Species	Population in millions
1.	Cattle	190.9
2.	Buffaloes	108.7
3.	Sheep	65.0
4.	Goats	135.17
5.	Pigs	10.29
6.	Poultry	729.2

(Livestock Census, 2012)

India continues to be the largest producer of milk in world. Government of India have initiated several measures to boost the productivity of livestock, which has resulted in increasing the milk production significantly from the level of 102.6 million tonnes at the end of the Tenth Plan (2006-07) to 127.9 million tonnes at the end of the Eleventh Plan (2011-12). Milk production during 2016-17 is 165.4 million tonnes respectively showing an annual growth of 6.27 . The per capita availability of milk is around 355 grams per day in 2016-17.

Agriculture and animal husbandry production is affected by natural disasters, such as droughts, floods, cyclones, storms, landslides and earthquakes, thus affecting the farm incomes of people. The susceptibility of these sector to these disasters is compounded by the outbreak of epidemics and man-made disasters, such as fire, sale of spurious seeds, fertilizers and pesticides, price crashes, etc. Livelihood systems of poor rural households are often so fragile that a small misfortune can destabilize households for years. Strategies for coping with risk include informal mutual aid agreements and/or formal micro insurance schemes. In developing countries, insurance markets are usually under-developed. Nevertheless, if the development path is supported by strong structures and institutions, anonymous markets will, over time, replace informal insurance networks, as they are more efficient.

The absence of off-farm investment possibilities further promotes investment in livestock production. Failure of an investment, especially when loan-funded, can leave a household in an extremely vulnerable position. Livestock death is considered to be a major factor contributing to poverty. Farmers using credit to purchase livestock face two risks at once: (1) loss of the livestock due to disease and subsequently

(2) failure of investment. Livelihood strategies will differ according to whether people have to deal with gradual changes or sudden shocks and crises. Coping strategies (e.g. sale of livestock) seek to minimize the impact of livelihood shocks and are a short-term response to sudden or periodic shocks.

The livestock sector is expose to many types of risks which detain its yields and reduce the returns from it. Therefore, protection of this sector is, in fact, protection of national income and ensure economic and social stability. Types of risks in the sector can be divided into natural hazard, institutional, economic and social risks:

1. The natural hazard risks are attributed to drought, irregular rainfall, high humidity, pests and diseases, floods, higher temperatures, storms, tornadoes, fires and all natural hazards that can not be controlled.
2. The institutional risks are related to the management, structures and systems used, weak agricultural/livetsock research and extension services, problems of holdings, the relationships of production and weak infrastructure.
3. Economic risks related to the macro policies of the economy, rate of inflation, policies of export and import, scarcity of financial resources and prices instability.
4. The social risks related to the problems associated with human and social relationships, the availability of public services and general understanding of advanced agricultural production, the possibility of transfer of technology, the degree of modern social harmony and the risks resulting from the war, displacement, social disturbance, environmental degradation and illiteracy.

The important risks that livestock can face are mortality due to diseases, theft risk, disappearance and escaping risks, natural hazards and loss of animal use. There are some tools or strategies farm operators can use to overcome these common risks, such as crop diversification, maintaining financial reserves, production contracting, marketing contracting, forward pricing, mutual fund and acquiring agricultural insurance. Risk perception can vary from farmer to farmer depending, for instance, on the farmer s own experience and on the degree of risk-aversion. Insurance is one method by which farmers can stabilize farm income and investment and guard against disastrous effect of losses due to natural hazards or low market prices.

Insurance is a financial tool to transfer risks associated with farming to a third party via payment of a premium. Insurance acts as a guarantee for investment and can serve as a form of collateral, allowing farmers access to credit services, investment opportunities, and protection from mild and severe shocks.

Risk Management is the process of measuring, or assessing risk and developing strategies to manage it. The strategies for risk management include transferring the risk to another party, avoiding the risk, reducing the negative effect of the risk, and accepting some or all of the consequences of a particular risk.

Triangle of rural finance

Savings, credits, and insurance products are closely related to each other, e.g. when loan defaults are tied to natural disasters, as in the agricultural sector, formal financial institutes (FFI) will either ration credit or build a credit premium to cover this risk (charging higher interest rates).

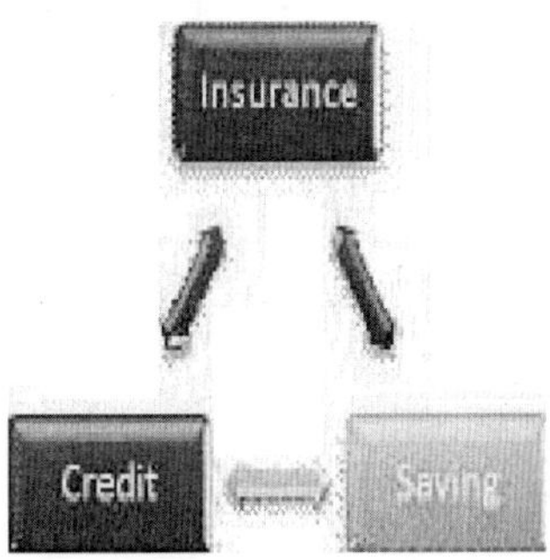

Agricultural insurance increases clients ability to repay their loans and therefore, has a positive impact on default rates in the sense of reducing them. Thus, farmers using insurance usually have also better access to credit with good conditions. For promotion of the livestock sector, it has been felt that along with providing more effective steps for disease control and improvement of genetic quality of animals, a mechanism of assured protection to the farmers and cattle rearers needs to be devised against eventual losses of such animals. In the event of an animal disease outbreak, the livestock sector suffers large or even catastrophic economic losses (Franks *et. al.*, 2001, NAO, 2002, Mangen and Burrell, 2003).

Hence, in order to check economic losses of the livestock sector, the Government launched a centrally sponsored scheme on Livestock Insurance, which was initially implemented on pilot basis during the 10th Plan.

Need of livestock insurance

Livetsock insurance provides coverage commonly known as Livestock mortality insurance, protects against livestock disease, old age or death by natural causes to the farmers. Insurance package provides Broad Causes of Loss protection for livestock, which includes the following:

i) Accidental shooting

ii) Attacks by dogs or wild animals (does not apply to sheep)

iii) Earthquake loss

iv) Electrocution

v) Flood loss

vi) Loading and unloading accidents

vii) Sudden and accidental collision damage causing death

viii) Covered cause of loss including fire, lightning, windstorm, drowning, flood, building collapse, vandalism, smothering caused by blizzard, and more. Coverage for the theft of covered livestock is also included.

Importance and benefits of Insurance

The main objective of Insurance is to stabilize and secure the needs of the farming community with a series of coverage to crops, livestock, farmer s property, himself and his family:

1. Insurance enable the farmer to expand production by attracting additional resources through credit.
2. Insurance work to create a minimum income for farmers and bring stability, this lead to sustainable development.
3. The insurance considered as a pillow to absorb shocks the farmers and breeders suffer, as a result of disasters.
4. Insurance helps in risks distribution over the years, which creates an atmosphere of stability in the economy, especially countries which depend on agriculture.

5. Insurance improve farmer s situation with regard to individual debt and helps institutions of co-operative financing to provide aid to them.
6. Insurance develop spirit of brotherhood and co-operation between farmers and push them to co-ordinating the efforts for the common benefit.
7. Insurance helps to reduce government appropriations earmarked for the prevention of the effects of disasters.
8. Insurance creates a real opportunity for a partnership between farmers and the private sector on one side and with the government on the other side.
9. Insurance contribute to raising productivity by specialization.
10. Insurance contributes to poverty alleviation of agricultural producers, who depend mainly on agriculture, especially in rural areas, and thus, achieve economic security of large segments of society.

Livestock insurance scheme

Livestock insurance scheme is a centrally sponsored scheme, which was implemented on a pilot basis during 2005-07 and in 2007-08 on a regular basis in selected 100 districts of the country. The scheme provides coverage to the crossbred and high yielding cattle and buffaloes, which were insured at maximum of their current market price. The premium of the insurance is subsidized to the tune of 50 per cent, which is being borne by the Central Government subject to a maximum of two animals per beneficiary for a policy of maximum of three years.

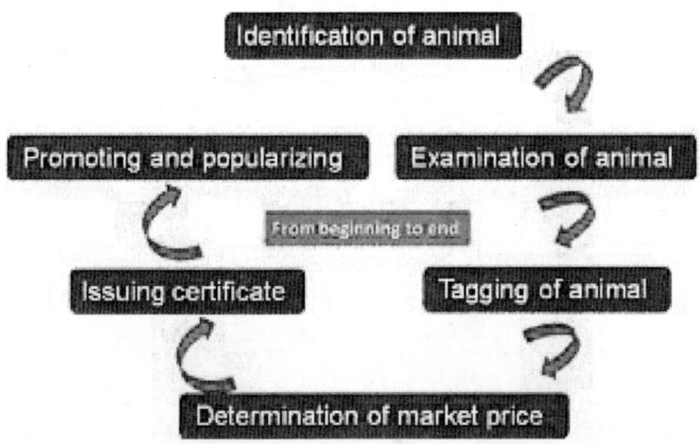

Role of Veterinarians in Livestock Insurance

The scheme provide coverage to all female cattle/buffalo yielding at least 1500 litres of milk per lactation, which are considered to be high yielding and hence, can be insured. Animals covered under any other insurance scheme/plan scheme will not be covered under this scheme. Benefit of subsidy is to be restricted to two animals per beneficiary and is to be given for one time insurance of an animal up-to a maximum period of three years. The farmers will have to be encouraged to go for a three-year policy, which is likely to be more economical and useful for getting the real benefit of insurance on occurrence of natural calamities, like flood and drought, etc. Animals covered under any other insurance scheme/plan scheme will not be covered under this scheme. Benefit of subsidy is to be restricted to two animals per beneficiary.

Objectives of livestock insurance scheme

The Livestock Insurance scheme has been formulated with the twin objective of:

- Providing protection mechanism to the farmers and cattle rearers against any eventual loss of their animals due to death as well as to demonstrate the benefit of the insurance of livestock to the people.
- Popularize it with the ultimate goal of attaining qualitative improvement in livestock and their products.

Premium rates

The premium rate of the scheme is subject to a maximum of 4.5 per cent for annual policies and 12 per cent for a three-year policy. The actual premium rate (Final Report 34) varies substantially from State to State. In 2007-08, the premium rate for a three years policy varied between 3.6 to 11.5 per cent across different insurance companies in different States.

Major Exclusions of Livestock Insurance

A. Common Exclusions:

a) Malicious or willful injury or neglect, overloading, unskillful treatment or use of animal for purpose other than stated in the policy without the consent of the Company in writing.

b) Accidents occurring and/or Disease contracted prior to commencement of risk.

c) Intentional slaughter of the animal except in cases, where destruction is necessary to terminate incurable suffering on humane consideration on the basis of certificate issued by qualified Veterinarian or in cases, where destruction is resorted to by the order of lawfully constituted authority.

d) Theft and clandestine sale of the insured animal.

e) War, invasion, act of foreign enemy, hostilities (whether war be declared or not), civil war, rebellion, revolution, insurrection, mutiny, tumult, military or usurped power or any consequences thereof or attempt threat.

f) Any accident, loss, destruction, damage or legal liability directly or indirectly caused by or contributed to by or arising from nuclear weapons.

g) Consequential loss of whatsoever nature.

h) Transport by air and sea.

i) Any non-scheme claim arising due to diseases contracted within 15 days from the date of risk are not covered.

B. Specific Exclusions

a) Pleuropneumonia in respect of Cattle in dew.

b) All the claims received without ear tag.

Documents of livestock insurance

- Proposal Form,
- Veterinary Health Certificate from a qualified Veterinarian giving the age,
- Identification marks,
- Health certificate, and
- Market value of the animal in the prescribed format.

Claim procedure

Claim procedure in the event of death: In the event any tragedy like death of an animal, immediate intimation should be sent to the

Insurers (Insurance company) and the following requirements should be furnished:

a) Duly completed claim form.

b) Dully filled death Certificate of animal obtained from qualified Veterinarian.

c) Postmortem examination report, if required by the Company.

d) Ear Tag applied to the animal should be surrendered. The condition of No Tag- No claim will be applied, if the tag is not surrendered.

Claim Procedure for Permanent Total Disability (PTD)

a) A certificate from the qualified Veterinarian to be obtained.

b) The animal will be inspected by the company s Veterinary Officer also.

c) Complete chart of treatment, medicines used, receipts, etc., should be submitted.

d) Admissibility of claim will be considered after two months of Veterinary Doctor/Company Doctor s report.

e) The indemnity is limited to 75 of Sum Insured.

Constraint for opting livestock insurance

- Illiterate and lack of awareness.
- Problem in claims settlements.
- Lack of delivery channels that provide access at the doorstep
- Low level of education
- Lack of complete knowledge about livestock insurance, etc.
- Premium rates
- Inadequate awareness program by Government Animal Husbandry department about livestock insurance.

SWOT analysis of the insurance scheme

Strength	eakness
1. Emphasis on promoting a partnership approach between Government and the private sector for export of quality goods.	1. To assure micro finance lenders and banks of the security of collateral-free loans, there should be provisions for community- based group-guarantee and group-monitoring of dairy borrowers.
2. Development of market and processing facilities under public-private partnerships	2. A large-scale livestock insurance system is yet to be developed. Subsidies should be coordinated with the Livestock Insurance Policy, and there is a need for a setting and monitoring mechanism in this regard.
3. The Policy is based on a long-term vision to encourage participation of public, private and co-operative sectors in dairy production.	3. Resource centers of improved livestock (dairy animal) breeds should be developed.
4. Objective is to increase production and productivity of milk in rural areas, which helps alleviate rural poverty.	4. A mechanism to ensure participation of smallholder farmers (backward linkage) at all stages of the value chain to retail products is essential.
Opportunit	**Threat**
1. To increase the production and productivity of crops and livestock products,	1. Limited human resources and implementation capacity,
2. To make crops and livestock products competitive and commercial,	2. Lack of continuity in leadership and insurance agents
3. To improvement in livestock and their products	3. Irregular and weak policy and program monitoring and evaluation,
4. Emphasis on promoting a partnership approach between Government and the private sector for export of quality goods.	4. Premium rate of livestock insurance

Livestock insurance scheme was introduced to provide adequate protection to cattle rearer against income losses due to death of cross-breed and high yielding cattle and buffalo by the Government of India in 2005-06 by paying a small amount of premium. The diffusion of the scheme was very limited and it was observed that the low level of education of farmers have negatively influenced the decision to purchase insurance. Farmers with higher level of education were more willing to participate in the proposed insurance scheme. However, farmers who were not willing to participate in proposed insurance scheme said that they did not want any insurance, were going to shift from risky dairy production system to less risky non-agricultural small and medium enterprises, and they did not have enough money to insure their animals.

R

Annual Report (2016-17). Department of Agriculture, Co-operation & Farmers Welfare Ministry of Agriculture & Farmers Welfare Government of India, New Delhi-110 001.

Annual Report (2016-17). Department of Animal Husbandry, Dairy and Fisheries, Department of Animal Husbandry, Dairying & Fisheries Ministry of Agriculture & Farmers Welfare Government of India, New Delhi-110 001.

Birthal, P. S., 2008. Livestock Sector of India: An Overview. Background paper prepared for India Livestock Review by the World Bank, Unpublished.

Franks, J., Lowe, P., Phillipson, J., Scott, C., 2001. The impact of foot and mouth disease on farm businesses in Cumbria. Land Use Policy 20: 159 168.

Livestock Census-2012Government of India Ministry of Agriculture Department of Animal Husbandry, Dairying & Fisheries rishi Bhawan, New Delhi-110001.

Livestock Insurance Scheme Government of India Ministry of Agriculture Department of Animal Husbandry, Dairying & Fisheries. http://www.newindia.co.in/Content.aspx pageid 76

Mangen, M.-J.J., Burrell, A.M., 2003. Who gains, who loses Welfare effects of classical swine fever epidemics in the Netherlands. Eur. Rev. Agric. Econ. 30: 125 154.

Mohd Ameer han, Mahesh Chander and D Bardhan 2013 Willingness to pay for cattle and buffalo insurance: An analysis of dairy farmers in central India, Trop Anim Health Prod 45: 461 468.

Sastry NSR and Thomas C . (2006). Livestock Production and Management, alyani.

Upendra B. Pradhanang, Soni M. Pradhanang, Arhan Sthapit, Nir . rakauer, Ajay Jha and Tarendra Lakhankar 2015 National Livestock Policy of Nepal: Needs & Opportunities in Agriculture 5: 103-131.

❑❑❑

Chapter 28

Disaster Management of Livestock

Sanjeev Kumar Singh Manoj Rathore and Amit Singh

[1] Department of Veterinary & Animal Husbandry Extension, College of Veterinary Science and Animal Husbandry, Uttar Pradesh Pandit Deen Dayal Upadhyaya Pashu Chikitsa Vigyan Vishwavidhyalaya Evam Go Anusandhan Sansthan, Mathura, [2] Deendayal Upadhyaya Institute of Rural Development, Agra University, Agra

I

Disaster is a hazard causing loss of life, injuries, disease outbreaks, negative effects on physical, mental and social well-being, damage to property, destruction of assets, loss of services, social and economic disruption and environmental degradation. No two disasters are exactly the same and their impact and consequences vary from region to region and community to community. India is one of the top four most disaster-prone regions in the world. Being a vast country with a tropical climate, India experiences all types of natural disaster, except volcanic activity. The frequency of droughts, floods, earthquakes and cyclones is increasing every year.

Disaster management is the systematic process of using administrative decisions, organization, operational skills and capacities to implement policies, strategies and coping capacities of the society and communities to significantly minimize the impacts of natural hazards and related environmental and technological disaster.

It may also be defined as the process of organization, planning and application of measures preparing for prevention, response and initial recovery from disasters. However, the World Health Organization defines disaster as any occurrence that causes damage, economic destruction, loss of human life and deterioration in health and health services on a scale sufficient to warrant an extraordinary response from outside the affected community or area .

Based on disaster affinity, our country can be categorised into five sub-divisions, as :

- The northern mountain region (including foothills) : mainly prone to snow storms, leading to landslides and cold waves, heavy rainfall, land and soil degradation. Massive snow avalanches occur in the Himalayan region, which have great destructive potential.
- The Indo-Gangetic plains : Floods are a common occurrence here.
- The Deccan plateau : This area is prone to drought and has erratic rainfall. Earthquakes of varying intensities have also been reported in this area.
- The western desert : This area, known as the Thar Desert, has limited and unreliable rainfall and is prone to drought.
- The coastal areas: The coastal areas are vulnerable to sea erosion, cyclones and tidal waves. Five to six tropical cyclones form in the Bay of Bengal and the Arabian Sea every year, two to three of these cyclones will be severe and will lash the densely populated coastal areas of India, causing extensive damage.

In India, approximately 70 per cent of livestock is owned by 67 per cent of small farmers, marginal farmers and landless people. These small holders generate milk, meat, wool, etc. for the community and contribute significantly to the GDP of our country. Although such small holders contribute merely 62 per cent of the total milk product. Approximately 60 per cent of livestock farming labour is provided by women and more than 90 per cent of work related to care of animals is rendered by womenfolk of the family.

Since the impact of disaster is always high on the weaker sections of the community and data reveals that vulnerability and impact of disaster is high, especially on the economically and socially marginalised sections of the community. Many developing countries are largely disaster prone. In India, nearly 22 out of 32 states and Union Territories are vulnerable to some form of disaster or other.

After the Gujarat earthquake, the Government of India (GOI), took the cognizance of Disaster Management as a national priority and set up a High-Powered Committee (HPC) in 1999 and a National Committee was constituted for making recommendations on the preparation of Disaster Management plans and suggesting effective mitigation mechanisms. The Tenth Five- ear Plan document had mentioned chapter on Disaster Management, whereas in twelth plan, the Finance Commission made financial arrangements for Disaster Management. On 23 December, 2005, the Government of India enacted the Disaster Management Act leading to the creation of National Disaster Management Authority (NDMA), headed by the Prime Minister and State Disaster Management Authorities (SDMAs) headed by respective Chief Ministers, to spearhead and implement a holistic and integrated approach to Disaster Management in India.

The vision of NDMA is To build a safer and disaster resilient India by a holistic, pro-active, technology driven and sustainable development strategy that involves all stakeholders and fosters a culture of prevention, preparedness and mitigation.

Types of Disasters

There are 30 types of common natural and man-made disasters, which can be classified into following 5 sub-groups :

Hydro- Meteorological Disasters

a) Cyclones

b) Droughts

c) Periodical floods/ Urban Floods

d) Hailstorm

e) Cloud Burst

f) Heat Wave

g) Coastal Erosion

h) Thunder

i) Lightening

ii) Geological Disasters

a) Landslides / Mud-flows

b) Earthquakes

c) Tsunami

NATIONAL DISASTER MANAGEMENT AUTHORIT

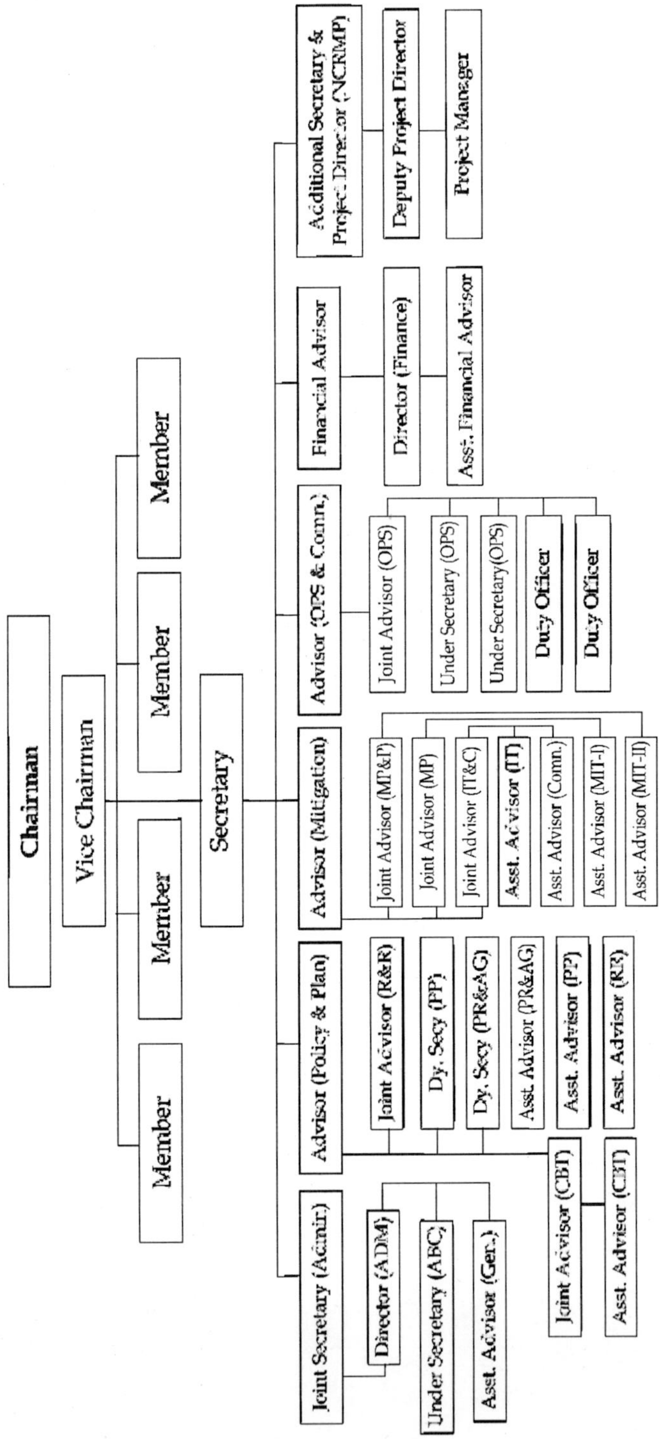

iii) Chemical, Industrial and Radiological Disasters

a) Industrial fires

b) Gas and Chemical Leakages

c) Nuclear Disaster

iv) Accidental Disasters

a) Forest Fires

b) Electrical Fires

c) Collapsing of Buildings

d) Urban fires

e) Oil Spills

f) Serial Bomb Blasts

g) Festival fire

h) Stampedes

i) Road/ Rail Accidents

j) Crash

k) Boat capsizing

v) Biological Disasters

a) Pest attacks

b) Food Poisoning

c) Water borne diseases

d) Cattle epidemics

Livestock's Role in Disaster

1. Animal can forewarn an incumbent disaster.
2. Animals, e.g., dogs are used for search and rescue operations.
3. People escape holding on to animals in case of flash floods.
4. They are the only available means of transport for injured people, when no other transport is possible.

5. Animals are also used for cleaning of debrises.
6. Animals, if salvaged, can provide food, energy, etc to the community.
7. Animals can be utilised for milk, manure, transport, fuel (dung cakes), etc. in the transit camps.
8. They are used for fetching water or for lifting water from the water sources, where machine or man power is not available.
9. Even the dead animals serve the community by providing material gains through their hide, bone, lard and carcass.
10. Partially damaged crops & grains unfit for human consumption can be gainfully used as animal feed.
11. Duck rearing or fish farming can be performed in flooded areas having slow drainage, which will help in clearing pests.
12. Pigs play an important role in clearing garbage, waste materials, etc. and they provide livelihood to economically weaker sections of the society, especially when other sources of food become scarce.
13. Dogs (pets and community animals) keep the creeping reptiles and straying wild animals at bay or at-least forewarn the community of their intrusion.

Disaster Management Plan for Livestock

A natural disaster is an unexpected event, which cannot be prevented, but its effect can be minimized through a well-developed plan. Since the disaster causes major threat to lives and property of livestock, hence the disaster management plan must be framed for the prevention of danger or threat of any disaster by mitigating or reducing the risk of any disaster.

Such protective measures includes installation of alarms, fire suppression systems, establishment of basic building security measures, the assembly of emergency supply kits and the organization of an in-village disaster response team involving farmers/livestock owners. The managemental planning can avert the disaster before it occurs, anticipating the future course of natural occurance, such as flood will reduce its vulnerability, to provide rehabilitation like construction of dwellings and other infrastructures, to undertake the liaison works, to protect and preserve the environment and to prevent the losses of life and property.

There are generally four recognized phases of emergency management, namely Mitigation, Preparedness, Response and Recovery. The table shows the main features of these four phases of emergency management as reported by the Emergency Management Institute (EMI). The same phases also applies to the management of animals, both, livestock and pets, during disasters.

Phase	Action
Mitigation Preventing future emergencies or minimizing their effects	Includes any activity that prevent an emergency, reduce the chances of an emergency happening, or reduce the damaging effects of unavoidable emergencies, e.g., buying food and fire insurance for homes.Mitigation activities take place before and after emergencies.
Preparedness Preparing to handle an emergency	Include plans or preparation made to save lives and to help response and rescue operations, e.g., evacuation plans and stocking food and water.Preparedness activities takes place before an emergency occurs.
Response Responding safely to an emergency	Includes actions taken to save lives and prevent further damage in an emergency situation. Response is putting preparedness plans into action, e.g., seeking shelter from a tornado or turning off gas valves in an earthquake.Response activities takes place during an emergency.
Recover Recovering from an emergency	Includes actions taken to return to a normal or even safer situation following an emergency, e.g., getting financial assistance for the repairs.

However, besides the aforesaid four phases of emergency management, a disaster management action plan can also be prepared by the animal husbandry departments for protection and rehabilitation of livestock, which shall essentially include the following stages:

1. Retrospective Epidemiological Study of Disaster

i) Collection, Interpretation and Analysis of raw data in order to conclude predictions.

ii) Disaster Vignetting is performed, i.e., mapping is performed on the basis of its incidence, frequency, magnitude, epicentre, vulnerable areas, etc.

iii) Profile of Herds in the area, i.e., total animal population, vulnerable livestock population as per their species, breed, age, sex, etc.

iv) Profile of the Community, i.e., total population, animal owning population, their age, sex, socio-economic status, education, cultural distribution, etc.

v) Livestock at risk, i.e., nature of hazard, the intensity of impact and mortality rate, etc.

vi) Risk factor analyses, i.e., analysis of type of risk.

2. Action Plan

The veterinary officers of the area should take necessary steps after disaster by rescuing the animals and shifting them in the relief camps, with the immediate objective to control and combat the outbreak of diseases. Such action plans should include:

i) Herd health care in terms of nutrition, caring of pregnant animals, care of new born and young animals, etc.

ii) Preventing risk through vaccination, pest/vector control, sanitary measures, etc.

iii) Early diagnosis and treatment of diseases. Many animals in which treatment is unlikely to be beneficial may have to be put to sleep, i.e., Euthanasia (mercy killing).

iv) Rehabilitation of livestock enabling them to recover from trauma or fear.

v) Timely disposal of dead animals.

3. Resource Management

i) Assessment of available man power, i.e., availability of veterinary doctors, para-veterinary staff, paravets, pashu-mitra, etc.

ii) Availability of medicines, surgical and medical appliances, diagnostics kits and life saving drugs and equipments, etc.

iii) Need to maintain supply chain management of fuels, lighting equipments, tents, sheds, grass bedding, trolleys, sanitation materials, storage houses for storing feed, fodder and water.

iv) Accessibility of ambulance for transporting animals, when they are sick or injured.

v) Veterinary medical facilities in effected and adjoining veterinary hospitals, mobile veterinary units, etc., a with grazing and watering facility.

4. Capacity Building Management

i) Capacity building is an ongoing process that equips officials, stakeholders and the community to perform their functions in a better manner during the disaster.

ii) Training of veterinary and para-veterinary staff, paravets, attendants, etc. before and during the disaster.

iii) Training of government administrators and other staff, i.e., block development officers, mobile & fire service personnels, civil defence police, sarpanch/village headmen, etc.

iv) Animal health awareness should be given to the trainees, such as social workers, volunteers, etc.

v) The National Institute of Disaster Management (NIDM) is the capacity building arm for the nation and the states have disaster management cells in the State Administrative Training Institutes, which performs the function of capacity building for effective and efficient disaster management.

vi) NDMA is running training capsules on the subject on a regular basis in the Lal Bahadur Shastri National Academy of Administration, Mussoorie and Sardar Vallabhbhai Patel National Police Academy, Hyderabad.

5. Organisational Management

i) To reinforce the political and administrative support in the disaster area.

ii) Involve all non-government organizations, media personnels, gaushala managers, animal welfare organisations and other volunteer groups of the disaster affected area.

iii) Eliciting commitment and allocation of funds through charity and government machinery.

iv) Formation of groups of veterinary service at block, district, state and central government level.

v) Organisation of district/block level bodies and assign them specific tasks and responsibilities in the disaster area.

vi) Establish regular communication through various channel means, alternate channels like community radios, etc. may also be used.

vii) Establish alternate source of power, energy, etc.

viii) Publicity and public relation activities should be maintained in the disaster area.

ix) Plan for mitigation and rehabilitation of animal owners along with animals must be established.

6. Execution Plan

The disaster management plan has to be executed to minimize the adverse impact of the multiple hazard with the broad context of sustainable development of the society.

Plan execution includes estimation of livestock affected and damage assessment due to disaster. Use of media is of utmost importance in locating remote areas, where often organisers attention may not easily be reached.

The sudden increase in deaths and causality of livestock naturally increase the demand for veterinary officers in the disaster area. Early relief period in disaster is always critical. It is important to understand animal behaviour, in each disaster situation, since with the passage of time the threat of diseases would also increase.

Recovery and Rehabilitation

All veterinary personnel s may not be required at the same time, hence it would be important to plan revolving shifts to avoid their mental and physical fatigue. Early phases would need more work force in all departments, viz., specialists like surgeons, anaesth-esiologists (pain managers), diagnosticians as well as taskforce like para-veterinary personnel and physical workers. Supervision and monitoring at this stage is of utmost importance and demands all qualities of leadership in veterinary officers, viz., confidence, competence, experience, patience, communication skill, etc. As soon as search and rescue operations are over, relief and rehabilitation would acquire importance.

The mental trauma of livestock due to the loss of a sibling or a partner where bullocks are used in pair, can be encountered and will have to be handled at appropriate stage. Certain extensive trauma cases that cannot be handled may have to be put to sleep (mercy killing). But doing such activities in full public view, where the public is already surcharged with losses of life and property may set in depression or even public outcry should be managed by the veterinary officers. Hence, the role for Veterinary extension specialists to conciliate such situations reveals the requirement of veterinary extension professionals in the animal husbandry department.

Control Rooms

A control room nodal centre for disaster management must be established at animal husbandry department for exchange of information and regular co-ordination with the duty officials for any veterinary support. The nodal centre must take regular feedback from affected veterinary hospitals, LEO s centres, veterinary dispensaries, key village centres, nodal centres established in villages, etc. of the affected area, vis- -vis must also keep link with the supply agencies for emergency supply of medicines, kits, equipments, vaccines, etc.

The task of a veterinarian after disaster is to check spread of diseases by taking complete care of diseased animals. The most major natural sequel of disaster is dumping of relief material without knowing what is required, shortage of space for operating various activities like laboratory, medical store, etc., uncontrolled demand for additional materials, improper or inefficient materials, like equipments that do not operate on battery, lack of trained staff (Veterinary extension and Public relation) to handle anxiety, lack of after-care facilities, lapses in co-ordination, duplication, absence of overall training for disaster management, etc. may hinder health and veterinary support.

The country s nodal agency, i.e., NDMA is the Incharge of disaster management (In India, it is the Ministry of Agriculture) should specifically draw its attention to disaster management in animals. A separate cell has to be established for the purpose in the department dealing with veterinary service. Disaster prevention measures and preparedness are to be organised by this department with the co-operation of their counterparts.

Animal population profile and distribution profile should be clearly drawn and plans for salvaging and rescuing the animals in major disasters, like cyclones and flood to be undertaken on the basis of this data.

It is suggested that agencies like gaushalas, dairy federations, non-government organizations and farmer producers organizations, etc. are organised in such a manner that their services can be better utilised at short notice for disaster management. Cyclone shelters are to be specifically devised for animals in cyclone prone areas of the country.

Drought relief programmes like arrangement of scarcity fodder, drinking water and subsidised food must be arranged as the stockpiles along with drugs and vaccines required to combat with allied disasters.

Each state should organise a disaster management unit in the Animal Husbandry Department dealing with veterinary services with technically trained staff having epidemiological data of their state and equipped with latest communication facilities. The required field staff should be kept in constant readiness throughout the vulnerable months of the year. During lean period, the team should undertake preparedness and relief exercise to test their efficacy and preparedness. There has to be a separate control monitoring cell attached to the Central Control Room dealing with Disaster Management of Livestock.

The epidemiological and statistical information collected before, during and after disaster should be compiled and discussed among the States of each zone on a scheduled timetable. Preventive actions taken or preparedness should be constantly monitored and lacunae thereof be frankly reported and corrected for future use.

R

1. Extension Disaster Education Network (EDEN). (2009). Preparing for an Agroterrorism Event. http://www.lsuagcenter.com/en/communications/publications/Publications Catalog/Disaster Information
2. http://www.aces.edu/pubs/docs/U/UNP-2099/UNP-2099. pdf.
3. https://www.growelagrovet.com/disaster-management-for-livestocks/ Disaster Management for livestock. Posted on May 5: 2015 by Growel Agrovet Private Limited
4. Sen, A. & Chander, M. (2003). Disaster Management in India : The case of Livestock & Poultry. www.researchgate.net, 22(3): 915-930.

5. http://www.vethelplineindia.co.in/role-of-live-stock-and-other-animals-in-disaster-management/
6. https://www.researchgate.net/publication/7557209_Disaster_management in India The case of livestock and poultry
7. Ganguli S. ., Urmil A.C. and Somiya P.A. (1993). Natural disasters: An Overview in Indian context. Ind. J. Commun. Med., 18(3): 110-113.
8. Unnikrishnan B. and Malavika A.S. (1998). Natural disasters: a public health perspective. In Proc. National Conference on Disaster and Technology, 25-26 September, Manipal, India.
9. Manipal Institute of Technology, Manipal, 110-112.
10. A.Chakrabarty. 2003. A textbook of Preventive Veterinary Medicine. alyani Publishers, West Bengal.
11. https://ndma.gov.in/en/about-ndma/evolution-of-ndma.html

❑❑❑

Chapter 29

Semen Collection and Evaluation Under ield Condition

Mukul Anand and Sarvajeet adav

Department of Veterinary Physiology, College of Veterinary Science and Animal Husbandry, Uttar Pradesh Pandit Deen Dayal Upadhyaya Pashu Chikitsa Vigyan Vishwavidhyalaya Evam Go Anusandhan Sansthan, Mathura

I

Sperms together with the glandular secreation is called *semen*. A single semen ejaculate contains large number of sperms embedded in the glandular fluid. Sperm are specialized motile cell or male gametes. They have special structural configuration for its movement and fusion with female gamete. Structurally, individual sperm can be divided into three parts *viz*. head, middle piece and tail, each with its specific functional role for the timely transport and fertilization. Head comparise of acrosome that contain enzymes. Middle piece contains high concentration of mitochondria that generate energy for sperm survival and sperm movement. The tail portion of sperm is flagellar that impart the motility to sperm. Each structure in sperm has its own physiological significance that contribute to successful fertilization. Acrosome contains enzymes (Acrosine and hyluronidase) that helps sperm to penetrate the cell surrounding ova (theca cell and granula cells). The timely release of acosomal content is critical of the sperm to reach ova and transfer of male genetic to the ovum during fertilization. The middle piece generates energy to maintain the metabolic processes of cell for its survival and movement. The tail imparts motility to cell for its timely transport for site of deposition to site of fertilization.

The semen contains million of sperm that are more that that are required for successful fertilization. Although the neat semen of bull contains 100-150 x 10^6 sperm per ml., but the minimum sperm require for successful fertilization range from 20-25 x 10^6 sperm per ml. that has been scientifically validated. This has opened new opportunities to utilize the single ejaculate from elite make for breed improvement. Now semen is artificially collected, diluted stored and inseminated in the female. Semen collection, cryopreservation and artificial insemination the three assisted reproductive techiniques that together help to utilize the single ejaculate as multiple dose for the long period of time. Semen collection and semen cryopreservation are two important process involved in determining the post thaw semen quality. Naturally semen is not exposed to environment and is internal to male and female reproductive tract. They are produced in male reproductive tract and release in female tract. In contrast to it, use of semen as insemination dose involves collection of semen through artificial means, dilution of semen and its cryopreservation in straws and thawing before its use as inseminate. During this process, sperm exposure to environmental stressors these stressors detoriate semen quality that starts from collection that continues upto freeze thawing. This make it important to understand the process of semen collection and its evaluation prior to its use as insemination does for improve the conception rate under field condition.

S

Semen collection involves collection of semen from male animal outside the female genital tract using artificial means. Collection of semen is an important process that requires precision and trained man power.The quality of ejaculated semen largely depends upon the method used. Also, the success of semen cryopreservation is influenced by the method adopted of semen collection. As per the need and requirement, different methods of semen collection are being employed which have their own merits and demerits. Generally, two common methods of semen collection are practised in goats:

1. Using Artificial Vagina
2. Electro-ejaculation method

1. Semen collection through Artificial Vagina (AV)

Use of artificial vagina (AV) is of the most widely accepted method of semen collection.An AV uses thermal and mechanical stimulation to stimulate ejaculation.The method is similar to natural service and is hygienic. Artificial vaginas are used to collect semen from many species that involves cattle, horses, sheep, goats, rabbits and even cats.However, the AV technique requires training of the bucks in the presence of a female on heat. In this method an artificial vagina is prepared to collect semen from animal.

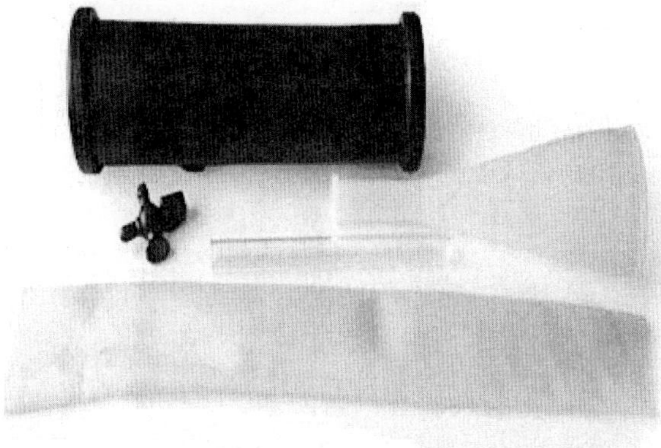

Atrificial Vagina

Artificial Vagina and Its Components

- Heavy hard rubber lose (length and diameter vary with species) open at both ends with a nostle for air and water in and outlet.
- Inner sleeve of rubber
- Semen receiving cone or rubber cone.
- Latex lining

Artificial Vagina

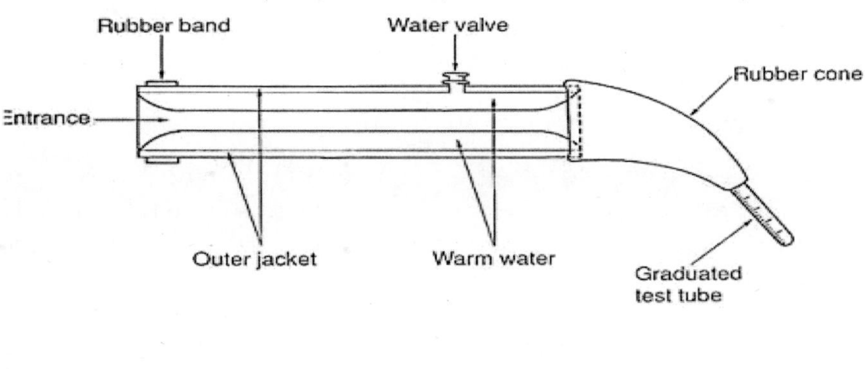

A

Before using for semen collection all the parts are washed thoroughly and sterilized properly, and assembled as artificial vagina, the rubber liner is inserted into the hose inverting both ends back by folding back from either side opening, and fastening with rubber bands. Now the space between the hard rubber hose and inner rubber liner forms a water tight compartment. The nostle at one end of the hose can be fixed.Turning through the threaded nut up or down. The water jacket of the Artificial Vagina is filled with hot water at a temperature of 42 C-45 C (depending upon the season) by opening the nostle. The graduated semen collection tube is fixed to the narrow end of the artificial vagina hose, and fastened by a rubber band. The inner side of the rubber liner on the anterior side of the artificial vagina is lubricated with sterile jelly to a length of 1 to 2 inches. Air is blown through the nostle into the water jacket, to create pressure in it, and the same is exerted at the rubber liner, to simulate natural vagina.The temperature of the artificial vagina is to be checked, at each collection, and it should fell like natural vagina at mounting time. To collect semen from male, the artificial vagina assembled, is held at 45 angle from the direction of penis. The artificial vagina is held with the left hand, when the male mounts the female goat. Penis is directed into the artificial vagina, and then male gives a thrust to ejaculate.

2. Electro-ejaculation method

Electro-ejaculation involves applying a series of short, low-voltage pulses of current to the pelvic nerves, which are involved in the ejaculatory response. It utilizes the electrical current to stimulate the local nervous system for errection and ejaculation of semen. It is less common and requires a high degree of precision. This method of semen collection is generally used for animals that are unable to mount or injured and is also useful for animals that reject the AV.

Three pieces of equipment are required for electro-ejaculation.

The electro-ejaculator itself is a power supply with rheostats to control the amplitude of the delivered current a collection tube, usually attached to a latex rubber cone (loving cup), in which semen is to be collected.

S

The probe is inserted into the rectum such that the electrodes lie within the pelvic cavity. Finally, the pulses of current are applied through an electro-ejaculator probe. The stimulation of nerve results in semen ejaculation. The advantage of electro-ejaculation is that it does not require a mount animal, and can be applied in the field using a battery-powered unit. Finally, electro-ejaculation can be used to obtain semen from animals that are physically incabable of mounting due to musculo-skeletal disease or injury.The techinique is uncommon and used under special circumstances in buck.

S E

The second important step for semen cryopreservation is semen evaluation. A pr cised evaluation of semen is very essential, as it is an important criteria to decide the use of semen for further processing. It is helpful to evaluate the quality of semen and determine the number of doses to be prepared from single ejaculate. Any mistake in the evaluation can drastically affect the conception rates. Number of tests are available to evaluate the semen quality. The test range from gross examination of ejaculated semen (volume, pH, colour, etc.) to microscopic examination (acrosomal integrity, capacitation, like changes,DNA integrity, TUNNEL, etc.). Different proteins present in the seminal plasma are also indicator of semen quality that can be evaluated through different test. Although precised but the majority of microscopic and biochemical test need sophisticated scientific instruments and reagent that are generally unavailable under field condition. But few of the test that form the basis of semen evaluation can be conducted at field level. These tests can present a picture about the quality of semen that is to be utilized for preservation and is also helpful to evaluate the quality of cryopreserved semen. The detail description of the test are as follows:

A. Macroscopic Semen Evaluation

Macroscopic semen evaluation included all evaluations performed with a naked eye, such as semen colour, volume and pH.

1. Volume

Volume of each ejaculate is directly measured in milliliters (ml) in graduated collection cup with an accuracy of 0.10 ml. Semen samples are observed for colour and consistency by direct visualization with naked eyes and any abnormalities in colour or consistency should be treated as abnormal and the sample should be discarded.

2. Semen pH

The semen pH can be determined using a :

t s a er: The litmus paper ranging from pH 5-8 is suitable to evaluate the pH of semen. To evaluate the pH of semen, a small drop of semen sample is placed of the litmus strip and evaluated for colour change. The change is colour is matched with the colour reference available and pH of sample is evaluated.

eter It is more precised method to evaluate the semen pH. pH meter should calibrated for species prior to its use. The electrode should be rinsed with sterile water and wiped with a sterile paper towel and then dipped into the semen sample for pH evaluation.

3. Mass motility

Mass motility of freshly collected semen can be assessed by placing a small drop of neat semen on a clean, grease free glass slide kept on thermostatically regulated stage at 37^{0}C and examined under low power objective (10) of the phase contrast microscope. Depending on the appearance of waves, swirls and vigor, the mass motility is graded on 0 to 5 scale as given in the following table:

G S

S.No.	Observation	Motilit score
1.	No motility	0
2.	No wave motion and only 10-20 per cent of spermatozoa were progressively motile	1
3.	Swirl s or wave motion absent but individual movement of spermatozoa was more evident with 20-40 per cent of spermatozoa progressively motile	2
4.	Swirls were slow and scattered in the field with 40-60 per cent of spermatozoa progressively motile	3
5.	Swirl s rapid and observed to move towards extremities with 60-80 per cent of spermatozoa progressively motile	4

6.	Very quick wave motion and it was difficult to trace the point of their formation and disintegration with 80-100 per cent of spermatozoa progressively motile	5

B. Microscopic Semen Evaluations

Microscopic semen evaluation includes all evaluations, which can be performed with a microscope, such as sperm concentration, motility, viability and morphology.

1. Progressive motility

The progressive motility of spermatozoa is estimated using a 10 objective of phase contrast microscope with thermostatically controlled stage. A small drop of diluted (50 x 10^6 per ml) semen is put on a clean, grease free glass slide kept on thermostatically controlled stage and a cover slip placed over it. Four fields are examined to obtain the average percentage of progressively motile spermatozoa by constant visual observation. The progressive motility of spermatozoa is then calculated as under:

$$\text{Progressive motility (\%)} = \frac{\text{No. of progressively motile spermatozoa}}{\text{Total number of spermatozoa observed}} \text{ x } 100$$

The number of progressive motile spermatozoa shoud be more than 80 in fresh diluted buck semen to be used for cryopreservation.

2. Spermatozoa concentration

It is estimated by the haemocytometer (Improved Neubauer s chamber) available in market. Prior to calculate of sperm concentration, semen is diluted using sperm diluting fluid. Although diluters are commercially available, they can be easily prepared at hospital.

S.No.	Ingredients	eight
1.	Sodium citrate	2.9 g
2.	Eosin (water soluble)	0.05 g
3.	Formalized distilled water	100 ml

P

Dilution of semen in a precised proportion is the first step to evaluate semen concentration.Semen is sucked into RBC diluting pipette upto 0.5mark and the diluting fluid was sucked upto 101mark. After filling up the pipette, it has to be held horizontally between the palms of hand and rolled for 2-3 minutes to ensure thorough mixing. The diluting pipette is shaken gently and discarding first few drops of diluted semen, a small drop is charged in the haemocytometer groove through capillary action. The haemocytometer is then left undisturbed for 10 minutes to ensure the settling of spermatozoa.The total number of spermatozoa were counted in five secondary squares, namely right and left top, right and left bottom and central squares. Each secondary square contain 16 tertiary squares, so total number of spermatozoa was counted in 80 tertiary squares. The average of the counts on both sides of haemocytometer chamber is taken for calculating the sperm density and the total number of spermatozoa per ml. of neat semen. The calculation was given as follows:

Area of 1 tertiary square	1/20 1/20 mm^2
Volume of 1 tertiary square	1/4000 mm^3
Number of spermatozoa in 80 tertiary squares	n
Volume of 80 tertiary squares	1/4000 80mm^3

Where, 80/4000 mm^3volume has n number of spermatozoa

Therefore, 1mm^3	n/80 400
	n 50
Total number of spermatozoa (undiluted)	50 n 200
Therefore, 1mm^3 of neat semen	10000 n
Neat semen contains (per ml)	10000 n 1000
	10n 10^6

3. Differential staining for live or dead spermatozoa

To ascertain the percentage of live or dead spermatozoa in semen sample, eosin-nigrosin staining technique was used as per the method described by Hancock (1952). It is an easy technique that can be utilized to evaluate the semen quality.

The composition of stain used was:

Eosin (water soluble)	1.67g
Nigrosin (water soluble)	10.0g
Sodium citrate dehydrate	2.9g
Double glass distilled water	100 ml

At the time of estimation, one small drop of neat semen is mixed with 5 to 6 drops of stain in a glass tube kept at 30^{0}C in a water bath and incubated for 5-10 sec. Smears are made on a clean, grease free slide and dried in air. At least 200 spermatozoa are counted and identified as live or dead under the oil immersion objective (100). The stained spermatozoa (eosionophilic) obtained a pinkish colour and are categorized as dead and the unstained ones against a dark background of nigrosin are counted as live. The percentage of live spermatozoa are calculated as follows:

$$\text{Live spermatozoa \%} = \frac{\text{Total number of live spermatozoa}}{\text{Total number of spermatozoa observed}} \times 100$$

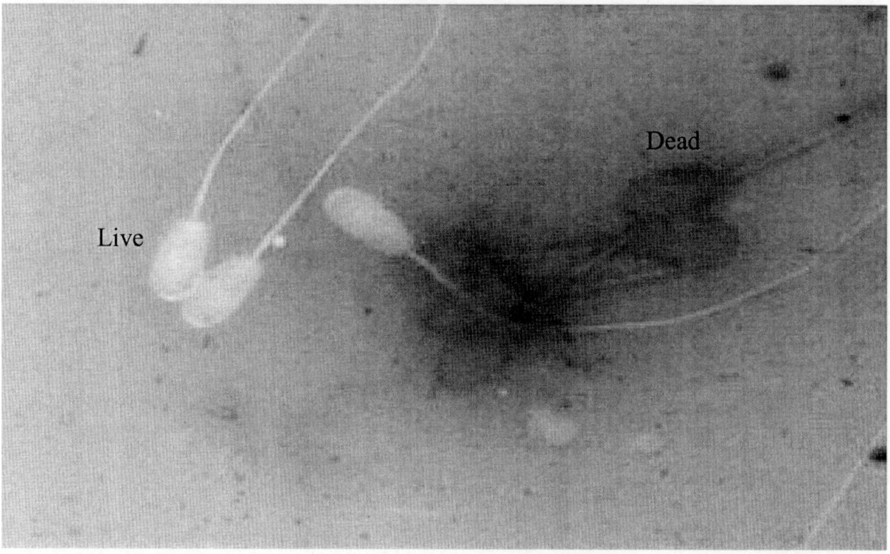

Showing live and dead spermatozoa (Eosin-Nigrosin stain, Magnification 100x)

4.Morphological Abnormalities

Live and dead count are also used for enumerating abnormalities based on classification as suggested by Lasley, 1951. The slides are observed under oil immersion using Phase Contrast Microscope. These studies are broadly classified into three groups as per abnormalities listed below:

S.No.	Head Abnormalities	Mid Piece Abnormalities	Tail Abnormalities
1.	Micro Head	Abaxial Attachment	Simple bent tail
2.	Macro head	Beaded	Coiled Tail
3.	Giant head	Proximal protoplasmic droplet	Loose tail
4.	Loose head	Distal protoplasmic droplet	Tail stump
5.	Detached head	Cork screw mid-piece	Double tail
6.	Pear shaped head (pyriform)	Bent Mid-piece	Corkscrew tail
7.	Bent head	-	-
8.	Knobbed acrosome detect	-	-

About 200 spermatozoa are counted in different fields and total abnormal spermatozoa are calculated as follows:

$$\text{Total Abnormalities (\%)} = \frac{\text{Total Number of abnormal spermatozoa}}{\text{Total number of spermatozoa counted}} \times 100$$

5. Hypo-osmotic swelling test (HOST)

To analyze the functional integrity of plasma membrane hypo-osmotic swelling test is performed according to the technique described by Jeyendran *et al.* (1984). The protocol is modified in reference to incubation time (1 hour) and osmolality required for goat semen. Hypo-osmotic solutions of 150 mOsmol g^{-1}should be prepared as follows:

HOST Solution	
Sodium citrate (g)	0.735
Fructose (g)	1.351
Ultra pure water (ml)	100
Osmolality (mOsm g^{-1})	150

P

One ml of hypo-osmotic solution, having an osmotic strength of 150mOsm/ g should be mixed with 0.1 ml. of semen and incubated at 37 C for one hour. Following incubation, a drop of well-mixed solution is taken on a clean dry glass slide and covered with a cover-slip. Sperm tail curling is recorded as an effect of swelling due to influx of water. A total of about 200 spermatozoa are counted in different fields under 40 phase objective under phase contrast microscope. These spermatozoa are classified into four different classes according to presence of following swelling pattern.

Patterns observed

A. No swelling, no membrane reaction

B. Swelling of the tip of the tail

C. Different type of hair pin like swelling or swelling of mid-piece

D. Complete tail coiling

Spermatozoa showing B, C, D type of pattern was considered to be HOST positive.

$$\text{HOST positive spermatozoa (\%)} = \frac{\text{Number of curled tail spermatozoa}}{\text{Total number of spermatozoa counted}} \times 100$$

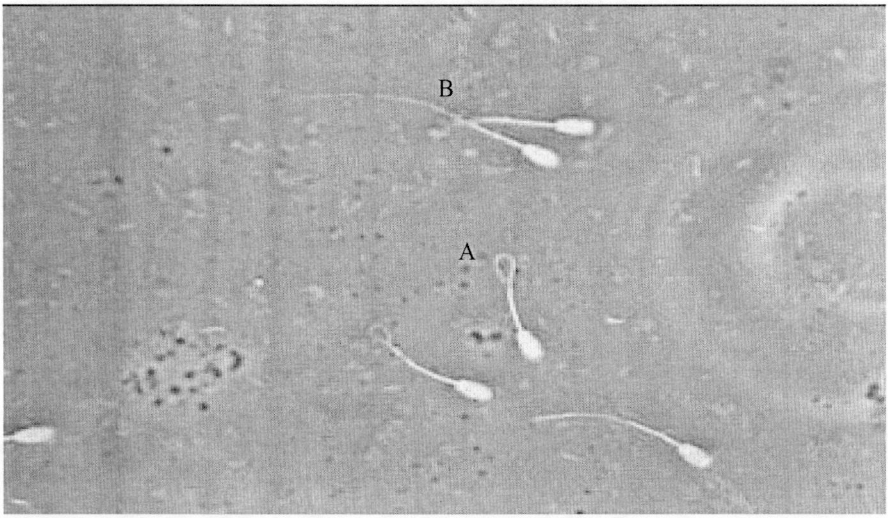

Showing HOST reactive (A) and non-reactive (B) spermatozoa (Magnification 40x)

6. Acrosomal integrity

Acrosomes play a vital role in the fertilization of ovum, hence percentage of intact acrosome is a good indicator in analyzing the fertilization potential of sperm. Acrosome integrity is judged by Giemsa staining technique as per the methodology described by (Watson, 1975).

Sorenson Phosphate Buffer

Solution A

Sodium phosphate, dibasic	11.876 g
Distilled water	1000 ml

Solution B

Potassium phosphate	9.08 g
Distilled water	1000 ml

0.1 M Sorenson phosphate buffer is prepared by adding, 33ml. of solution A and 17 ml. of solution B

i ative

5 Formalin solution was used for fixation of spermatozoa

orking Solution

Giemsa stain	3ml
0.1 M Sorenson phosphate buffer	2ml
At pH 7	
Distilled water	35 ml

S P

A thin smear of diluted semen drop is made on a clean, grease free slide. Smear is air dried and kept in 5 formaldehyde solution for 30 minutes at 37^0C. The slides are washed in double distilled water and air-dried. Then, the slides are kept in the staining jar solution for 4 hours at 37^0C in the incubator.The stained slides are washed with distilled water, air-dried.the acrosomes that stain dark purple are evaluated for status. A 200 spermatozoa per slide are examined under high power (100x) of phase contrast-microscope:

$$\text{Intact acrosome spermatozoa (\%)} = \frac{\text{Number of normal acrosome stained spermatozoa}}{\text{Total number of spermatozoa counted}} \times 100$$

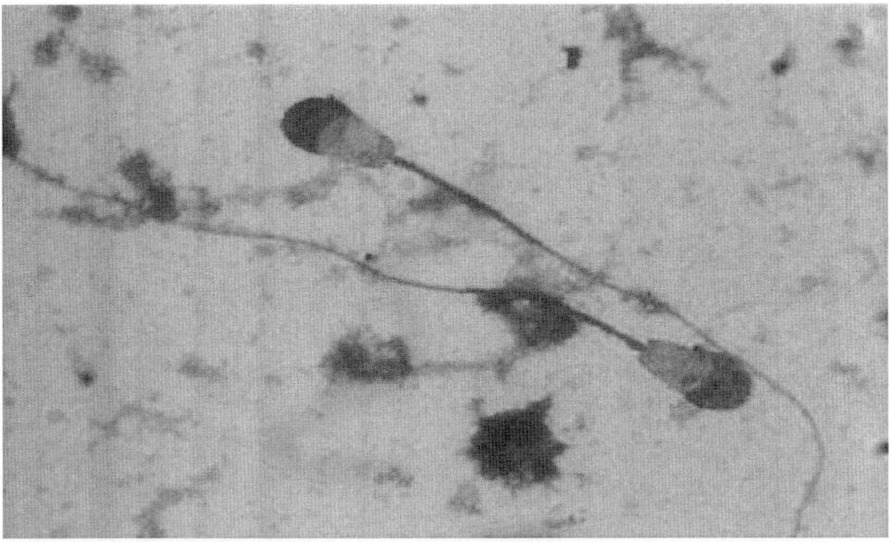

Showing stained acrosome in spermatozoa head (Giemsa stain, Magnification 100x)

7. Capacitation status and acrosome reaction status: Chlortetracycline (CTC) assay (Collin *et al.*, 2000)

Capacitation status and acrosome reaction were assessed using chlortetracycline (CTC) staining, as described by Collin *et al.* (2000) with a little modification. Chlortetracycline (CTC) binds with membrane calcium, whose distribution appears to change through capacitation, and is readily visualized by fluorescence microscopy. Thus, CTC distribution pattern seems to be related to the capacitation stage.

P

Semen sample was washed in phosphate buffered saline (PBS), pH 7.4 and centrifuged (1500 rpm, 15 minutes) with 200 x 10^6 spermatozoa/ml.

The CTC stock solution containing 750 M CTC-HCl (Sigma), 130 mM NaCl, 5 mM L-cysteine, 20 mM Tris acid (pH 7.8) was prepared daily, wrapped in foil to protect against light, and stored at 4°C until required. Ten microlitres of sperm suspension were mixed with 15 L of CTC solution on a slide at room temperature. Then, 0.3 L of 12.5 glutaraldehyde in 2.5 M Tris base was added as a fixative. Samples (in duplicate) were covered with coverslips and stored in the dark at 4°C.

A total of 200 sperm per slide were observed within 24 hours using a Nikon Eclipse TE 2000-S microscope with phase contrast and epifluorescence optics under blue-violet illumination (excitation at 400 440 nm and emission at 470 nm).

Sperm were evaluated according to 1 of 3 CTC staining patterns (Fraser *et al.*, 1995). Three different forms of CTC pattern found were:

orm I:	Even distribution of fluorescence over the entire head (uncapacitated sperm pattern F).
orm II:	Fluorescence-free band in the post-acrosomal region (capacitated, acrosome intact sperm pattern B), fluorescence in anterior portion of the head.
orm III:	Fluorescence free head except for a thin bright fluorescent band along the equatorial segment (acrosome-reacted cells, pattern AR)

In all the cases, fluorescence in the middle piece of the flagellum was observed as well. At least 150 spermatozoa per slide are scored.

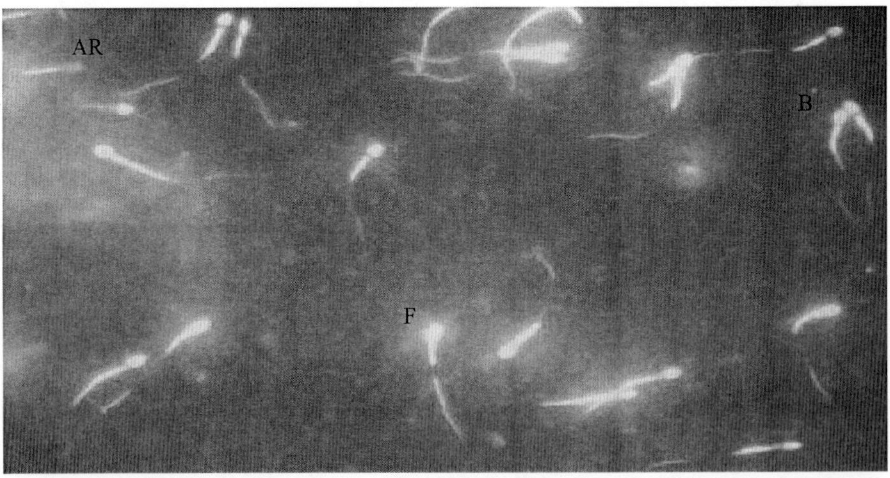

Showing various patterns of chlortetracycline (CTC) Fluorescence assay (Magnification 10x)

a) Pattern F b) Pattern B c) Pattern AR

8. Computer Assisted Semen Analysis (CASA)

The motility patterns and kinematic characteristic of spermatozoa were evaluated through computer assisted semen analyzer using sperm counting chamber, negative phase contrast and 10 x objectives. Following parameters were studied in the study:

Parameter	Unit	Description
VCL	m / sec	Curvilinear velocityDistance travelled by sperm head (actual curvilinear trajectory) divided by time.
VSL	m / sec	Straight Line velocity Distance between the first and last tracked points divided by time.
VAP	m / sec	Average path velocity Distance of averaged path of the sperm head trajectory divided by time. Average path is derived by smoothening the actual curvilinear path.
LIN		Linearity: The Linearity of the curvilinear trajectoryRatio (VSL/VCL) x 100.
STR		Straightness: The straightness of the average path Ratio (VSL/VAP) x 100.
WOB		Wobble: A measure of the oscillation of actual trajectory about its averaged path.Ratio (VAP/ VCL) x 100.
BCF	hz	Number of times the curvilinear trajectory crosses the average path trajectory per second.
ALH	m	Amplitude of Lateral head displacement.max ALH: Is the maximum value of the displacement of the sperm head from its average path multiplied by 2.
DNC	m /sec	DANCEDNC VCL x ALHmeanA measure of the pattern of sperm motion. Area swept by the head during its actual movement. Where ALH mean is the mean of the peak displacement values of the sperm head from its average path.

Settings of the CASA system (Biovis CASA 2000, Version 4.6, India) designed using algorithm based on size, shape, detection of sperm head were as follows: Frames/s - 60, number of frames acquired - 61, max velocity (for tracking): (um/s) - 150 motility min, curvilinear velocity (VCL): (um/s) - 25 motility min, average path velocity: (um/s) - 10 motility min, straight-line velocity: (um/s) - 1 min, track length (of frames) - 51, aspect - 0-99,999, area - 2-20, axis (major) - 4-20, axis (minor) - 2-10, compact- ness - 0-50, perimeter ratio - 0-99,999, minimum cell size on major axis - 20, minimum cell size on min axis - 10 magnification - 10 phase, calibration (pixels/unit) - 1.905 , (pixels/unit) - 1.905 , size of image - 1280 960 pixels. Semen was diluted and adjusted to a concentration of about 50 106 spermatozoa per ml for computer aided motility analysis. A 4 l of diluted semen sample was loaded in metallic sperm counting chamber with surface graticule of 100 x 0.01 sqmm (sperm processor, Welcomenagar, India) and a range of 3-6 fields were acquired for motility analysis.

R

Hancock, J. L. (1952). The morphology of bull spermatozoa. J. Expt. Biol., 29: 445-453.

Jeyendran, R. S. Van, H. H. Perez-Pelaez, M. Crabo, B. G. and Zanevald, L. J. D. (1984). Development of an assay to assess the functional integrity of the human sperm membrane and its relationship to other semen characteristics. J. Repro. and Fert. 70: 219-228.

Watson, P.F. (1975). Use of geimsa stain to detect changes in acrosomes of frozen ram spermatozoa. Vet. Res. 97:12-15.

Collin, S. Sirard, M. Dufour, M. and Bailey, J. (2000). Sperm calcium levels and chlortetracycline fluorescence patterns are related to the in vivo fertility of cryopreserved bovine semen. J. Androl. 21: 938-943.

□□□